ONLINE EDUCATION 2.0

Evolving, Adapting, and Reinventing Online Technical Communication

Edited by

Kelli Cargile Cook
Texas Tech University

and

Keith Grant-Davie
Utah State University

Baywood's Technical Communications Series
Series Editor: Charles H. Sides

Baywood Publishing Company, Inc.
AMITYVILLE, NEW YORK

Baywood Publishing Company, Inc.
26 Austin Avenue
P.O. Box 337
Amityville, NY 11701
(800) 638-7819
E-mail: baywood@baywood.com
Web site: baywood.com

Library of Congress Catalog Number: 2012022522
ISBN: 978-0-89503-805-0 (cloth : alk. paper)
ISBN: 978-0-89503-806-7 (paper)
ISBN: 978-0-89503-807-4 (epub)
ISBN: 978-0-89503-808-1 (epdf)
http://dx.doi.org/10.2190/OE2

Library of Congress Cataloging-in-Publication Data

Online education 2.0 : evolving, adapting, and reinventing online technical communication / Edited by Kelli Cargile Cook and Keith Grant-Davie.
    p. cm.
  Includes bibliographical references and index.
  ISBN 978-0-89503-805-0 (cloth : alk. paper) -- ISBN 978-0-89503-806-7 (pbk. : alk. paper) -- ISBN 978-0-89503-807-4 (epub) -- ISBN 978-0-89503-808-1 (epdf) 1. Education, Higher--Computer-assisted instruction. 2. Internet in higher education. 3. Communication of technical information. I. Cargile Cook, Kelli, 1959- II. Grant-Davie, Keith, 1957-
  LB2395.7.O55 2012
  378.1734--dc23
                                            2012022522

Table of Contents

SECTION III: REINVENTING COURSE CONTENTS AND MATERIALS

Introduction

Keith Grant-Davie and Kelli Cargile Cook

Ten years have passed since we first solicited chapters for *Online Education: Global Questions, Local Answers*. During this time, the scope of online instruction in professional and technical communication has more than doubled. When our first book was published in 2005, we reported that 22 U.S. colleges and universities offered online courses or degrees. An informal survey of members of the Council for Programs in Scientific and Technical Communication in 2009 revealed that the number had increased to 56 institutions offering programs or individual courses online. A total of 40 U.S. programs offered at least one degree completely online of those 56. Considering this growth, we wondered how online pedagogy and learning have changed since we collected the essays for *Online Education: Global Questions, Local Answers*: how have faculty, students, online courses, and programs evolved in the last 10 years, and what have we learned about online education in technical communication that can sustain and improve these programs over the next 10 years? Specifically, we set out to answer a number of questions in our second collection, *Online Education 2.0: Evolving, Adapting, and Reinventing Online Technical Communication*:

1. Have we moved beyond the theory-building stage we described in our first book to a more theory-based instruction? If so, what theories are we using, and which ones work best in application?
2. The recession of the last few years has had a profound impact on higher education, bringing reduced funding and staff cutbacks from which we are given little hope of relief in the near future. How is online education responding to what we call this "new austerity?"
3. The technological context in which we teach online has simplified online instruction through the use of standardized and institutionalized classroom

1

management systems, but it has also complicated our work if we choose to employ social networking, virtual worlds, or mobile technologies. Why and how are we using these newer developments in our classes, and to what end?

These questions were the prompts we used initially to call for contributions. Our contributors' essays address these prompts both directly and indirectly. As a whole, the essays demonstrate that the answers to these questions are as situational and complex as they were 10 years ago when we first began our study of online technical communication instruction. We have chosen not to synthesize our contributors' answers to these questions here in the new collection's introduction. Rather, we focus the introduction in two ways: as a comparison of the two collections and with overviews to the new collection's parts and their contents. At the end of the collection, we include an Afterword in which we reflect on the status of online technical communication instruction as illustrated through these essays and predict where we expect the next 10 years will take us.

A COMPARISON OF THE TWO COLLECTIONS

Unlike the first collection, this one begins with two assumptions about online education: it is a viable medium of instruction, different from but not inferior to face-to-face instruction; and most of us will, at some point, teach online. On these assumptions, we do not feel the need to debate, ponder pros and cons, or make the case. We believe the case has already been made: online education is here and, for the foreseeable future, it is here to stay. As evidence, we need only look to our field's conferences and journals, to the diversity of scholars who responded to our initial call for this second collection and their programs.

When we began developing our first collection in 2001, we took a deductive approach, targeting well-known scholars in online technical communication instruction and asking them to help us articulate and address the questions that program directors, professors, and instructors faced when developing programs and courses for online delivery. We asked these scholars to examine the challenges of initiating an online program or course—what we called global questions—and then to provide a description of the solutions they or their institutions had developed to answer these questions. In contrast, with our second collection, we took a more inductive approach. To learn how faculty, students, online courses, and programs have evolved since 2001, we solicited contributors broadly rather than targeting specific scholars. With this collection, we wanted to reach out to a wide variety of institutions and instructors.

The result is exactly what we wanted: We have contributors from established programs in technical communication, such as Arizona State University, University of Nevada-Las Vegas, Utah State University, Texas Tech University, the University of Memphis, and Old Dominion University, to name a few; but we also notably have chapters from urban and rural institutions (University of Cincinnati, University of Minnesota-Mankato), technological and career colleges (Texas State Technical College, Davenport College), and private and for-profit universities (Davenport University, Kaplan University). Contributors are geographically dispersed across the United States from Anchorage, Alaska, to Orlando, Florida, and from Mankato, Minnesota, to Harlingen, Texas. Our authors hold positions from full professors to adjunct instructors to graduate students. As a group, they represent the breadth and the scope of online education in technical communication as it currently exists. We are pleased to be able to provide such a diverse group of scholars with the opportunity to discuss their online work.

The diversity of the collection's authors provides a wide-angle snapshot of online technical communication. We have organized these perspectives around three central topics: (a) how programs and faculty experiences have evolved, (b) how faculty and their courses have adapted to students' changing needs and abilities, and (c) how course design and activities have expanded, given new technologies and delivery methods. Our authors examine topics of interest for readers with online teaching experience, such as the economic recession in the United States and its impact on online programming, multimodal course material design, privacy and intellectual property issues, and faculty development and training. We have also included chapters we think will attract newcomers to online education. These contributions also build upon the first collection's consideration of instructional design topics, such as scaffolding, and of online students' abilities to access student services. The new collection's authors describe their experiences using familiar course delivery technologies, including Blackboard and Design2Learn, as well as cutting-edge pedagogical options, such as Second Life and online games.

Readers of our first collection will recognize some familiar themes and arguments that return in this second collection: that pedagogical aims should drive the use of technology, not vice versa; that online education is neither better nor worse than traditional, face-to-face education, but different; that the larger questions raised in these pages do not have uniform answers but must be answered within the constraints of individual institutions; and that technical communication scholars continue to be particularly well-qualified as leaders in online education. We think these observations are as true today as they were in 2005. However, this 2.0 collection has its own set of themes that several chapters address in different ways: what to do when resources are constrained; how to build programs that can be sustained through the inevitable changes in resources, personnel, and technology; how to train and mentor the increasing numbers of faculty (both full and part time) teaching online for the first time; and how to achieve consistency across multiple sections and multiple instructors in a program. Notably, this collection also has more emphasis on teaching technical communication online at the undergraduate level—a rarity when we developed the first collection but much more common now.

As a whole, the essays in this collection reflect the growing popularity of online education and the challenges and rewards of such work. In contrast, the previous collection articulated common questions and concerns of early online work, and it encouraged online instructors to dialogue with others to discover local answers for developing and promoting online programs. This collection extends that conversation, describing the next steps that can be taken to sustain online programs and the students and teachers who comprise them and highlighting the dramatic increase in faculty and students engaged in online education.

Its chapters describe the experiences of diverse and geographically dispersed contingent, adjunct, and graduate student instructors who have joined more permanent faculty teaching online. Online instructors' need for training, mentoring, or communities of practice is a common theme. At the same time, our contributors note that student populations within online classes have grown more diverse with older, nontraditional students, students from a wide variety of majors, and international students common in their classes. The diversity of student ages, geographic locations, interests, majors, and access to technology adds to the mix of challenges in online courses.

To teach online is not an easy or automated transfer of face-to-face instructional strategies; like any good teaching it requires thoughtful experimentation and reflection. So, while our first collection was largely about developing and promoting online programs and courses, this second collection is about creating communities and collaborating with others to sustain online programs and courses. As we edited this collection, we noted that online education should not be a solo act, even if instructors are the only people in their departments doing it. Each instructor will need help from others—choosing and using the technology, learning to adapt to the particular demands of online teaching, or interacting with colleagues who may not share a common vision. We hope both our collections will engage readers in a conversation with the virtual community of online educators—people who are already doing this work and sharing what they have learned or done that has been successful. Both collections offer support and ideas to anyone who has taught online or is thinking about teaching online.

Section I: Evolving Programs and Faculty

The first section of the book explores issues of freedom versus constraint and creativity versus consistency in programs characterized by large numbers of instructors and limited resources. The section opens with a story of survival and adaptation in face of challenges. In "What Do You Do When the Ground Beneath Your Feet Shifts?" Barry Maid and Barbara D'Angelo describe a situation that we suspect may be common around the country: a large writing program staffed mostly by a diverse, continually changing, part-time faculty at a state university. Maid and D'Angelo were charged with improving consistency and quality of instruction while at the same time facing a series of administrative upheavals and funding cuts. They describe how they created a second-generation online program with courses designed from the outset for online delivery (rather than converted from face-to-face delivery). These courses feature a common syllabus and modularized assignments. Maid and D'Angelo recount the challenges of trying to motivate and engage faculty by allowing them some input in curricular development through a social networking site.

Chapter 2, "Theoretically Grounded, Practically Enacted, and Well Behind the Cutting Edge: Writing Course Development Within the Constraints of a Campus-Wide Course Management System," presents a different take on the challenge of capitalizing on limited resources. Denise Tillery and Ed Nagelhout share how they learned to make the most of a low-tech, university-sponsored, off-the-shelf course management system in a large business-writing program. Like the authors of the first chapter, their program is staffed largely by adjunct instructors. They use templates to achieve consistency across classes and to enable assessment, but at the same time they try to allow instructors some individual freedom and foster a sense of community through an expanded view of the rhetorical canon of delivery. In this view, they focus on the course management system as a site of delivery where all stakeholders—administrators, teachers, and students—are encouraged to take part in the ongoing development of the course. Participants, therefore, form a community of practice collectively invested in and responsible for the course.

Chapter 3, "Creativity and Consistency in Online Courses: Finding the Appropriate Balance," also discusses communities of practice and consistency as Keri Dutkiewicz, LuAnne Holder, and Wayne Sneath report on faculty opinions about creativity and uniformity in course design. Their study was conducted at Davenport University, a private, nonprofit university in which 50% of the courses are online, the faculty is largely adjunct, and both faculty and administrators are widely distributed geographically. The university ensures consistency across multiple sections of the same course largely by using predesigned courses. The study looks at faculty and student responses to these courses and to opportunities to customize them. The authors recommend that faculty be involved in communities of practice dedicated to the development and management of such courses.

The value of creating communities of practice in online education is further developed by Lisa Meloncon and Lora Arduser in Chapter 4, "Communities of Practice Approach: A New Model for Online Course Development and Sustainability." The authors argue from their own experience that forming communities of practice (COPs) can be a good way for technical communication instructors to develop and teach online courses with limited resources. COPs also help make courses sustainable in the face of continually shifting technologies, teaching practices, and course content. Contrasting them with other kinds of collaboration, Meloncon and Arduser argue that COPs promote the kind of formal interaction that helps create, share, and retain the community's knowledge capital. It also helps alleviate the isolation associated with online teaching and mitigates "the challenges of time, economics, culture, and increasing workloads."

The first section of the book concludes with Chapter 5, "Training Faculty for Online Instruction: Applying Technical Communication Theory to the Design of a Mentoring Program," in which Janie Jaramillo-Santoy and Gina Cano-Monreal describe a way to meet the challenges of sustaining an online writing program in the face of massively increasing demand for classes, reduced funding for teacher training, and changing skill requirements for online teachers. Their solution, like Meloncon and Arduser's, involves collaboration, in this case using the skills inherent to technical communicators when creating a peer mentoring program to train teachers new to online instruction. They describe how the Mentor2Mentor program at Texas State Technical College was developed and how it operates. Through their case study, Jaramillo-Santoy and Cano-Monreal illustrate how a well-designed mentoring program can create a support network that assures the long-term success of an online program, even when challenged with financial and personnel limitations.

Section II: Adapting to Changing Student Needs and Abilities

While the first section of the book looks at online education in technical communication from the perspective of teacher-administrators charged with developing and maintaining strong online programs in the face of difficult circumstances, the second section asks how faculty and courses have adapted to students' changing needs and abilities. Emily Thrush and Susan Popham's Chapter 6, "Teaching Technical Communication to a Global Online Student Audience," discusses some ways we can expect our classes to change, arguing that technical communication teachers will face more online teaching and increasing numbers of international students. This change will oblige us to learn how to respond to (and reap the benefits of) very diverse online communities. While cautioning that these challenges are still too new to have clear solutions, Thrush and Popham raise the questions we will need to answer as technical communication instruction becomes more globalized, suggesting that we will need to reconsider the design of our courses and assignments and the kinds of language skills we need to teach.

In Chapter 7, "Students in the Online Technical Communication Classroom: The Next Decade," Angela Eaton replicates the survey of online students that she reported in our first book. In keeping with the expansion of online education nationwide, her second survey represents more schools—12, as compared with the 6 in the 2002 survey. Students responding to the 2010 survey were, on average, older, but they represented a wider age range. They chose online degree programs for much the same reasons as students in the first survey—to fit their working schedules, to have access to a program not available where they live, and to improve their skills. Skill development and job retention appeared to be more important to them in 2010 than in 2002, perhaps reflecting the economy. As in 2002, online students still place particular value on well-structured courses and instructors who are proficient with the technology and maintain an active presence in the class. Although the two surveys yielded largely similar responses, we think it's important to periodically update our understanding of how and why students choose online education in technical communication and what they like and dislike about it.

In Chapter 8, "From Gamers to Grammarians: How Online Gaming is Changing the Nature of Digital Discourse in the Classroom," Virginia Tucker argues that participation in online gaming communities (more than in social media) does not harm students' ability to write, but rather it eases their transition into online classes and encourages them to lead and participate in online class discussions. This surprising essay presents evidence from a replication study to demonstrate that students who have participated casually in gaming communities come to an online class already understanding the value of working together, within agreed rules, toward a shared goal. Furthermore, she argues that the rhetorical value placed on good grammar and verbal expression in online gaming community discourse (enforced by peer pressure) may improve the quality of their writing. Tucker writes,

> It is becoming clearer that serious gamers do not condone nor facilitate the dumbing-down of language. The text-dependent nature of online gaming invites conversation among community members about grammar and language, indicating that these issues of verbal intelligence are important to online communities. . . . Essentially, when writing is all one has, then credibility depends on eloquence and precision in language. . . . Thus, in online discourse, ethos is dependent upon one's writing ability.

In Chapter 9, "Cybergogy, Second Life, and Online Technical Communication Instruction," Lesley Scopes and Bryan Carter describe the kind of communities of practice that can develop when online classes take place in Second Life, which they argue is not a game but rather an unscripted, "social centric 3-D immersive virtual world." Games have goals and conclusions, whereas environments like Second Life persist in the absence of individual participants. Scopes and Carter see virtual environments as being good places to enact constructivist learning theories, where the focus is on student creation of meaning in collaboration with others. Drawing on Scopes' Cybergogy of Learning Archetypes, the authors describe five different types of activity that can be used in virtual environment classes. For technical writing, they explain two assignments that take advantage of the virtual environment. The first involves creating and writing about "machinima"—short videos involving characters and locations within the virtual environment. The second is simulation writing, which invites students to explore Second Life locations and propose additions to these locations.

While Scopes and Carter advance the technological frontier in online education, Keith Gibson and Diane Martinez in Chapter 10, "From Divide to Continuum: Rethinking Access in Online Education," conclude this section of the book by sounding a more cautionary note, pointing out that the students who populate online classes are not necessarily digital natives. They argue that our enthusiasm to adopt new technologies should not blind us to the fact that our students are, and probably always will be, spread along a digital continuum between those who have rapid, unlimited access to the Internet and those who do not. Age and socioeconomic factors account for this continuum. Gibson and Martinez discuss the potential advantages and disadvantages of using four current technologies in online education: mobile applications, social networking, interactive videoconferencing, and massively multiplayer online games. They urge thoughtful examination of the risks and rewards of using these technologies.

Section III: Reinventing Course Contents and Materials

In the final section of the book, our chapter authors share some ways that online education has led them to make innovations in their teaching materials or in the way they interact with students. In Chapter 11, "Adapting Instructional Documents to an Online Course Environment," Jacqueline Cason and Patricia Jenkins ask what it means to adapt teaching materials (they focus on assignment instructions) for use in online classes. They describe three phases through which their own practices have evolved, each phase representing further movement away from sole reliance on print-based documents. In the first phase, Replacement Practice, they used the online environment more as a site of transfer for existing print-based materials than as a site of interaction. In the second phase, Sequential Learning Units, they repackaged materials in screen-view format to fit the structure of their course management system, embedding links to additional materials. In the third phase, they turned to multimodal composing, re-creating their materials using audio and video tools like Keynote, Screenflow, and QuickTime, which liberate their materials from the confines of the course management system. Cason and Jenkins discuss the textual features, composing practices, reading practices, and social roles that characterize each of these three phases. They argue that the phases are not exclusive. They still use print-based documents and sequential learning units when appropriate, in addition to multimodal text. Cason and Jenkins lead us to think about the ways our course materials may constrain and enable our pedagogical intentions and about ways technological choices, made by us or by our institutions, may constrain and enable our students as well.

In Chapter 12, "Expanding the Scaffolding of the Online Undergraduate Technical Communication Course," Dan Jones suggests three methods for using scaffolding to establish a strong instructor ethos in online undergraduate technical communication courses. First, he describes a system of folders that he argues have some advantages over the typical walk-through modules used in Webcourses. Second, he argues that well-designed evaluation rubrics are an essential element of any good online course, an important point overlooked by some while they build their online courses. Finally, he discusses techniques for establishing and projecting instructor ethos and building a sense of community within the classroom. Throughout the chapter, Jones argues that instructors who expand the scaffolding of their online courses while also applying these and other best practices are providing their students the best online learning experiences.

Lee Tesdell argues in Chapter 13, "Innovation in the Distributed Technical Communication Classroom," that viewing the online classroom as a distributed activity system provides an opportunity for teachers of technical communication to innovate and engage in creative pedagogy. He discusses distributed learning in the light of activity theory as a way to detail the relationship among the human actors, the goals of the teaching/learning, and the technology in the activity system that is the online classroom. Throughout this discussion, he identifies benefits and challenges that online instructors encounter, and he provides multiple examples of innovative opportunities that occur within an online course.

In Chapter 14, "Library Services for Online Students," we are glad to include the perspective of a librarian. Britt Fagerheim describes how libraries are revising their collections and services in response to the increasing numbers of students studying at regional campuses and through distance education. Fagerheim outlines the issues facing librarians in their work with distance education students and faculty members, such as the poor representation of library resources in some course management systems. Using examples drawn from technical communication, she describes how libraries are developing new policies and procedures, modifying collections, and developing online instructional materials such as LibGuides and "embedded librarians" to support the work of students and faculty in the realm of distance education, just as they do with on-campus students.

Section III ends similarly with Chapter 15, "'Keeping it Real': Contextualizing Intellectual Property and Privacy in the Online Technical Communication Course." Natalie Stillman-Webb observes that teaching online can bring new pedagogical strategies and, with them, different forms of communication, collaboration, and information distribution. Yet with the potential for easier distribution of information online come questions of ownership of that information and ethics in its digital transfer. Her chapter addresses the limits of textual sharing—legal, ethical, and practical: What space exists in theories of collaboration and peer review for discussions of intellectual property and privacy? How have inter-pretations or conceptions of intellectual property and privacy changed with the proliferation of digital texts and online education? How can instructors of such courses negotiate intellectual property issues while taking advantage of com-munication technologies that support effective teaching of technical writing? What aspects of intellectual property beyond "fair use" or the educational context need to be considered in light of the types of work done in technical writing courses? To answer these questions, the author presents strategies for negoti-ating between "keeping it real"—encouraging students to gain technical writing experience by composing with and for outside organizations—and addressing intellectual property and privacy issues in theory and practice within the online technical communication course.

We strongly believe that effective instructors reflect and learn from their instructional interactions in whatever environment they occur. The contributors to this collection have affirmed our belief. Throughout this collection, their chapters demonstrate that learning communities emerge when their participants—students, teachers, and support personnel—collaboratively consider how to achieve common goals or solve instructional challenges and then share these experiences with others. Such learning communities, we have discovered, can extend beyond physical or virtual boundaries or even a printed page. By reading and considering the stories in this collection, we have already begun to learn from our contributors' experiences and experiments, and what we are learning we are sharing in conversations and correspondence with others. We hope that you will find their stories as engaging and informative as we have, and that their stories will shape your own conversations and activities as you evolve, adapt, and reinvent technical communication online.

http://dx.doi.org/10.2190/OE2C1

Section I: Evolving Programs and Faculty

CHAPTER 1

What Do You Do When the Ground Beneath Your Feet Shifts?

Barry Maid and Barbara J. D'Angelo

What do you do when institutional and economic forces produce seismic shifts in what appeared to be a stable and growing online technical communication program? In this chapter, we propose to answer that question and to explicate the evolution of the design, delivery, and assessment of a second-generation online program and its courses as a way to survive the shaky ground of the "new austerity" faced by the academy.

In the fall of 2008, the program in Multimedia Writing and Technical Communication (MWTC) at Arizona State University (ASU) was a small independent applied writing program—stable and growing. Our only degree program was a BS degree offered entirely online. We were being courted by the ASU administration to create an online Master of Science degree. A new dean came on board and thought the program needed to grow and was talking about finding ways to increase full-time faculty lines. All seemed well, and then just after the beginning of 2009, the ground shifted.

ASU reorganized, and our independent writing program was placed in a larger quasi-unit called Interdisciplinary Humanities and Communication. Compounding the organizational change, the number of our majors grew from 30–35 to well over 100. Also, the number of students enrolled in our service courses increased significantly. We, and ASU, are still trying to figure out what all of this means given the wide variety of programs in the new unit that have little disciplinary affinity. However those of us in the newly renamed program of Technical Communication (TC) decided that we needed to rethink how we design, deliver, and assess our online courses in order to best serve our students.

11

Like most universities facing the results of the economic downturn, ASU is currently trying to cope with severe cutbacks in state funds. In addition, ASU's Provost believes in large rather than small programs. We used to be termed a "niche program," which was good. She now refers to programs like ours as "boutique programs," which is bad. This administrative view compounded the fact that the TC program was significantly underfunded and understaffed. How we have coped with the realities of our situation has resulted in our evolution toward being a second-generation online program.

We have had to find ways to accommodate more students and work within the vagaries of institutional change and limited resources, and so we must have an effective and efficient way to deliver our courses online. We decided to move to a second generation of online delivery (Online 2G) to ensure that we maintain quality within the constraints posed by seismic institutional shifts. We see the first generation of online courses as essentially being face-to-face courses that have been tweaked so that they can be delivered online. In the best-case scenario, and what we initially attempted, the online versions deliver the same content, and students meet the same outcomes. For us, Online 2G are courses that are specifically designed for online delivery. These courses have course outcomes that map to larger program outcomes. The course structure incorporates a common syllabus and set of modularized assignments. Instructors for each section of the course are expected to follow the syllabus and assignment set. This maintains consistency across sections; however, instructors have the flexibility to use teaching strategies and approaches suited to their expertise. We also always request instructor feedback in order to incorporate instructor-based changes after every semester.

Presently (spring 2010), nearly 82% of our classes are taught by part-time faculty. We expect that percentage to increase. By making sure our program is delivered entirely online, we recruit the best part-time faculty from anywhere. The modularization of courses allows us to maintain curricular consistency with this potentially shifting faculty pool as well as to leverage online delivery mechanisms.

All of this gives us an interesting opportunity to function in a difficult institutional moment and to use shifting grounds as exigence to develop the next generation of online course delivery. We expect that, though our solution is institution-specific, much of what we are doing can be scaled to other programs facing institutional and economic changes.

HISTORY

The history of the program originally called Multimedia Writing and Technical Communication (MWTC) at ASU, especially with regard to the development of program outcomes, curriculum, and assessment, has been chronicled in several places (D'Angelo, 2009; D'Angelo & Maid, 2004; Maid, 2005).

However, up to this point, we have not yet discussed how the program moved to an entirely online means of delivery and how we are now moving toward what we see as a second generation of online delivery of courses.

Very briefly, ASU hired Barry Maid in January 2000 to create the MWTC program housed on what is now the Polytechnic campus (ASU Poly). The original concept that ASU presented to Maid when he arrived was that this program would prepare writers to work in what people in the Phoenix metro area hoped would be a growing software industry. Despite the "interesting" program title, the general sense was that graduates would work writing software documentation. From the beginning, Maid understood that doing so would significantly limit the potential of the program and perhaps even doom it. The curriculum Maid created during spring of 2000 and approved by the Arizona Board of Regents on June 30, 2000, was one he has regularly called "vanilla." He expected students from the program would be able to move into any applied writing position and be comfortable working in both print and digital environments. Barbara D'Angelo, who had been teaching part time for the program since 2002, was hired as a full-time contract faculty in 2004, and in 2006 we hired Claire Lauer as a tenure-track assistant professor.

We have then been running a full-fledged undergraduate degree program initially with two (now four) full-time faculty members, only three of whom teach program courses. In addition, the program employs a number of part-time faculty that ASU calls Faculty Associates (FAs). When Maid arrived at ASU, FAs who taught the existing service courses under the program's prefix (TWC) were people with English degrees who needed work. Courses were basically staffed the way many programs staff First Year Composition—individuals without any real field or applied expertise. Maid changed the way FAs were hired by looking for people with at least the minimal academic credential (a master's degree) and who either had experience teaching technical or business communication or workplace experience as a practitioner.

While changing who was hired helped to ensure that the applied writing curriculum would be taught, it also made the FA pool significantly smaller. At the same time, it became clear that the large number of potential FAs in the greater Phoenix area were people with full-time jobs. That meant that finding FAs to teach daytime classes became highly unlikely. It also meant that the geography of the Phoenix metropolitan area made it difficult to find FAs for night classes. (The Poly campus is located 23 miles southeast of the Tempe campus and 34 miles from downtown Phoenix. The distance is not that far in terms of Western cities, but the drive is lengthy in evening rush hour, and it is difficult for people who work in downtown Phoenix to drive to the Poly campus for evening classes.) In addition to the issue of geography, the reality is that students who are attracted to technical communication programs are usually not 18-year-old first-year students. Rather, technical communication students tend to be older and have some workplace experience, and they are likely to have at least some credits from another institution. In fall 2009, ASU's Institutional Studies reported that the average age of our undergraduate majors was 33.6 and that 87.5% of our majors transferred in 12 or more hours. We were clearly a bad fit for an institution that wanted to attract local, 18-year-old students. As described later, this "bad fit" would become exacerbated when reorganization of the campus took place in 2009.

THE EARLY DAYS:
FROM ON-CAMPUS TO ONLINE

Initially, all the classes were face-to-face. Indeed, ASU's original model was that the program would be delivered face-to-face to residential students who lived on-campus. When Maid first arrived at ASU, there was some original discussion about online delivery of coursework in the MWTC program. It was natural to think about delivering online classes since Maid had experience with distance learning using both interactive video and online for most of the decade of the 1990s. Still, in the initial stages of the program creation and development, Maid consciously decided not to jump into online delivery. He had several reasons for this decision. First of all, he wanted to make sure the program had clear and understandable outcomes and a curriculum that helped students meet those outcomes. Method of delivery was initially irrelevant. With solid outcomes and ultimately, curriculum mapped to those outcomes, method of delivery could be modified. What mattered were the outcomes and the curricular consistency.

However, significant underfunding caused us to be creative in terms of delivering courses to an increasing number of students. That led to delivering courses online before the initial plan, to moving the entire program to an online-only delivery. In order to allow this to happen, in the spring of 2002, Maid wrote an internal ASU grant that allowed him to hire two people—Julia Ferganchick and Michael Moore, both of whom had solid applied writing expertise and online teaching experience—to help prepare the existing curriculum for online delivery. Using good first-generation thinking, the courses that Ferganchick and Moore developed were simply online versions of the original curriculum. Their task was to ensure that while they were changing the method of delivery, the outcomes for the four courses they moved to online delivery and curriculum would remain intact. They simply ported the content. As Rude has pointed out, individuals typically try to understand something by comparing it to something familiar, including online education (Rude, 2005), and so it is no surprise that the first conversion of our courses to online format followed the familiar pattern of traditional on-site courses. And in many ways, the courses were consistent with the type of course that Cargile Cook (2005) calls first-generation distance courses constrained by technological boundaries. In the fall 2002 semester, the MWTC program offered its first two online classes. Over the next 2 years, the remainder of TC courses were converted to online delivery.

REVERSING THE DISTANCE MODEL
AND CHANGING WORLDVIEWS

Offering sections of the program online solved multiple problems. First, it significantly increased the size of the potential FA pool. No longer would the program be forced to look for qualified local FAs who could make it to campus to teach when the course was scheduled. In addition, students who lived and worked a great distance from campus could take courses. By fall of 2004, all courses we taught were offered online, making it possible for a student to complete the major without ever stepping foot on the ASU Poly campus. While we continued to offer some service courses online or in hybrid format, those were also converted to an online-only format by 2009.

This experience turned out to be exceptionally important, because the fact was that online delivery of our courses became normal. Online was not special. It did not have a special curriculum. Neither the students nor the faculty were evaluated in any other way. FAs are hired with the expectation that they teach online. As ASU faculty, FAs may take advantage of the university's workshops (offered on-campus and online) for distance learning (primarily focused on software and course management system use) and teacher development. However, the TC program has not offered any additional training other than an initial meeting with the instructor to discuss course outcomes and purpose, and to explain previous versions of syllabi or assignments. Our expectation has been that as professionals, FAs would understand and meet the expectations of teaching online as well as TC program outcomes. Teaching and learning online was plainly and simply the way business was done in the TC program and prepared us to move toward what we call the second generation of distance education in technical communication.

As conversion to online-only evolved, instructors made decisions about delivery method. The majority of courses were and are delivered using Blackboard, the course management system supported by ASU. A couple of instructors, more comfortable with building Web sites and systems, developed their own course sites using content management systems and integrated wikis, blogs, podcasts, and video lectures. Instructors also had the flexibility to adapt course content. Clearly, as technological boundaries shifted and evolved, pedagogical experimentation was taking place in ways that benefitted the TC program but that also began to place the original vision at risk.

THE BEGINNING OF TECH COMM ONLINE 2G

The freedom and flexibility to make decisions about course content and online delivery mechanisms had several advantages. It allowed instructors to develop the course in ways that suited their teaching styles and comfort levels. In addition, it allowed for creativity and experimentation in both course design and delivery. However, this freedom and flexibility also resulted in disadvantages that emerged over time. First, curricular flexibility allowed for creativity, but over time it also tended to evolve into some instructor-based idiosyncrasies instead of a consistent programmatic focus. While all TC courses are assigned outcomes, the tendency appeared to be that instructors were losing sight of the original purpose and required outcomes as assignments and delivery methods evolved. Since instructors were located across the country and working online only, there was little opportunity for curriculum or other meetings to ensure that programmatic goals and outcomes were communicated. Second, as enrollment grew, so did the number of sections for individual courses. Flexibility in course design for these courses resulted in inconsistency across sections, which eventually began to impact the effectiveness of the course. And so the programmatic cohesion based on outcomes and the curricular consistency that Maid sought when he started the TC program was beginning to erode. Rude declared that "Program designers need a clear vision of their goals and target student group" (Rude, 2005, p. 70). That vision was clear when Maid created the TC program, but the initial foray into online education had started to derail it. This first became apparent in our business communication course, and our solution became our first foray into Online 2G.

One of the original charges of the MWTC program was to provide a service course in business communication for students of what was a new general business program at ASU Poly. Several years later, it quickly became apparent that the course was problematic. Many of the problems were similar to any course that is offered in multiple sections and taught by multiple instructors, all with their own ideas about pedagogy and course content. Some problems related to content or pedagogical issues as identified by the faculty in the business administration program: inappropriate assignments that were better suited to a first-year composition course, inconsistent assignments across sections (approximately 5–7 per semester taught by different part-time instructors), lack of rigor, and complaints about the textbook. Course and programmatic integrity were of concern as it became clear that many sections were not adhering to intended outcomes. In the summer of 2007, D'Angelo was assigned to address these problems; she used a research process to engage stakeholders (TC faculty teaching the course, faculty from the business program, advisory board members for the business program) and to collect data to make decisions about course redesign (D'Angelo & White, 2008).

As a result of the research and resultant analysis, the course was renumbered and renamed TWC 347: Written Communication for Managers, with a new design with a standardized syllabus incorporating core units and assignments. D'Angelo worked with one of the FAs for the course to do an initial redesign of the syllabus and assignments; however, the intent of the redesign was to engage all instructors in course development. To do this, we created an online instructor site for posting of course-related documents for easy access; a forum for instructors to share ideas and common questions or problems while teaching the course; and "extra" materials such as handouts, Web sites, and tutorials to help teach the course. In addition, we developed a Web-based assignment bank so that instructors could contribute a variety of assignments for each of the core units of the course. Although we decided upon a standardized and modular approach to this course, our intent was not to impose one set of assignments on instructors. Rather, the vision was to standardize course structure to meet a set of outcomes across sections and use an assignment bank in which assignments would be tagged by unit and by outcome so that instructors could build their section of the course within the course structure, but with some variety and choice.

This model of creating a structured and standardized course was designed to effect a compromise between the need to maintain integrity across a number of sections, all taught by FAs, and the need to motivate and engage FAs to be effective instructors with some control over their teaching. Given that the course was our first attempt at employing this model, we can now, 3 years later, see some successes and some areas that could be improved upon.

One success that emerged during the first semester of the redesign is that many of the instructors appreciated the freedom the course structure gave them to spend less time on course design and more time on directly working with and helping students. During the first semester of the redesign, for example, several of the instructors reported having more time to answer student email or spend in writing conferences with individual students because they didn't have to worry about finding time to create assignments.

The course design itself was also a success. The structure of the course revolves around a role-playing scenario in which students create their own business. Each of the modularized units consists of assignments in which students compose documents within the context of the role-play. In addition, discussions are run as student-led meetings in which students are required to organize and run, complete with agenda, discussion, and minutes. In our assessment of the course, students overwhelmingly commented that the role-playing structure not only made the course enjoyable for them but also provided them with practical experience with communicating in a way that was applicable to their jobs and careers.

On the other hand, the assignment bank never took off. It's not clear why this was the case; however, many of the instructors did contribute assignments and suggested revisions to course activities and tasks by emailing them to D'Angelo. Whether this was due to instructor reluctance to post assignments publicly is unclear. But as a result, by the third semester of using the new course design, nearly all assignments were instructor-contributed. Maintaining this level of contribution has, though, been a challenge. Over time, FAs have contributed less than during the initial couple of semesters. This decrease in participation by FAs is potentially due to any number of reasons. However, it coincides with the reorganization that the MWTC program and ASU Poly has undergone, external economic problems that resulted in funding cuts to ASU and furloughs, and the stress of rapidly increasing enrollment numbers stretching an already thin resource base.

Another problem area turned out to be the online instructor support site. The forum quickly became an area in which FAs tended to complain and gripe about students rather than offer support or share ideas. Why the forum was not more successful is not completely clear since instructors had welcomed the idea as a way to bridge geographical distance to share experiences and ideas. As with the assignment bank, timing may have played a role. However, as a strategy for a more full-fledged approach to modularization, we think some sort of online forum or social network is needed.

Lastly, technology problems created another problem. During initial redesign of the course, a common Blackboard shell was adopted to ensure that all sections would have access to all course resources. However, ASU's centralized course request system made the use of a common template across sections difficult and resulted in problems with section enrollment. Since we were not able to resolve those technical issues, we ended the use of a common shell. Given reorganization and the financial situation at ASU, the technology issues surrounding the use of Blackboard are not currently resolvable.

Despite problems, based on experiences with this course design, Maid and D'Angelo realized a model had emerged for a more standardized curriculum that was intended to be taught by an ever-changing cadre of FAs. This structure simply made more sense as more and more of the program's curriculum needed to be taught and assessed in multisections classes. Not only was enrollment beginning to skyrocket, it was becoming increasingly clear that hiring new full-time faculty would simply never happen under current ASU policies and financial strain. In addition, the fact that the program was exclusively an online program that attracted a particular demographic allowed Maid and D'Angelo to start thinking of slightly different ways to deliver the program more effectively to more students. Despite storm clouds on the horizon, we were, after all, still a young and rapidly growing program willing to do things differently to meet the needs of students, within the constraints of our situation. But then, as we alluded to at the beginning of our narrative, the bottom fell out from under us.

THE END OF NORMAL

Beginning July 1, 2008, we began to see change that ultimately resulted in several reorganizations. Eventually the MWTC program was folded in the School of Letters and Sciences (SLS), merged into a unit called Interdisciplinary Humanities and Communication and renamed Technical Communication. These organizational shifts created several problems for us. Although we continue to be a degree-granting program, we are no longer an independent unit but instead part of a larger unit with programs that are, unlike us, primarily designed to deliver lower-division general studies courses. Our relationships with our closest collaborators were undermined by the reorganization as they too were merged with other schools or colleges and in some cases moved to other ASU campuses. The TC program's faculty have historically worked with faculty in business, engineering and technology, applied psychology, applied health fields, and external constituencies in business and industry; the result of the reorganization into a humanities unit has made those partnerships and collaborations difficult to impossible. Further, administrative changes took place so that D'Angelo's position was reduced from 10 to 9 months, curtailing most curriculum development and assessment efforts. Lastly, since we were no longer an independent unit, we lost control of our budget. Now, all decisions related to spending—from the minutest purchase of office supplies to larger expenses on salary and equipment—must be approved by the Director of SLS.

Ironically, reorganization did not impact growth of the TC program. Majors more than doubled from what seemed to be a constant number between 30 and 35 from the program's inception in about 2008 to approximately 140 as of summer 2010. Yet for ASU, the TC program continues to be a "boutique program" and as of summer 2010, one without clear leadership or definition. Since ASU would no longer support a program head position with a 12-month salary, Maid decided to return to 9-month faculty status once his administrative contract ended.

WHAT TECH COMM ONLINE 2G NOW MEANS FOR US AND FOR OTHERS

We are certainly not the only program or institution to be facing hard times and shifting priorities. We report our plans for what we would do if we could continue and hope others might be able to benefit from our experiences and plans to move to the next generation of online delivery. Based on what we learned from our early ventures into TC Online 2G with our business communication course, we would take a twofold approach. The first is in curriculum development. The second is in recruitment of FAs.

Two approaches are needed for Online 2G curriculum development. The goal in curricular reform is to develop an outcomes-based curriculum that is assessable and can be modularized. The need for outcomes to create an assessable writing program is well-discussed in the literature, including the technical communication literature (Allen, 2004; Carter, Anson, & Miller, 2003; Huot, 2002; White, 1994). The need for programmatic outcomes is equally valid for online programs, perhaps even more so. What we propose, based on our experience, is using outcomes as a basis to ensure programmatic integrity and consistency while taking advantage of technologies to find a balance between standardization and flexibility in a way that is pedagogically sound and is comfortable for our FAs. In our redesign of TWC 347, for example, we were able to incorporate a role-playing scenario and assignments and discussion that fit the outcomes and purpose of the course: to teach business students how to communicate as managers in managerial contexts. If we were to redesign our introductory course, TWC 301: General Principles of Multimedia Writing, the course structure would be very different in order to meet different outcomes and purpose.

Our sense is that the key to achieving this is to be as inclusive as possible on the front end and then create options for all faculty teaching the course to engage in ongoing curricular development. Based on what we learned with the redesign of our business communication course, classes that are regularly taught in multiple sections need both consistency of outcomes and learning, and some flexibility to allow for instructor pedagogical preferences and expertise. In our business communication course, instructors with MBAs and business experience contribute assignments and discussion topics that are relevant to the purpose of the course. Similarly, we would expect that instructors with technical writing expertise and industry experience would contribute assignments and pedagogical practices that are appropriate for our technical communication courses. In addition to our business communication course, two other TC classes are most in need of attention—TWC 301: General Principles of Multimedia Writing, and TWC 401: Principles of Technical Communication—both of which are offered in multiple sections each semester. Using a similar research model as with TWC 347, these courses would be redesigned to incorporate a common syllabus and modular approach to assignments. We would also develop a social networking site and learn from our previous failure with an assignment bank and instructor forum to develop an instructor network focused on sharing information and improving the course over time. This effort, however, requires both time and administrative support as well as a financial commitment to ensure success.

While we are clearly referring to our own situation, what we intend to convey is that the use of standardized modular course structure in which instructors are part of the redesign and continual development process, we think, is a positive step toward Online 2G delivery. Such a course design is defined by a curricular integrity that provides a structure in which all sections are taught so that there is consistency in outcomes and delivery regardless of who teaches the course. At the same time, instructors are engaged in the design of the course and encouraged to contribute assignments or other pedagogical approaches and techniques, allowing for flexibility in terms of teaching style. In addition, since many of the FAs in the TC program are practitioners, we are able to tap the strengths of academic curriculum design of our curriculum and assessment from our more academic faculty as well as the real-world expertise of our FAs.

The second approach would be to create a full-blown national, and perhaps international, search to find new FAs. There are multiple potential pools of qualified instructors. Unfortunately, most institutions don't have a recruitment strategy for part-time faculty beyond the local market, especially if we are looking for academically qualified practitioners as well as career academics. In combination, finding a better way to engage faculty in development activities and draw them in as stakeholders in the program would be an important aspect. We are fortunate to have had a group of FAs who have not only taught their courses but have contributed in our efforts to support students, develop curriculum, and help with assessment. Again, this approach requires programmatic leadership and administrative support, neither of which the TC program currently enjoys. Though we have curtailed our efforts, we believe they are key if Online 2G is to be successful.

Lastly, part of Online 2G is the need to create an environment in which students and faculty may interact with one another outside of courses. This type of interaction is important, particularly in an online program such as the TC program, in which students and faculty reside anywhere in the country (and in which students in the military may even be stationed overseas while taking classes). We currently use a Ning site for our capstone course and invite all TC faculty and students to view and comment on student portfolios at the end of each semester. However, this level of interaction is minimal; unless students take initiative to interact with one another and with faculty, there is no mechanism or structure for them to do so. Although we do not currently have such a structure, if we were to fully implement Online 2G, we would create a social networking site for students and for faculty. We might choose to create two different Ning communities. (Social networking services are a very fluid environment, and by the time we might be ready to implement this feature, the landscape may have changed significantly.) Ideally, it might be nice to have one community with a faculty or a student subcommunity option.

In particular, an online community may help FAs feel more engaged with one another and with the TC program. Currently, FAs are assigned and teach their courses in a somewhat isolated fashion. The fact that they are geographically dispersed means there is no time or physical place for us to have them meet, interact, and collaborate. Using a social network would alleviate this problem. Not only would it allow us to engage FAs' expertise as practitioners in curriculum development efforts, it would allow them to engage with one another and to develop their own support networks for teaching or professional collaborations.

Equally, unless majors make an effort to engage with one another outside of classes, there is currently no mechanism for them to socialize or interact with one another. In the past, students have requested that the TC program organize or offer opportunities for student engagement with one another. Individual students and one of our alumni have, on occasion, attempted to organize such events. However, individual efforts are difficult to sustain over time, and each of these efforts died out. We know anecdotally that current students engage with one another outside of class by phone, instant messaging, and chat. However, we believe that a formal TC program site is needed to allow students to interact with one another as majors and to allow nonclass and less formal interaction with faculty and program alumni. Such a site is important to allow students to network and to allow for a good introduction to the discipline.

What we have learned then, and what we believe is portable to other programs with a small cadre of full-time faculty who need to deliver an assessable online program, is the following:

Programs need to create an outcomes-based curriculum for every course. For all courses that involve multiple sections with different instructors, that curriculum needs to be standardized, though not inflexible. Doing so allows for modularization—the ability to plug diverse instructors into multiple courses and expect that they and their students will succeed. At all stages, there needs to be the potential for inclusion and engagement. Staffing of these programs must be serious. Even if resources allow for only part-time faculty, those faculty must be academically qualified, with workplace experience when appropriate, and be comfortable in working and teaching in virtual environments. And of course there must be programmatic leadership from a disciplinary expert and both administrative and financial support from the institution.

Currently, the TC Program is without either so that our biggest concern is that the integrity of the curriculum will be undermined. Since both authors no longer have administrative responsibility for the program, we are considering a stopgap measure until the economic situation improves and/or the institution brings new disciplinary leadership on board. D'Angelo's position as a clinical faculty member means she will continue to coordinate the business communication course so that the modular approach will be maintained at least for that course. Since Maid is returning to faculty status, we are considering the creation of a unit-based service role in which he will chair a program curriculum group that can begin to look at modularizing or developing our courses and most importantly, maintain the integrity of the current curriculum. Clearly this is a stopgap and limited approach, and one that we do not yet know will be accepted by the person overseeing the program. It cannot be maintained over time, but we hope we can maintain the evolution of Online 2G until a more long-term solution can be found.

We don't mean to imply that what we suggest is revolutionary. We've put pieces of many things together and attempted to learn from our experiences and how to improve upon them. However, we are specifically targeting technical communication programs that are historically small and underfunded. We have seen some success in the modularization of TWC 347 which, while it has a standardized syllabus and textbook and has approved assignments designed to meet course outcomes, is not inflexible. The key is getting the right instructors, getting them to buy into the concept, and then getting them to become part of the curricular process. What we have tried to develop with what we call Tech Comm Online 2G is an efficient and effective model for delivering a degree program. While institutional constraints may not allow us to continue to implement Tech Comm Online 2G at ASU, we believe that what we have learned may help others to shape their own programs based on their own institutional needs and constraints.

REFERENCES

Allen, J. (2004). The impact of student learning outcomes assessment on technical and professional communication. *Technical Communication Quarterly, 13*(1), 93–108.

Cargile Cook, K. (2005). An argument for pedagogy-driven online education. In K. Cargile Cook & K. Grant-Davie (Eds.), *Online education: Global questions, local answers* (pp. 49–66). Amityville, NY: Baywood.

Carter, M., Anson, C. M., & Miller, C. R. (2003). Assessing technical writing in institutional contexts: Using outcomes-based assessment for programmatic thinking. *Technical Communication Quarterly, 12*(1), 101–114.

D'Angelo, B. J. (2009, November 4–7). Using portfolio assessment to discover student learning. *Proceedings of the 74th Annual Convention of the Association for Business Communication*, Portsmouth, VA.

D'Angelo, B. J., & Maid, B. M. (2004). Moving beyond definitions: Implementing information literacy across the curriculum. *Journal of Academic Librarianship, 30*(3), 212–217.

D'Angelo, B. J., & White, O. (2008, November). *Learning from our stakeholders: Using research to redesign a business writing course.* Paper presented at the Association of Business Communication Annual Conference, Lake Tahoe, NV.

Huot, B. (2002). *(Re)articulating writing assessment for teaching and learning.* Logan: Utah State University Press.

Maid, B. M. (2005). Using the outcomes statement for technical communication. In S. Harrington, K. Rhodes, R. Overman Fischer, & R. Malenczyk (Eds.), *The outcomes book. Debate and consensus after the WPA outcomes statement* (pp. 139–149). Logan: Utah State University Press.

Rude, C. (2005). Strategic planning for online education: Sustaining students, faculty, and programs. In K. Cargile Cook & K. Grant-Davie (Eds.), *Online education: Global questions, local answers* (pp. 67–85). Amityville, NY: Baywood.

White, E. M. (1994). *Teaching & assessing writing* (2nd ed.). San Francisco, CA: Jossey-Bass.

http://dx.doi.org/10.2190/OE2C2

CHAPTER 2

Theoretically Grounded, Practically Enacted, and Well Behind the Cutting Edge: Writing Course Development Within the Constraints of a Campus-Wide Course Management System

Denise Tillery and Ed Nagelhout

Over the last 10 years, students have become more comfortable with different types of electronic communication, and delivery systems have proliferated: social networking sites, blogs, and online forums have all become familiar means of communication. Building courses programmatically means taking advantage of that familiarity to create a uniform system of delivery that will maintain consistency between sections, facilitate teacher training and communication, and help us collect meaningful data for assessment. Moreover, as universities come under increased pressure to assess student performance accurately and to offer more online courses to meet student demand, a university-sponsored course management system (CMS) is becoming an increasingly common course environment. Some programs have responded by developing cutting-edge technologies, incorporating a wide range of applications for both courses and assignments. But what happens when circumstances put you well behind the cutting edge? When you lack the resources and expertise to develop a customized CMS, how do you take advantage of technological sophistication from the margins?

25

In this chapter, we argue for a rhetorical awareness when using any CMS, grounded in the canon of delivery and the concept of user-centered technology, especially if that CMS is used to facilitate teacher training and data gathering as well as student learning. We begin with a brief history of our program development, showing the process of working with an external vendor in an ultimately unsuccessful attempt to bring the online and face-to-face sections into closer alignment, and then abandoning that system in favor of the campus-wide CMS, which enabled a more consistent delivery of content and communication across multiple sections and formats. We conclude with rhetorical choices made at three levels: administrator, instructor, and student. These choices ideally allow users agency to fulfill their responsibilities, foster communication across all levels of the program, and enable meaningful assessment information to circulate throughout the program and initiate improvements at all levels.

Our program, like every other program in the country, is shaped not only by our choices but also by our institutional constraints, primarily constraints of resources, infrastructure, and technological sophistication (both ours and our information technology department). In this respect, we are the first to admit that we are less concerned with cutting-edge technologies and more concerned with how users apply and think about available technologies. We want our CMS in particular to provide accessible modes of instruction and resources. We want to encourage teachers and students to actively engage with technology rather than be passive users. To do this, as we will describe throughout this chapter, we focus on delivery as a much more sophisticated and diverse part of our rhetorical canon to the extent possible with our CMS. But we must work within the confines of the current system, and "dance with the ones that brung us." As we will show, delivery in our program is a "long-term, comprehensive, and complex" process that offers "the beginning of new work and even the motive to produce it" (Rude, 2004, p. 273) at all levels of our program. In order for our CMS to allow for agency, foster communication, and enable assessment, we supplement our imperfect system with multiple points of contact for students, teachers, and administrators. Delivery thus expands beyond the CMS to unify elements of our program and deliver our programmatic goals while achieving a balance between instructor autonomy and consistency among sections.

PROGRAM BACKGROUND

The University of Nevada, Las Vegas, is an urban university located in a state where education is poorly supported. Rarely rising above 49th in any measure of educational spending (well behind the cutting edge), the state is dominated by the casino and mining industries, neither of which place much emphasis on an educated workforce. Despite these limitations, UNLV still wishes to be recognized locally and nationally as a "premier metropolitan university."

However, while UNLV seeks to enable a very traditional academic structure, the university itself is primarily a nonresidential commuter campus with a student population of approximately 26,000 students. Similarly, the student population reflects a more nontraditional make-up, growing toward a new majority: single parents, older and returning students, students from multi-ethnic and multicultural backgrounds. On top of that, the vast majority of students work from 20 to 40 hours per week while taking a full course load, and since Las Vegas is a 24-hour city, students work a range of shifts; in fact, it is commonplace for at least a few students in the early morning sections to come from a graveyard shift to class before going home to bed. Our business writing program was born within this environment.

In 1996, the College of Business moved all sections of business writing (about 20 per year at that time) to the English Department as a result of an accreditation review. To assist in the administration of these courses, the English Department received two faculty lines. The first hires to administer the program discovered that the course had no standardized curriculum, and content did not reflect current research and pedagogy on workplace communication. Moreover, there was little administrative structure that ensured the continuity of instruction across sections, making the development, implementation, and assessment of common outcomes difficult. Designed originally based on writing program administration scholarship (e.g., Rose & Weiser, 1999, 2003), our business writing program began with an assumption that our students need to develop multiple literacies: rhetorical, visual, information, computer, and ethical (Nagelhout, 1999). Since 1999, our program has had a united vision for teaching and learning in the writing classroom, one that stresses the importance of a consistent student experience through the use of common outcomes, a common syllabus, common readings, and a core set of assignments.

Some of our initial thinking about course development was influenced by Robert Kramer and Stephen Bernhardt's (1999) report on Glyph, a Web-based instruction environment at New Mexico State, which shows how moving instruction to online spaces facilitates the development of multiple literacies. Because we wanted to use technology to grow our program and foster teacher support, we sought to develop our own locally constructed electronic textbook and instructional Web site. We realized immediately, however, that our IT skills put us well behind the cutting edge, so we chose to outsource its development. We began initial discussions with publishers in March of 2000, explaining our vision to various publishing representatives.

A representative from Kendall/Hunt's custom publishing division showed us an original Web site design, created by one of the company's own designers, which resembled Kramer and Bernhardt's (1999) Glyph site more than anything we had seen before. This representative also assured us that we could make all manner of changes at our discretion, ranging from fixing typos and broken links to adding new content. This ability to make frequent changes, we believed, was essential to a dynamic teaching and learning resource. We piloted this "electronic textbook" in fall 2001 in 20 sections with the intention of conducting formative assessment on its usability for students and instructors. Unfortunately, we spent most of the semester editing content. Our initial assessment of usability was mixed. In spring 2002, we revised the Web site with graduate student teaching assistants who wrote projects and other curricular materials, compiled a detailed index, and researched and annotated links to supplemental Internet resources (for a more detailed account, see Jablonski & Nagelhout, 2010).

Despite our commitment to revision and upgrades, Kendall/Hunt was looking for something much more stable (like Porter, Sullivan, & Johnson-Eilola, 2009) and much less work intensive on their end. By 2005, they pulled much of their support and strongly intimated a desire to recast and reformat the site. Eventually, the "electronic textbook" was revised as a traditional paper textbook (Jablonski, 2006), and we had to look for a new environment to meet our technological needs. So beginning in fall 2006, we began to migrate our materials to support all of our business writing sections and teachers into the less-than cutting-edge WebCampus platform approved by the UNLV administration. (UNLV uses Blackboard/WebCT's most recent product, Vista, but refers to the CMS as "WebCampus" to avoid confusion with Windows Vista. We use UNLV's terminology of WebCampus in this chapter.)

Our application of a more traditional CMS like Blackboard and WebCampus initially mirrored uses described, especially in various surveys of higher education (see in particular, Harrington, Gordon, & Shibik, 2004; Morgan, 2003). But as our program has grown, we have had to adjust. When we first began administering the course in 1999, all courses were taught face-to-face in computer classrooms, which met two days per week. We soon began to offer online sections as well. Then in 2007, we added hybrid sections, which met one day per week face-to-face and did the rest of the work online. We currently offer approximately 70 sections per year (20 face-to-face, 30 hybrid, and 20 online) to nearly 1,500 students. Administrators are tenured or tenure-track faculty responsible for, among other things, scheduling sections and making sure that WebCampus is available for all teachers. Teachers are a balance of part-time instructors and graduate students responsible for course preparation and course delivery.

To maintain program consistency, we, the administrators, initially provided materials to teachers on CD along with instructions for uploading the appropriate files to their WebCampus sections. As this proved much too cumbersome, we next tried using a Master Course approach in fall 2008, with all teachers downloading the course through WebCampus at the beginning of the semester. Again, wholesale changes were difficult to administer, so we have most recently taken advantage of the template function in WebCampus.

DELIVERY AND THE WEBCAMPUS
TEMPLATE

The embodied material aspect of delivery helps us describe how we have managed to maintain consistency across different platforms, both in the physical and virtual classroom. Delivery, starting with Cicero, has been associated with the embodied physical component of rhetoric; it is the point of contact between the speaker and the audience. Although delivery had been largely neglected in rhetorical theory throughout much of the 20th century, recent work on document design and visual rhetoric has identified delivery with the rhetorical aspects of page and screen design (Connors, 1993; Dragga, 1993; Trimbur, 2004). But delivery can include even several steps beyond design. Carolyn Rude, in arguing for an expanded notion of delivery, suggests that instead of stopping at the moment a text is published, we extend our concept of delivery to include related rhetorical acts over a period of time, including recursive processes of revising after interacting with readers (2004).

We also find this expanded concept of delivery works hand-in-hand with the idea of user-centered technology, as described by Johnson (1998). In a user-centered view of technology, the user is conceptualized as "an integral, participatory force in the process" of system design (p. 30). This design process requires that designers interact with actual users, not just mental constructs of users; thus, the user is an active participant in technology design and use (p. 33). Johnson argues for a rhetorical understanding of user-centered technology, seeing users as agents and producers of knowledge, not simply passive receptacles of know-how (p. 57). The users in Johnson's user-centered system would participate in system design and maintain their agency within their organizational and cultural constraints, which would allow for the extended delivery that Rude (2004) describes; both would result in a recursive process whereby the audience uses the point of delivery as a means of responding to and shaping the message.

With the majority of our students living off-campus and working from half-time to full-time, we wanted to emphasize multiple points of contact for all stakeholders, where students in particular can interact with the instructor, with individuals, with small groups, and with the whole class. And we wanted this to occur consistently in our face-to-face, hybrid, and online platforms, a recursive process within a CMS environment that we believe enables administrators, teachers, and students to participate in the process of shaping and delivering the program.

Our program views writing as a complex, reflective, social activity. From this perspective, the delivery of the course itself, as the primary point of contact for all stakeholders in the program, must reproduce this complexity and sociability. We want our students to become more flexible users of technology and recognize the constructed nature of information media and understand the implications for their use. In short, we want students (and teachers) to think rhetorically when using technology. Therefore, a CMS can never be "invisible" and must provide more than just a repository for content.

We chose to use the template function in WebCampus for a variety of reasons: the delivery of content was stable and consistent across sections; administrators could revise/update/upgrade the content at the template level, with changes automatically updating in all sections, even during the semester; and teachers can download the course content quickly and easily into their sections and have complete control over their individual sections. While WebCampus is far from perfect, the flexibility afforded by the template function allows numerous points of contact for all user-levels in our program, and we have tried to design the template for a consistent and coherent delivery.

As we have implied, our template is the virtual space that unifies all 70+ sections of the course for all users across our three platforms (online, hybrid, and face-to-face). The template is designed and maintained by the administrators, working closely with our distance education staff, the instructional designers who provide us (the course administrators) with technical expertise. While we would certainly like more robust tools in our CMS, especially for collaboration, we decided early on that with our mostly itinerant staff (primarily part-time instructors and graduate students), we wanted to keep the learning curve as level as possible, especially for new teachers with little experience using technology in the classroom. In this way, our template relieves teachers of the responsibilities for creating assignments, discussion boards, and project modules themselves; they simply copy the template into their own course shells and modify it as they wish. Those with more experience teaching the course might make more modifications; those teaching the course for the first time (up to one-third of our staff) can work quite easily from the template alone, so they can spend their time thinking about their teaching, and not reinventing the wheel every semester. The template structures the interactions between teachers and students, and we hope that as instructors get familiar with the CMS and course content, they can gain autonomy by modifying the template. And as we receive feedback from teachers and students, we can use that information to make improvements so our template delivery is (ideally) recursive, although the process is limited by our own time and technology constraints. Maintaining all content within a single CMS seemed the most prudent option, despite constraints imposed by WebCampus, so we constructed our template around three primary areas: projects, instructor's documents, and assessment (see Figure 1).

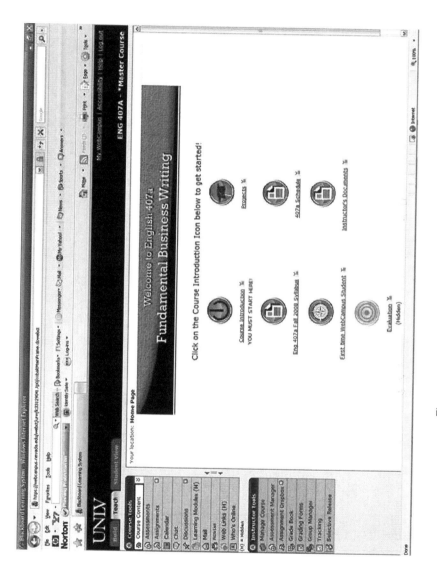

Figure 1. Template home page for instructors.

The projects area contains all materials for the four major projects. Each project contains multiple options for teachers and multiple deliverables for students:

Introductory Project (3)
- Informal Personal Profile
- Professional Formal Introduction
- Introductions Analysis Memo

Case Project (3)
- Internal Document
- External Document
- Project Assessment Memo

Employment Project (4)
- Job Analysis Memo
- Résumé
- Cover Letter
- Project Assessment Memo

Major Collaborative Project (5)
- Research Design Plan
- Progress Report
- Oral Presentation of Findings
- Final Recommendation Report
- Final Project Assessment Memo

The projects are organized to follow a fairly conventional process: invention/planning, drafting, peer review, revising, teacher response, revising/editing, evaluation. The template includes discussion boards for each stage of the process for all projects, reinforcing our commitment to the social nature of writing in a business context. Because these discussion boards are already in the template, teachers don't have to spend a lot of prep time building these features each semester; more importantly, students who are comfortable with the WebCampus format and online communication can begin participating immediately.

Also included are the grading criteria and evaluation sheet for each assignment, which are used by all instructors. This information helps the students understand the expectations for each project and how the instructor's responses to their writing will be structured.

Even in the face-to-face sections, students are required to submit assignments electronically, and instructors use the evaluation sheets for grading electronically. In these ways, our template is the virtual embodiment of the several points of contact between students themselves and between students and teachers (see Figure 2).

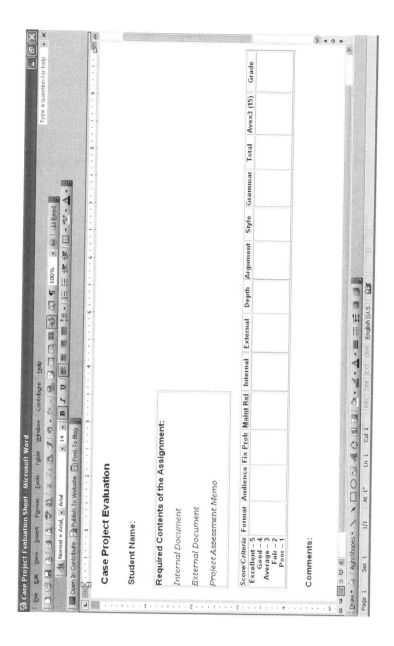

Figure 2. Case Project evaluation sheet.

Our projects are designed to help students meet course objectives while allow-ing instructors some freedom of choice. There are three individual projects and one group project. All but one of the projects has multiple options for instructors to choose from. The initial Introductory Project has two options, both of which require students to demonstrate mastery of memo conventions and provide an opportunity to learn different features of WebCampus. The Case Project has four different alternatives; each case presents a scenario of a conflict or error in a professional context. The Case Projects teach students to analyze complex social, organizational, ethical, and rhetorical contexts, and to draft and revise documents for multiple audiences. The final individual project, the Employment Project, is a typical job-search project taught in many business and technical writing service courses. Our program takes a rhetorical approach to this project, asking students to research not only the industry but also the target company and shape the cover letter and résumé to the needs of the reader. The Major Collaborative Project has three alternatives. Each asks student teams to draft proposals, research design plans, progress reports, oral presentations, and final reports. They learn how to determine goals; organize the workload; perform, evaluate, and synthesize research; negotiate collaborative writing projects; and develop reports that meet the needs of their readers.

Each project includes multiple deliverables along with a project assessment memo to establish how the student not only met the requirements of the project but also fulfilled the goals of the course. These multiple deliverables are all drafted, peer reviewed, commented upon by the instructor, and evaluated through the WebCampus system, even in face-to-face classes. Students thus learn how to navigate the online system: use the readings, discussion threads, and e-mail function to clarify the assignments; ask for help if needed; and communicate with each other and the instructor. They find themselves acting as agents within a system that structures their roles for them, as workers in a knowledge economy may find themselves working within a system that both enables and limits their actions. The students often find ways to complement the online system; for example, it is not uncommon to see students pull out cell phones (with the instructor's permission) and text missing classmates to discover whether the teammate has completed a promised portion of the project.

The second primary area of our template is instructor's documents (see Figure 1). This folder is kept hidden from students and includes our 10-hour-per-week schedule, which offers a way for instructors to manage their workload; "mentor materials" for teacher use in the classroom, including required course materials (like the syllabus, schedule, and project evalu-ation sheets), supplemental classroom materials (like project handouts, Power-Point slides, and project notes), sample materials (student drafts, minilectures, and samples of daily messages), suggestions for course preparation, additional readings, and a discussion of the theoretical assumptions of the course designers.

All of these materials have been collected by teachers in the program over the past 15 years.

Our program philosophy includes a strong belief that strong teacher support structures are imperative to successful course delivery and assessment, which leads to more effective and more efficient teachers. Some of our initial thinking on teaching support structures was influenced by the Texas Tech Online-Print Integrated Curriculum (TOPIC) system, which demonstrates ways that electronic technologies can facilitate teacher professionalization (Kemp, 2003; Nagelhout, 2007; Salvo, 2001). The points of contact for teachers, designed to value teachers as legitimate stakeholders in the program, include organizing, delivering, and facilitating mentor groups, teacher workshops, norming sessions, focus groups, and staff meetings. Most importantly, expectations for teacher interaction are always tempered by our 10-hour-per-week commitment. In our program, we believe that if four courses are considered a full-time load, then no teacher should spend more than 10 hours per week per course. This would include time in class, time in office hours, time preparing for class, time responding/evaluating student writing, and time in staff meetings or professional development. Thus, our template serves as both a teacher training tool and set of resources, one that can be updated and altered from semester to semester. The template contents are necessarily supplemented with these ongoing training meetings and subsequently revised and updated in a recursive delivery process that relies on student and teacher engagement.

The third primary area of our template is for assessment, which is actually inside the instructor's documents folder. This is the main point of contact for the administrators. From the beginning, the administration of our business writing program has been a collaborative affair. A goal of the program has always been to avoid an "individual" approach to administration that too often collapses into turf wars and battles of "ownership"; instead, program development has been viewed more as a complex adaptive system (see Jablonski & Nagelhout, 2010). This collaborative approach leads to a more stakeholder-friendly environment, one in which everyone has a voice and everyone is expected to participate in the development of the program.

While our template has simplified the task of maintaining consistency across sections and keeping schedules, assignments, and grading standards as uniform as possible, we also rely on the template to structure the delivery of written feedback from students to other students, from teachers to students, and from teachers back to administrators. In other words, our template incorporates a process for collecting data for assessment: instructors paste copies of randomly selected student grades for the projects into a spreadsheet at the end of each semester and send those to the administrator. As a result, we have a robust source of data for assessment purposes, enabling us to see where students might be struggling so that we can adjust course content and emphasis.

There are some drawbacks to the way this delivery system structures communication patterns. When student discussions take place online, the asynchronous discussion threads can lack some of the immediacy of face-to-face interaction in which comments can be challenged by other students as soon as they are made. Less engaged students may not read posts made by other students, so they may not respond when their ideas are challenged. A lack of engagement in discussions can lead to weaker drafts because those disengaged students are not forced to think through ethical contexts thoroughly; this can be a particular problem in the case project, described below. Nevertheless, the online and hybrid course formats demand that students engage with ideas while simultaneously learning and acquiring skills in digital environments, which is where workplace communication often occurs in the professions to which these students aspire.

A CASE PROJECT EXAMPLE

We would like to offer an extended example of a particular assignment to show where points of contact occur as part of the delivery of our CMS for all levels and to show how these points of contact allow agency, foster communication, and enable assessment.

As we described earlier, our case project offers four options for teachers. Each case project seeks similar ends, using similar documents. Students must solve a problem that has arisen within an organization that was caused by someone in their company. Using their communication skills, they must author (individually) an internal document (an e-mail or memo) and an external document (e-mail or formal letter) written to an appropriate person in the other organization. The internal document is written to superiors in their company and explains the problem, provides criteria for analyzing the situation effectively, offers possible solutions, and concludes with a recommendation for action. The external document is the first step in solving the problem. This document is written to a person in the other organization who can effect change and must maintain good relations with the other organization. The final "deliverable" for the Case Project is a project assessment memo that students use to explain their thinking, justify their choices, reflect on their writing process, and show how they have met the course outcomes.

Project Criteria

An important point of contact between student, teacher, and administrator is the set of criteria defined for each project. With all of our projects, we provide criteria for evaluating student writing that are tied directly to our course outcomes, and we spend a good bit of time defining all criteria for each assignment. For example, we have six general criteria and four project-specific criteria for the Case Project:

General Criteria
- Format
- Audience
- Depth of Thought
- Argument
- Business Style
- Grammar and Correctness

Project-Specific Criteria
- Fix the Problem
- Maintain Relations
- Quality of Internal Document
- Quality of External Document

The criteria list establishes the basis for expectations for students and teachers (and administrators) in the program. Our goal, of course, is transparency in evaluation, which is not only good assessment practice, but empowers everyone in the program by structuring peer reviews, teacher responses, and assessment. Defining criteria provides everyone a voice.

Project Delivery

The assignment reaches the classroom through the CMS. The traditional processes of invention/planning, drafting, review, and revising are all mediated through the CMS. We try to take advantage of as many of the CMS tools as possible in order to foster communication as fully as possible, although we realize that the CMS does not adapt as neatly as we would like.

The invention/planning stage occurs in both whole-class and small-group formats. Whether face-to-face, hybrid, or online, the larger whole-class discussion is vital in order for students to begin to understand the complexity of the case project. There is always much more going on than students will see on a first read. A lively discussion about the evaluation criteria generally grows out of these initial discussions of the case as well. To help push student thinking even further, many of our teachers also create small-group discussion boards. We try to track student participation by both quantity and quality of post in order to assess the value of this part of the process. We have found that the students who engage with the discussion boards produce more effective writing, and we bring that message back to the classroom, reminding students to take responsibility for their learning. As with our staff meetings, the CMS cannot stand alone; its delivery must be supplemented with face-to-face activities or direct e-mails from the instructor in an online setting.

Our CMS is not necessarily ideal for the peer review stage of the process. The face-to-face and hybrid sections tend to offer better experiences for the students because they get the benefit of both talking and responding in writing through small-group discussion boards. The online sections tend to suffer since the comments are primarily in-text. Some teachers have tried to use the chat function of the CMS as a means for enhancing the peer review experience, with only limited success. Students who enroll in online courses generally choose that option because of schedule restrictions, and they typically find it virtually impossible to use a synchronous chat function.

The teacher-response stage of the process functions within the CMS through the assignment dropbox feature. This allows students to submit a draft to the teacher who can then offer comments, most often using a "Track Changes" feature, and return the draft through the assignment dropbox. The CMS at least allows for drafts to be submitted and returned multiple times if necessary. Teachers, having participated in the staff meeting, can offer a pointed response to the most important areas of concern in a student draft. As a program, we believe that students will learn to write most effectively if they receive feedback in-process rather than only at the end. But if teachers are to stay within the 10-hour-per-week expectation, then they must respond as efficiently as possible.

Finally, the evaluation stage is to "grade" the project only. At this point in the process, students receive an evaluation sheet only (see Figure 3):

Students receive evaluation only and comments designed to help them improve individually as writers in the future. Since most students in Business Writing arrive with meager experience in teacher response to their writing, we find it important as a program to define for students (and teachers) the ways we use criteria and the ways we interact with student writing. We spend a good bit of time in each of our sections (and in staff meetings) explaining the difference between response and evaluation. Since all students have multiple opportunities to receive feedback on their drafts, there are no opportunities to "revise" after the project has been evaluated. As we explain to our students, "If you are in a business setting, and you send a letter to a client, you will not get an opportunity to revise the letter if the reader does not like it." We want them to develop good habits of mind for writing and use the tools available to them (as afforded by our CMS) to improve a particular product as much as possible before the deadline.

After all projects have been returned, our CMS only offers to average numerical scores within the gradebook function for comparing scores. This of course is quite limited in terms of allowing agency, fostering communication, and enabling assessment. To meet these goals and enhance our CMS, we ask teachers to enter the scores for all of the criteria for all students on a spreadsheet (see Figure 4).

A quick analysis of the spreadsheet will show teachers exactly where students were most successful and least successful in completing the assignment. Armed with that information, we ask teachers to review the assignment with the students, especially in terms of the general criteria that will more than likely show up in a future assignment.

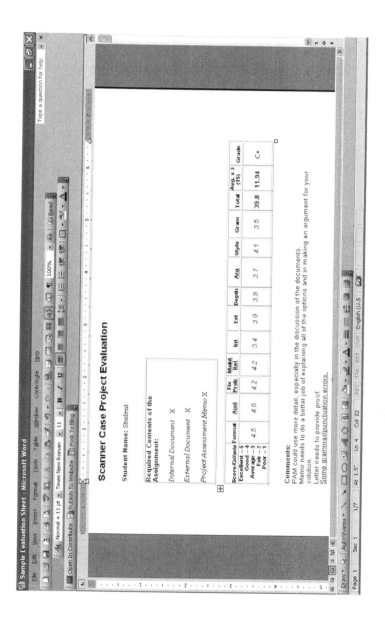

Figure 3. Scanner Case Project evaluation example (complete).

Microsoft Excel - 407A-008 Individual Course Assessment

A1: Intro Project

Intro Project

	Format	Audience	Info.	Access	Rhet.	Org.	Style	Detail	Visual	Grammar	Total	AVE1(5)	Grade
Student 2	3	4		4	4	5	4	5	4	5	43	4.3	B-
Student 6	3				3	4	3	3	3		34	3.4	C
Student 10													
Student 14	5	5	5	4		5	5	5	5	5	49	4.9	A
Student 18													
Student 22													

Case Project

	Format	Audience	Fix Prob	Maint Rel	Internal	External	Depth	Argument	Style	Grammar	Total	AVE3 (15)	Grade
Student 3	3	4	4	4	3	3	3	4	4	4	38	11.4	B
Student 7	4	4	4	4	4	3	3	3	3	3	35	10.5	C-
Student 11	4	4	4	4	4	2	2	2	2	3	28	8.4	C
Student 15	4	3	3	4	3	3	3	4	4	3	35	10.5	C
Student 19	3	3	1	3	2	2	2	1	3	3	25	7.5	C-
Student 23													

Job Project

	Format	Audience	Resum 1	Resum 2	Resum 3	Resum 4	CL 1	CL 2	CL 3	Grammar	Total	AVE3 (15)	Grade
Student 4	3	3	4		3		3	2	2	2	27	8.1	C-
Student 8	3	3	3		3		2	4	3	4	30	9	D-
Student 12													
Student 16													
Student 20													
Student 24													

Progress Report

	Format	Audience	Info.	PR Cont.	Rhet.	Org.	Style	Detail	Visual	Grammar	Total	AVE1(5)	Grade
Student 1	5	5	5	5	4	5	5	5	5	5	48	4.8	A
Student 5	4	4	3	3	2	4	4	4	2	3	33	3.3	C
Student 9	5	3	5	5	5	5	5	4	3	3	41	4.1	B
Student 13													
Student 17													
Student 21													

Design Plan

	Format	Audience	Info.	Detail	Strategies	Materials	Schedule	Style	Grammar	Total	AVE2(10)	Grade
Team 1												
Team 2												
Team 3												
Team 4												
Team 5												
Team 6												

Oral Presentation

	Format	Audience	Info.	Oral	Outline	Points	Linked	Org.	Visual	Grammar	Total	AVE2(10)	Grade
Team 1	3	4	4	4	2	3	3	3	3	3	30		C
Team 2	5	5	5	5	5	5	5	5	5	5	49	9.8	A
Team 3	5	5	5	5	5	4	4	4	4	4	46	9.2	A
Team 4													
Team 5													
Team 6													

Sheet1 / Sheet2 / Sheet3

Figure 4. Individual course assessment file (complete).

For example, a teacher might have determined that all students scored lower than expected on formatting. This use of assessment provides an immediate opportunity to have a conversation with the students about good formatting, what formatting means in different rhetorical situations, and what students need to consider for future assignments. The teacher might also spend a bit more time discussing formatting for the invention/planning stage in the next assignment. This also provides the students with specific opportunities for asking questions about the work and for communicating with the teacher in more concrete ways.

Program Analysis

Finally, at the administrative level, we gather a spreadsheet of randomly selected students from every section (see Figure 5).

Our CMS does not allow us to customize the gradebook or the evaluation sheets so that we might gather this information more efficiently, so we require all teachers to send their spreadsheets as attachments. Once all of the spreadsheets are combined for a specific semester, we can begin to assess programmatically. By creating spreadsheets based on the evaluation criteria, we can analyze the data in a variety of ways, limited only by our imagination. We can analyze by outcome, by criterion, by a single project, across projects, by course platform, by section, across sections, and so on.

For example, if we assessed for our course outcome, "Design documents for both content and visual appeal," we can examine the findings for a particular criterion like formatting. In spring 2008, the overall average for all projects across all sections was 4.23/5. The lowest Format scores occurred in the Case Projects (3.98/5 average) and the highest occurred in the Employment Project (4.39/5 average). Using numbers like these, we can have conversations about student learning, teacher effectiveness, teacher support, and program effectiveness. But our CMS lacks the tools for initiating these conversations effectively across the program at all levels.

CONCLUSION

As we have illustrated throughout this chapter, we see the CMS and our master template as an extension of a set of texts delivered across space, time, and course formats. The delivery of our 70+ sections of business writing per year encompasses not only the rhetorical acts of each instructor as he or she manages each section, but also the related acts of teacher training, student development, administration, and data collection. Each step in our process of developing the course, from creating the master course template, to training the teachers in how to load and use the template, to orienting students to the online environment, represents a point of contact, an opportunity for our set of texts to interact with its intended audiences or set of actors.

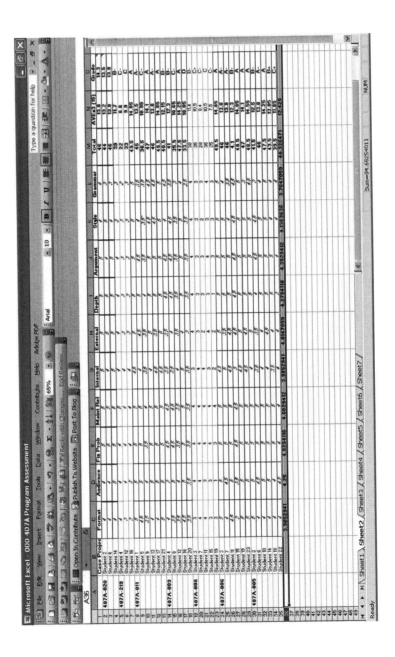

Figure 5. Program assessment file (complete).

In 2009, these points of contact were increased institutionally when UNLV mandated that all freshman- and sophomore-level courses make midsemester grades available to students through WebCampus, so our students and teachers are gradually becoming more familiar with the CMS even before they start our classes. This increased experience has helped us by cutting down on the initial orientation for both students and teachers, but it has hurt us in terms of WebCampus's already poor reputation for unexpected outages, difficulties with different platforms, and other sources of frustration. We try to put these frustrations into a professional context for the students and teachers both, reminding them that workers rarely get to choose their tools; in addition, reflexive conversations about WebCampus in teacher-training sessions as well as in the classroom (or virtual classroom) serve the purpose of making the technology visible. As long as the CMS is developed and owned by a third-party vendor, we will fall short of Johnson's (1998) ideal of user-centered design, because neither we nor our instructors, nor our students have access to the actual software designers. But we can use the ideal as much as possible when developing and revising our template.

We represent a program that is well behind the cutting edge of innovation in information technology and course management software. Our lack of resources has forced us to adapt work-arounds. Like the students who prefer to use text-messaging instead of WebCampus's chat function, we look for ways to take advantage of technology from the margins. For example, to fix the problem of lack of aggregate data on different scoring categories within assignments, our work-around requires instructors to take several extra steps to copy data from a table in MS Word and paste it into Excel spreadsheets, which the administrator must aggregate into a single programwide workbook. The time invested by both instructors and administrators on this work-around is repaid by the huge amount of data we've collected that we can use for different types of research. Our solutions are not always smoothly incorporated into the CMS, but with some creativity and many compromises, we meet our program's goals.

REFERENCES

Connors, R. J. (1993). *Actio*: A rhetoric of written delivery (iteration two). In J. F. Reynolds (Ed.), *Rhetorical memory and delivery: Classical concepts for contemporary composition and communication* (pp. 97–111). Hillsdale, NJ: Lawrence Erlbaum.

Dragga, S. (1993). The ethics of delivery. In J. F. Reynolds (Ed.), *Rhetorical memory and delivery: Classical concepts for contemporary composition and communication* (pp. 79–95). Hillsdale, NJ: Lawrence Erlbaum.

Harrington, C. F., Gordon, S. A., & Shibik, T. J. (2004). Course management system utilization and implications for practice: A national survey of department chairpersons. *Online Journal of Distance Learning Administration, 7*(4), 1–13.

Jablonski, J. (2006). *Business and technical writing at UNLV*. Dubuque, IA: Kendall/Hunt.

Jablonski, J., & Nagelhout, E. (2010). Assessing professional writing programs using technology as a site of praxis. In J. Allen & M. Hundleby (Eds.), *Assessment in technical and professional communication* (pp. 171–187). Amityville, NY: Baywood.

Johnson, R. (1998). *User-centered technology: A rhetorical theory for computers and other mundane artifacts.* Albany, NY: SUNY Press.

Kemp, F. (2003, September 30). *Instruction manual for TOPIC.* Retrieved from http://ttopic.english.ttu.edu/manual/manualreadall.asp?typeof=manual

Kramer, R., & Bernhardt, S. A. (1999). Moving instruction to the Web: Writing as multi-tasking. *Technical Communication Quarterly, 8,* 319–336.

Morgan, G. (2003, May). Key findings: Faculty use of course management systems. *EDUCAUSE Center for Applied Research.* Retrieved from http://www.educause.edu/ECAR/FacultyUseofCourseManagementSy/158560

Nagelhout, E. (1999). Pre-professional practices in the technical writing classroom: Promoting multiple literacies through research. *Technical Communication Quarterly, 8,* 285–299.

Nagelhout, E. (2007, Fall). Faculty development as working condition. *College Composition and Communication FORUM, 59*(1), A14–A16.

Porter, J., Sullivan, P., & Johnson-Eilola, J. (2009). *Professional writing online, version 3.0.* New York: Longman.

Rose, S., & Weiser, I. (Eds.). (1999). *The writing program administrator as researcher: Inquiry in action and reflection.* Portsmouth, NH: Heinemann.

Rose, S., & Weiser, I. (Eds.). (2002). *The writing program administrator as theorist: Making knowledge work.* Portsmouth, NH: Heinemann.

Rude, C. (2004). Toward an expanded concept of rhetorical delivery: The uses of reports in public policy debates. *Technical Communication Quarterly, 13,* 271–288.

Salvo, M. (2001). Ethics of engagement: User-centered design and rhetorical methodology. *Technical Communication Quarterly, 10,* 273–290.

Trimbur, J. (2004). Delivering the message: Typography and the materiality of writing. In C. Handa (Ed.), *Visual rhetoric in a digital world: A critical sourcebook* (pp. 260–271). New York: Bedford/St. Martin's.

http://dx.doi.org/10.2190/OE2C3

CHAPTER 3

Creativity and Consistency in Online Courses: Finding the Appropriate Balance

Keri Dutkiewicz, LuAnne Holder,
and Wayne D. Sneath

Davenport University (DU) is a private, nonprofit university serving approximately 13,000 students at multiple locations across Michigan. Students earn degrees in health care, business, and technology. DU uses predesigned courses (PDCs) in most of its online offerings. These courses offer a consistent navigational structure across the institution and help to ensure pedagogical consistency across multiple concurrent sections of the same course. This desire for consistency mirrors in-seat practices (such as using a common textbook) designed to ensure students across multiple sections are given equal opportunity to meet learning outcomes. Davenport implemented PDCs with the goal of enabling instructors to focus expertise on teaching rather than the "click and wait" component of building an online course.

This chapter examines how faculty teaching professional writing online at DU perceive the use of these predesigned courses. Based on a study of instructor and student perceptions of PDCs, the chapter reports how instructors balance course consistency among multiple sections, creativity to address unique needs of a particular class, and autonomy in professional contributions to these courses as well as their sense of support and belonging to a community of practice consisting of peer instructors and administrators at DU. Also explored are the reported effects of faculty customizations and personalizations of these courses on student perceptions of learning. The study indicates that a balance of faculty

45

autonomy in customizing courses with the inclusion of required predesigned elements best serves to meet instructor expectations in meeting the unique needs of online learners. These findings can guide other institutions using, or considering using, predesigned courses being taught by multiple instructors, particularly adjunct instructors.

BACKGROUND OF ONLINE INSTRUCTION
AT DAVENPORT UNIVERSITY

As of fall 2009, just under 50% of all DU credits were delivered online using Blackboard. Many of these online sections, including English 311: Professional Writing, are on a 7-week accelerated schedule. However, staffing of full-time faculty and staff dedicated to online academics remains significantly lower per credit delivered than comparable in-seat staffing levels. A large percentage of online courses are taught by adjunct faculty, and most online department coordinators supervise greater numbers of sections than their in-seat counterparts. In addition, the online adjunct faculty are located around the globe. The English and Communications faculty teaching online live across the United States as well as in China, India, Greece, and Korea. The full-time online academic team at DU is also a geographically dispersed team located across the United States. This team is composed of department coordinators, instructional designers, faculty development professionals, and administrative staff.

In general, the online academic team has largely embraced master courses, or PDCs, as one way to improve quality and ensure alignment across sections given limited resources. During the 2006–2007 academic year, the online academic team made the decision to develop and maintain PDCs for any online course offering more than 7 sections per year. In the English department, which has fewer courses but offers at least 8–14 sections of each course per 7-week term, this decision precipitated the need to develop PDCs for nearly all courses. Of particular relevance is the fact that these PDCs were implemented with a group of faculty who had been accustomed to teaching individually developed sections; most faculty included in the study were not hired with the expectation that they would be teaching a predesigned curriculum. This study therefore offers insights into instructor attitudes toward PDCs as a new approach.

The PDC model at DU provides a consistent navigation template that is used throughout the institution for online courses. The PDC model builds consistency for students across different courses; online Math, English, Management, and information technology (IT) courses all use the same navigational template. Within a specific multisection course, the PDC also provides consistent content, pedagogical approaches, and workloads across all sections. However, even with consistent lessons, assignments, and due dates, instructors do have some autonomy to customize their classes. Using the PDC model, this chapter explores ways to balance consistency with instructor creativity in customizing courses to meet his/her own teaching style as well as the individual needs of student learners in a specific section.

DU PDCs are not "off the shelf" content purchased from third-party providers; every PDC is developed by a DU team of subject matter experts including department coordinators, faculty, and (ideally) instructional designers. This cross-functional team works to implement a particular course using the PDC navigational template that spans the entire university. Stewart, Bachman, and Babb (2009) agree on the importance of cross-functional development teams. While few faculty members have the instructional design or technical background required for effective online course development (Oblinger & Hawkins, 2006), they serve as subject matter experts who ensure that student learning is prioritized over technical design (Gerber & Scott, 2007). The navigational template is determined by the full-time online academic team, with instructional design taking the lead. Once set, this university-wide navigational template cannot be changed by individual instructors or for individual classes without diminishing one key benefit of PDCs, consistent navigation across courses. This consistent navigation allows students to focus on course content rather than engaging in time spent on a new learning curve to discern the navigation structure for each new course taken.

Currently the PDC template used in online classes at DU contains the following menu elements: Announcements, Syllabus, the e-textbook, Weekly Materials, Discussion Board, and Resources/Help (see Figure 1).

The Announcements is the default opening page. Announcements are customized by individual instructors who decide on content and frequency of announcement postings. The other two links that are most frequently visited by students are the Weekly Materials and the Discussion Board. Lessons, resources, objectives, and assignments are housed in the Weekly Materials link. Each week contains a new module of materials (see Figure 2). Each weekly module is unique and may contain rich-media elements and/or links to resources outside the courseroom. While every course uses the same weekly materials structure, individual courses populate this core area of the course with different kinds of assignments, readings, and activities.

The Discussion Boards are also organized by weekly modules. Generally, classes pose several questions or other online activities each week; some PDCs enable instructors to create their own discussion questions while other PDCs prepopulate the course with specific topics (see Figure 3). Discussion board assignments vary in focus and may prompt application of new material, evaluation of an approach, or analysis of a document.

Furthermore, at DU most large, multisection online classes that use a PDC are staffed by at least one course coordinator. The course coordinator role is similar to the lead instructor role outlined in Kearsley and Poitras (2007). Course coordinators develop the pedagogical strategy and course content for individual

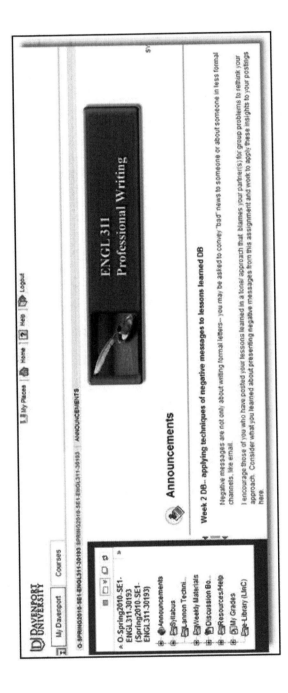

Figure 1. PDC template menu for English 311: Professional Writing.

Week 3 Overview & Learning Outcomes

Overview:
This week we will focus on defining technical terms to various audiences. We will also continue work on the Professional Language and Culture report by completing a Report Design Worksheet

Learning Outcomes:

- Demonstrate ability to compose detailed technical definitions for a non-expert audience

- Compose detailed report planning document

- Develop greater understanding of planning for professional writing

Making the Connection:
Defining terms so that all parties understand the meaning can be very important in a professional setting. As we look at creating expanded definitions this week you will look at terms that you are quite familiar with in your field, yet try to look at that term from the perspective of someone unfamiliar with that term. Often in looking at a concept from the eyes of a novice, an expert can see details of that concept that are otherwise overlooked.

Week 3 Agenda.doc

Week 3 Preparation: Readings & Resources
Click on the folder link to access information regarding reading and lecture assignments for week three

Week 3 Tasks: Discussion Board & Assignments
Click on the folder link to access information regarding week three discussion board and assignments.

Week 3: Assignment Submission Folder
Click on the folder link to submit your assignments for week three. Identify the appropriate assignment link and submit as an attachment. To add more than one attachment, use the 'Add another file' feature that is located below the text box. When you have successfully submitted your assignment, an exclamation mark (!) will appear in the grade book

Figure 2. Sample Weekly Materials page of the PDC for
English 311: Professional Writing.

Week 2 Forum 2: Reflection on Feedback

Last week you engaged in peer reviews. This week you will will be reviewing each others' work in pairs. What kinds of information do you hope to receive when a fellow student reviews your work? What can you do to provide the best feedback to other students? What kinds of feedback on your work do you give or receive in your profession? How can being skilled in providing quality feedback shape your professional reputation?

Week 2 Forum 3: Tone and persuasive techniques

Read the three documents posted under Weekly Materials-- Week 2-- Discussion Boards and Assignments. Then, select ONE of the three documents provided to evaluate in depth via this DB.

What tone does the writer use? What persuasive techniques are used? Who is the intended audience and how do you know? Is the document effective for this intended audience? Why or why not? Could it have been improved?

Respond to the postings of at least two other learners. You can respond to postings for any of the documents.

Week 3 Forum 1: Two definition versions

Post two versions of a concise (2-4 sentence) definition of the term you will use for your expanded definition. Version 1 should be written for an audience of experts in the field. Version 2 should be written for a non-expert audience. What are the differences between the two?

Then, respond to at least 2 other students' concise definitions. What further questions do you have about this term? Do you agree that the non-expert definition clearly presents the concept/ term even to people with no knowledge of this field?

Figure 3. Sample Discussion Board questions for
English 311: Professional Writing.

master course templates, building courses within the university-wide navigational template. This faculty role involves being a formal mentor/coach for faculty teaching the class, a subject matter expert, and the lead online instructional designer responsible for maintaining the PDC. Course coordinators are most often experienced instructors for the course; they leverage their expertise teaching the course to provide rapid turnaround on instructor questions and help department coordinators complete routine course checks that monitor consistent use of PDC elements and quality of student-instructor interaction during weeks 3 and 5 of the 7-week accelerated term.

Prior to the adoption of the PDC format, online courses at DU tended to be labeled as poor quality or lacking in rigor by some faculty and administrators. According to the Sloan Consortium's 2009 survey of online education in the United States, the perception that online courses are not as valuable as in-seat courses is common. Administrators in less than one third of the institutions surveyed indicated that their faculty value online education (Allen & Seaman, 2010). To address this issue, the online academic team used the development of quality PDCs to help improve not only the perception of quality in online classes within the institution but the actual quality of education delivered to students. The PDC development teams continue to work hard to ensure that the PDCs are at least as rigorous as in-seat classes.

Finally, DU elected to use PDCs to streamline the administrative processes of course copying and course management. With a PDC approach, all sections of a large, multisection course are populated with the same core PDC content. Being able to batch copy courses reduces the set-up time required every term. Instructors, too, save time; they have minimal course preparation before classes start. This time savings is important given limited resources and the rapid turnaround between 7-week accelerated terms. At times, the online team at DU has less than one week between the end of one term and the start of the next.

While the benefits of consistency and alignment are strong, and while the online team needed a streamlined approach to course copy and administration, questions and concerns about PDCs remain. These questions, which we identify in the next section, led us to conduct the research study reported in this chapter.

A CASE FOR USING PREDESIGNED COURSES

This study is a preliminary attempt at evaluating the success of PDCs in terms of instructor engagement and student perceptions of learning. Specifically, the following research questions were investigated:

1. How can PDCs maintain core areas of consistency while enabling instructional flexibility and autonomy through the inclusion of appropriate instructional elements?

2. What strategies of faculty communication, structure, and professional development support maximum consistency as well as creativity and autonomy in online course development?
3. To what extent do students notice instructor customizations to the PDC? Do students perceive that these customizations improve their learning?

Online course consistency and quality across sections, as well as the numerous means for monitoring and assessing these factors, have been investigated in previous research. Faculty members' reactions to prescribed course elements and their subsequent engagement and motivation in course construction and delivery have been explored in some detail (Kearsley & Poitras, 2007; Herrington, Herrington, Oliver, Stoney, & Willis, 2001). Course templates and checklists, consistent faculty training, lead course instructors, and standardized assessment tools for assignments have all been used to align multiple sections of online courses. Other studies have reported generally positive faculty reactions to these kinds of course standardizations (Stewart et al., 2009). Specifically, according to studies by Bonk (2001) and Herrington et al. (2001), instructors prefer a consistent course design that is easy to use as long as the design maintains a professional look and some flexibility (Bonk, 2001). Once created, these PDCs allow instructors to reuse and tweak existing course features instead of independently creating similar elements.

Studies also indicate that students indicate a preference for consistent design. Poor design is often stated as a contributing factor in student dissatisfaction with the quality of an online course (Hathaway, 2009). In one study, more than 90% of the students surveyed indicated that online courses should be organized in a consistent structure as opposed to each instructor designing a completely customized course. However, more than 90% of students in this same study also indicated that the quality of an online course was dependent on customization gained through high levels of interaction between the instructor and the learners (Young & Norgard, 2006). Additionally, when the learners received personalized feedback, as opposed to collective feedback, they indicated a higher level of personal satisfaction as well as an increased perception of enhanced learning (Hathaway, 2009).

According to current research, faculty embrace the advantages of predesigned elements as long as they maintain some level of autonomy to personalize courses. Additionally, faculty favor PDCs that model constructivist approaches to student learning and engagement focused on problem solving and not on rote memorization or skill practice, as these constructivist strategies encourage the production of new knowledge and provide less opportunity for student cheating and plagiarism (Liaw, 2004; Stewart et al., 2009). The administrative burden of individual instructors designing courses from scratch is also removed with the consistently delivered structure and content of a PDC (Stewart et al., 2009).

While current research begins to explore faculty perceptions of the balance between autonomy and creativity in PDCs, this study focused on identifying the ways institutional context impacts this balance. Existing literature helps to identify and frame ideas relating to faculty perceptions of PDCs, but further examination of the issues of communication and collaboration is needed to better understand the ways PDCs impact faculty communities of practice. In one study of online instructors, respondents overwhelmingly (82%) indicated an interest in participating in a community of practice where they could share pedagogical approaches, discuss problems, and offer advice (Bonk, 2001). This study investigates how the PDC model can address this need for community to support the correlations that exist between autonomy, creativity, and consistency, all of which remain core goals for the implementation of PDCs. It also explores student perceptions of learning in online courses in which instructors make customizations and personalizations to prescribed content. The findings can be used as one resource for institutions using a large adjunct faculty population in making policy decisions concerning which courses should be designed as PDCs and how those PDCs should be implemented and maintained. Additionally, this study can serve as one resource in developing policy for adjunct faculty support and collegiality.

BACKGROUND OF THE COURSE FOCUS, ENGLISH 311: PROFESSIONAL WRITING

This study focuses on online sections of English 311, the capstone English course required for graduation by all DU majors. As a result of the university requirement, enrollment in the class is consistently high. Students come from multiple majors and demographic groups, and as may occur with other required writing courses, the class seems to strike fear and loathing into the hearts of many students.

The official description from the *Davenport University Academic Catalog* describes English 311 as follows:

> This course develops the written and presentation skills necessary for success in professional, supervisory, or managerial positions. Students learn to present information in document and oral styles appropriate to diverse workplace audiences and situations, including team writing. As a team, students create a major professional document. Students also learn to use a variety of formats, styles, and delivery systems to achieve the clear, concise, and professional communication required by the global economy.

Approximately 65–80 sections of the course are offered online each academic year and only in the 7-week accelerated format. While the English 311 team must manage the course using a PDC and must adhere to the official university-wide navigational template in Blackboard, developers are offered a great deal of flexibility with the instructional content of the PDC.

The first draft of the English 311 PDC was built by Dr. Keri Dutkiewicz, the department coordinator for online English and Communications, and contributing author to this study, who is located in western Michigan. She reviewed all existing sections of the course, talked to each instructor via phone, and then compiled best practices from multiple sections to design the first PDC. Dutkiewicz piloted the new PDC for one term, during which time feedback from faculty, administrators, and students was collected and used to make course changes. She maintained all English PDCs, including English 311, for approximately one year, until course coordinators were in place to help maintain the PDC. When Dr. LuAnne Holder, another member of this research team from eastern Michigan, moved into the role of Course Coordinator for online English 311, she continued the collaborative process of regularly updating the class based on instructor and student feedback. At the time this study took place, the PDC had been through several major revisions and numerous "tweaks" based on student and instructor feedback, including that from Dr. Wayne Sneath, the final member of this research team, who is located in Grand Rapids, Michigan.

The English 311 course uses the same standard navigational template used across the institution. However, while the PDC menu remains consistent, the content within each link continues to evolve. New items are added to provide additional resources. Current items are edited based on faculty and student feedback. Some items are deleted and some are rearranged. However, these changes are not made by individual instructors, but by course coordinators who collate faculty feedback into a master course template for English 311. Then this master course template is copied each term to all sections, thus providing consistent course material across all sections each term.

Methodology and the Research Process

The 49 participants in this research study included all faculty teaching English and Communications courses online at DU during the summer and fall terms of 2009. These faculty participants represented a diverse population—part-time online-only faculty, full-time in-seat faculty who teach one or two classes per year online, novice teachers, experienced online faculty, and experienced faculty new to the online environment. Additionally, input from students enrolled in English 311 during both fall 2009 sessions was solicited.

As mentioned earlier, when DU began the process of launching PDCs in 2007, the leadership of the online English program worked to develop and launch the course collaboratively with faculty input. However, from this beginning point, faculty opinions of the PDC approach remained divided. Some faculty at DU appreciated the instructional assistance, while others resented the control PDCs exerted over teaching. Rather than focus on the purely affective dimensions of faculty satisfaction with PDCs, this study sought to better understand how faculty were working with PDCs and the impact of PDCs on student perceptions of learning and success. To this end, a survey was designed to obtain the faculty perspective of the PDC process, specifically concerning the ways they customized instruction within the PDC and the ways they wished they could customize the course (see Appendix A). This survey was delivered online using a free online survey tool, SurveyMonkey.

Feedback was also gathered via Web-based meetings conducted using Wimba Live Classroom, an online meeting space that enables presenters and audience members to share PowerPoint slides, respond to onscreen questions, chat, and talk via headset and microphone in real time. Other sources of data included a review of student evaluations and reflections as well as data gathered through reviews of ongoing courses and the customizations made in them.

The research team met weekly via Wimba Live Classroom during data collection to sort through feedback and locate potential trends, correlations, and disjunctions. The data was coded according to strengths and weaknesses of the PDC, successes and failures of customizations, and suggestions for improvement to the PDC process as well as for collaboration among instructors. The input from these sources initiated revisions to the PDC model that demonstrated a shifting perspective on the appropriate balance between consistency and creativity in online course design, as well as the development of communications initiatives to promote an improved faculty community of practice.

Finally, a survey of student perceptions of learning, online course customizations, and personalizations was conducted using Survey Monkey (see Appendix B). Additional student input was gathered, such as feedback on evaluations and reflection exercises. This data provided insight into the impact of course design and delivery on students' perceptions of learning as well as on their level of engagement with the instructor and the course.

Survey Data Results and Analysis

The study gathered four sources of data: faculty survey, student survey, review of student course feedback, and review of faculty course content. The faculty survey gathered responses from 26 of the 49 instructors engaged in teaching English 311 online for a 53% response rate. These instructors were invited via e-mail to participate in an anonymous survey presented on Survey Monkey. Students were invited to participate through communication within their English 311 classes. Of the approximately 200 students enrolled in English 311 for the fall 2009 term, 43 students responded to the student survey for a 21.5% response rate. They were assured anonymity and provided access to a URL linking them to a separate student survey on SurveyMonkey.com.

FACULTY PERCEPTIONS: TIME, AUTONOMY, CUSTOMIZATIONS, AND COLLABORATION

One issue queried through the faculty survey concerned attitudes regarding the relationship between autonomy and the time investment needed to customize a course. The English 311 PDC is designed to significantly reduce the amount of time an instructor must invest in course preparation and in course maintenance. Since many of the faculty are part-time instructors, often with other full-time jobs, most survey respondents indicated that they appreciated the time advantage of teaching a PDC. One faculty respondent indicated that using a predesigned course allowed more time for engaging directly with students. However, more than 80% of the faculty also indicated that they wanted some autonomy as well. One respondent noted that room for instructor personality, expertise, and style is beneficial to students.

While some respondents indicated they would be willing to give up most or all autonomy in exchange for little or no preparation and maintenance time, the majority indicated that the current balance of time and autonomy was appropriate (53.8%), and more than a quarter of the respondents (26.9%) indicated a willingness to invest more time in customization and personalization of the course. No respondents, however, wanted to develop a completely customized course on their own.

One hypothesis of the study was that perhaps faculty felt restricted in making changes to the PDC because they were unclear about what changes were permissible. When PDCs were first introduced at DU, faculty were encouraged to teach the PDC "as is" in order to have a shared experience and begin to build consistency in workload, course focus, and community of practice across sections. Over time, department leadership and course coordinators began to enable greater levels of customization. However, the survey revealed that communication of this shift in expectations to faculty was insufficient. For example, narrative comments on the survey indicated that many faculty were still not clear about what constituted "acceptable parameters for changes or customizations."

However, when asked to identify the acceptability of modifying specific elements on a Likert scale, a large percentage of respondents correctly identified elements that they were encouraged to customize (announcements 96%, adding resources 70%, providing synchronous sessions 91.7%, and discussion board interaction 96%). Likewise, the faculty correctly indicated elements that should not be modified such as the agenda and the assignment details. In other words, while faculty felt they had an unclear understanding of how a PDC could and should be customized, they intuitively knew what the parameters were. The online English and Communications Department encourages customizations to discussion boards, adding resources, using announcements, and such, with the belief that instructors should have the option to engage students in ways that make sense to their instructional philosophy, as long as any changes do not impact the larger structure and approach of the course. Agendas and course calendars that shape the structure and timing of the class, as well as major paper/project assignments, however, should not be changed if consistency is to be maintained across sections.

Stamatis, Kefalis, and Tsadiras (2006) explain that academic professionals tend to engage in collaboration for research purposes more than for sharing teaching ideas. While teaching-focused institutions like DU prioritize student engagement over scholarly research, and while composition has long enjoyed a collaborative culture, perhaps the DU faculty were not as comfortable collaborating around teaching as had previously been assumed. Several survey respondents included comments indicating that while they had seen the PDC increase collaboration among instructors, this collaboration could continue to be enhanced. For example, faculty felt frustrated that their suggestions for improvement were not immediately implemented. Educating faculty about the logistics of course modifications addressed this immediate concern; however, the conversation indicated that faculty, while willing to collaborate in theory, may not always actively engage with colleagues using asynchronous communication tools.

Learning how to collaborate within a geographically dispersed, cross-functional team is not a skill administrators can assume faculty possess. As Oblinger and Hawkins (2006) remind us, participating in this kind of course development team may be a new experience for many faculty. Continuing to offer synchronous Live Classroom sessions that reinforce other methods of communicating and collaborating with PDC development teams may help faculty more effectively participate in PDC discussions.

Student Perceptions

The majority of student respondents (88.1%) indicated that their instructors did not use innovative customizations outside the standard online course. The few customizations noted focused on small group discussion boards, chat rooms, and personalized e-mails from the instructor. However, the majority of students (83.7%) did feel that the instructor's personality was at least somewhat evident in the course. Individual student comments indicated that an instructor's personality was made evident through responses to questions, discussion board postings, e-mails, and feedback on assignments.

When students were asked which customized elements improved their learning, individual guidance and help from instructors (55.8%) and links to outside sites (54.7%) rated the highest. Standard PDC elements received much higher ratings with the following predesigned elements selected as significantly or somewhat improving learning: text lectures (62.5%), textbook (67.5%), and detailed assignment sheets (76.2%). Just over 60% of the students indicated that small group collaboration sites also contributed significantly or somewhat to their learning. While these collaboration sites are established within the PDC, most of the activity is unique to the specific group of students collaborating.

Students did not seem to distinguish between predesigned elements and customized elements in their courses. Most of the students used predesigned elements to support their learning, yet they saw collaboration as a significant contributor to their educational experience. Interestingly, one of the customized elements that the students found most beneficial, the small group collaboration sites, is an element customized to a large extent by the students themselves.

Student survey data supported the findings from the faculty survey. The majority of the customization and personalization in English 311 takes place within elements that are predesigned in the PDC. The customization of these elements by instructors, through personalized responses and feedback, seems to be seamlessly integrated as an augmentation of the basic PDC. Such customizations were viewed by both students and faculty as beneficial to a successful learning experience.

DISCUSSION BOARDS: KEY INSTRUCTIONAL ELEMENT AND UNRECOGNIZED METHOD OF CUSTOMIZATION

After analyzing survey data regarding instructor attitudes, preferences, and self-identified levels of customization, these results were compared with an independent review of actual course content. One element of the PDC, the discussion board, was identified by both students and faculty as an efficient approach to promoting learning. In addition, a review of individual sections indicated that the discussion board was the most frequently modified instructional space within the PDC.

The discussion board assignments are predesigned elements of the PDC. As such, instructors receive their courses with these questions prepopulated. However, faculty personalize discussion boards in their encouragement of student participation, responses to posts, and interaction on the discussion board in ways that reflect individual personalities and pedagogies. For example, Keri Dutkiewicz uses the virtual café discussion board to provide supplemental minilectures on key aspects of effective persuasion in professional documents. Her posting on using a feature-benefit-impact approach in the final persuasive proposal is not a part of the PDC content, but it helps to reinforce textbook and PDC content.

Sample DB post:

I just read through all the executive summaries that have been posted. Comments are posted in the whole class DB so everyone can benefit from and engage in the conversation.

Overall, keep working on the persuasive appeal of your executive summaries. Your goal is to persuade, to convince someone first to keep reading and second to do what you want, whether that is donate money, support a new initiative, etc.

Some problems I saw in the executive summaries include:

- Listing "facts" with no detailed explanation does not make a strong case. You have to interpret and contextualize facts to help readers understand why/how these facts are important.
- Lack of clear project focus and advantage—Clearly state what problem you are solving and why your solution is the best one. Is your solution the most cost-effective? The most humane? Both?
- Lack of clear competitive advantage—Why is your approach and/or organization unique? Why should your project or idea be supported when others may not be?

While faculty may not explicitly recognize their participation in discussion boards as course customization, this student interaction is in fact a primary way that instructors customize the course content to meet the learning needs of individual students. Instructors also use discussion boards to personalize the course through the tone they select, through sharing personal stories, and through the ways they may incorporate graphics or emoticons into their discussion board posts.

For example, starting the above sample post with questions reflects a desire to engage students and help them make connections between this post and the document students are currently writing. The instructor's tone is direct and reminds students that the goal of the class is to help everyone improve. The post proceeds to explain the feature-benefit-impact approach with several examples then concludes with the following:

> Your final projects are a real "capstone" project asking you to bring together what you've learned about citing sources, persuasive writing, formatting documents for the professional realm, and tailoring your message to a specific audience.
>
> I encourage you to work with your group to discuss the ways you can tailor your proposal to your specific audience in order to make a stronger, more persuasive argument.
>
> As always, let me know what I can do to help ;-)
>
> Keri

Here again the instructor establishes her personality, pedagogy, and expertise through a custom message. This instructor values tailoring writing to a specific audience and uses the post to remind students of something that has been discussed repeatedly—they are expected to adjust the style, tone, and content of every assignment to address the intended audience. The concluding smiley face and first name signature adds a touch of informality and approachability. Other instructors do not discuss feature-benefit-impact, so the content of this post is unique. Across sections, variations in instructor positioning via discussion board tone, activity, and level of formality work to customize and personalize course content based on instructor perceptions of student learning needs.

In course feedback and in responses to survey questions, students indicated that the discussion board interaction provided exposure to alternate perspectives, presented key course ideas, encouraged critical thinking, and focused on real-life application of content. They indicated that the discussion boards were a way for an instructor to reveal his/her personality. Interestingly, on the survey question that asked students which elements affected their learning, only slightly more than half (67.5%) indicated that large group discussion boards affected their learning significantly (23.3%) or somewhat (44.2%). Alternately, 100% of the faculty indicated that large group discussion boards supported learning significantly or somewhat. Faculty noted that they used the discussion boards as a vehicle for clarifying assignments, providing additional resources, and encouraging students as well as a means for revealing personality and teaching style. This discrepancy between student and faculty perceptions may simply be attributed to faculty having a more nuanced lens for perceiving student learning. Students may not always be aware of the ways their online discussion boards impact their learning, or they may perceive required discussion board participation as busy work "outside" the core work of the major class assignments.

CLARIFYING FACULTY EXPECTATIONS
THROUGH ONLINE MEETINGS

The faculty survey illustrated that while new-hires were completing a recently revised and enhanced 4-week online faculty training and assessment program that carefully explained additional nuances of the PDC approach, longer-term faculty were not receiving this same message effectively. As a result of the data gathered from the survey, the need to clarify expectations regarding customization via Web meetings became evident. Web meetings were essential because DU's online faculty are located around the globe; no faculty member should be disenfranchised from the process simply because of geographical distance. The resulting web-based sessions were designed to help faculty better understand what types of customizations were required, which ones were encouraged but not required, and which changes should not be made. Faculty needed assurance that they were not required to invest a great deal of time during the course set-up process. In addition to these tactical goals, larger strategic goals for the sessions were established, specifically to

- Help faculty take time to reflect on how far our department has come with PDCs and to recognize the advantages this approach has delivered;
- Reinforce the community of practice among the faculty teaching English and Communications classes online for DU;
- Motivate faculty to reengage in conversations about PDC design and development in order to continually improve the courses; and
- Reassure faculty that they are valued and respected as academic professionals—they are more than the "facilitators" of the predesigned class, they are the instructional experts who help students to learn and make the PDCs a success.

To achieve these goals, the department coordinator solicited faculty participation in the online meetings via e-mail. Her e-mails to faculty were designed to communicate that their survey responses yielded valuable results, that these results had been carefully reviewed, and that the department wanted to propose course changes and offer key clarifications based on the data. Sharing the survey results with faculty provided a way to express to them that their time was appreciated and that their investment was not wasted on yet another administrative fad. Instead, the purpose was to thoughtfully review the PDC model with the goal of improving instructional design and quality at the university.

Two synchronous Live Classroom sessions were held to provide faculty with survey results and to provide guidelines for effective customization. One session was offered in the morning, and one was offered in the evening to accommodate the greatest percentage of faculty. Through these sessions, faculty were encouraged to use

- The comments section on the faculty check-in evaluations that take place twice each term. The comments section is an effective means of gathering ideas from faculty concerning customizations that have worked well in their courses. The discussion during the Web sessions revealed that many faculty perceived the check-in process as more of a supervisory routine designed to gather data on their performance than an opportunity to engage in meaningful conversations about teaching.
- Announcements to post a recap after an assignment, post a kickoff for the next assignment, and/or post fun announcements to give students a sense of the instructor's personality. Faculty were, by and large, using announcements, but many of them used announcements to share key deadlines, reminders, etc. rather than using the announcements to teach, build community, or motivate students.
- The Copy File functionality in Blackboard to utilize effective customizations in subsequent or multiple sections. By teaching faculty how to copy materials from a previously taught section to a new section, we helped

overcome one barrier to effective customization—time. Once faculty customize a class, they can replicate these same customizations by copying them over to the new section. By using the copy feature to copy specific elements, the administrative course copy process remains the same, and all faculty get the newest version of the PDC every term, while effective customizations do not need to be re-created each term.

Several faculty respondents indicated a concern that their feedback on PDC improvements took many terms to implement. To help clarify the administrative process of copying and managing sections, the Live Classroom sessions provided an overview of the PDC process, including course copy procedures. Two areas were discussed that impact the timing of changes. First, the course copy occurs during the midpoint of the previous term. Therefore, if updates are not made to the PDC prior to midterm, the changes would not appear in the next term. Also, suggestions for major changes need to be piloted in a small number of sections for at least one term in order to work out problems with implementation before the change is released to all sections.

At the beginning of the Live Classroom session, participants were asked to self-identify which of the following phrases best described their current approach to teaching with the PDC (the percentage of participants selecting a specific phrase is indicated next to each term). Participants also could choose more than one term.

- I prefer to make very few customizations and personalizations in order to minimize time required for course set up—25%.
- I would prefer to invest significantly more time in exchange for greater instructional autonomy—0%.
- I would prefer to invest just a bit more time to have a little bit more autonomy in key areas—62%.
- I participate in Live Classroom sessions with my Course Coordinator to share ideas about PDCs—50%.
- I use the course check-in form to share ideas about the PDCs with my Course Coordinator—75%.

This data reinforced earlier anonymous data from the faculty survey; most DU faculty do not want to spend a great deal of time with course set-up, even if it means they would have full instructional autonomy. With a heavy dependence on adjunct faculty working multiple positions, the respondents in this study indicated that they valued the time-saving elements of the PDC approach over the autonomy to create their course independently. In terms of communication, a relatively low (50%) percentage of participants regularly participated in sessions with course coordinators to share ideas about PDCs. However, in the conversation that followed this introductory poll, faculty indicated that they greatly appreciated the invitations to share ideas. In many respects, the invitation to share had a significant impact on feeling valued, feeling part of the community, even if the individual chose not to participate.

At the conclusion of the session, 71% of participants in the Live Classroom sessions indicated that they had a better understanding of the PDC goals, processes, and approach after attending. Interestingly, only 42% of participants also indicated that they would be significantly more likely to use discussion boards or announcements more effectively to customize the PDC. This relatively low rate may be due to faculty believing they were already effectively using discussion boards and announcements.

In response to another question, 57% of participants indicated that they would be more likely to communicate and collaborate with the course teaching team and course coordinator(s) to improve the PDC and share their teaching expertise. Willingness to collaborate coupled with increased understanding of expectations, constraints, and technical/administrative realities is essential to continual quality improvement. Kearsley and Poitras explain, "Quality is not achieved in a vacuum or by instructors working in isolation. It takes a team to ensure a quality classroom experience and it takes a team to achieve the ultimate goal of providing high quality online courses" (2007, p. 4). Only time will tell if faculty participation in conversations about teaching with the PDC increases, but preliminary observations indicate that faculty engagement has improved as a result of the Live Classroom sessions about PDCs.

CONCLUSIONS, IMPLICATIONS, AND RECOMMENDATIONS

Constructivist pedagogy attempts to move students from knowledge confirmation to knowledge construction with a certain degree of necessary discomfort. Effective online course design and management should move faculty to do the same. The tension between knowledge confirmation and knowledge construction mirrors the tension between consistency and creativity in online courses. Faculty teaching online should be able to use predesigned components, yet we still expect that faculty will continually adapt this content within appropriate boundaries to meet learners' needs. The following section summarizes conclusions from our research and makes recommendations for improved faculty engagement with PDC course construction, communication about the instructional design process, and strategies to improve student perceptions of learning that confirm the benefits of existing practice and allow for growth, change, and improvement.

PDC Consistency and Autonomy: How can PDCs maintain core areas of consistency while enabling instructional flexibility and autonomy through the inclusion of appropriate instructional elements? Data from the faculty survey and Live Classroom sessions clearly supports that DU faculty appreciate the reduced amount of time invested in course preparation and maintenance that PDCs provide, which can allow for more deep and frequent engagement with students. Results would also indicate however that some autonomy is highly valued; instructors want the freedom and means to express their personality, expertise, and style.

The following are recommendations that can help online programs using a large percentage of adjunct faculty maintain this effective balance between course consistency and faculty autonomy in PDCs:

• Work with faculty to identify discussion board threads that can be changed. Additionally, alternate threads could be offered, and instructors could select from a pool of threads to minimize the time investment needed to customize the discussion board.
• Add supplemental resources to the PDC using the File Availability function in Blackboard to hide the element until the instructor chooses to make it available, if desired.
• Build a repository of learning objects that faculty could use as needed. Such a repository would enable reduced time investment during course set-up while still allowing for variation across sections.

Communicating with Faculty and Effective Course Development and Management: What strategies of faculty communication, structure, and professional development support maximum consistency as well as creativity and autonomy in online course development? The 2-part methodology of surveys followed by Web meetings enabled the research team to evaluate not only faculty perceptions of the PDC but also methods of communicating about PDCs to faculty. Both the faculty surveys and Web meetings revealed that not all faculty were receiving current and consistent information about required PDC elements versus components open to customization. This disparity was particularly apparent in a comparison between new online faculty members hired in the past 12 months and those who had completed an outdated version of DU's required online faculty training. However, one of the primary ways that consistency was maintained and encouraged was through frequent and ongoing communication between all faculty and their course coordinators, either through the course feedback form, online discussions and blogs, or personal correspondence. Dedicated course coordinators were perceived as essential to ongoing administration and maintenance of the PDCs as they helped to create a sense of cohesion among faculty teaching a particular PDC.

Also essential to supporting creativity and consistency was the use of in-house professional development opportunities to build communities of practice while sharing strategies for customizing PDCs. Observations of online discussion boards about teaching the PDC revealed that faculty will generally not take the time to participate in these forums, but that they will attend focused, time-bound, Web meetings facilitated by a colleague and dedicated to a particular topic of interest.

Recommendations for improved communication with faculty to support more effective course development and management suggest that

- Faculty mentors need additional training on how to introduce new faculty to the ways PDCs are used at DU. Course coordinators who serve as mentors should be compensated to complete the newest version of the training so they can understand exactly what information new-hires have and what they are lacking.
- Departments should create mentor guides that detail required PDC course components. These guides could include topics such as rubrics, strategies for commenting on student papers, and methods for customizing PDCs to meet differing student learning styles.
- Investments in additional resources for training, support, and compensation should be initiated to ensure that course coordinators have the tools and skills they need to do their jobs, as well as the compensation required to minimize turnover. With a large pool of adjunct instructors, consistency among course coordinators is crucial to maintaining a sense of community.
- Course coordinators must make extra efforts to reach out and ask for feedback from faculty and to implement reasonable changes to the PDCs in a timely manner. Even if faculty do not respond, simply receiving the e-mails asking for feedback makes faculty feel as if their opinions are valued.
- Department coordinators, faculty, and course coordinators should all be encouraged to develop Web sessions on topics of interest, including APA format, incorporating classroom assessment techniques into online classes, using announcements effectively, etc. Engaging greater numbers of faculty in these presentations will continue to solidify our communities of practice.
- Faculty development must continue to work hand-in-hand with departmental leadership to ensure that the online faculty training reflects the realities of current online teaching technologies and pedagogies, including approaches to PDCs.

Student Perceptions of Learning and the Impact of Course Customizations: To what extent do students notice instructor customizations to the PDC? Do students perceive that these customizations improve their learning? This study did not address actual student learning in PDC versus non-PDC courses. However, the analysis of student perceptions of PDCs indicated that they perceive improvements to their learning experience when they personally engage with the instructor. Students want personalized communication from their instructor regardless of the type of course modifications or relative level of innovation that instructors use when working with PDCs. Frequency and quality of personal interaction between the student and the instructor via the discussion boards, e-mail correspondence, chat rooms, and comments on assignments were perceived by students as most important to their learning. The student survey data also clearly indicated that students appreciate instructors who convey a sense of their personality online. Students believe they learn better when instructors personalize their classes. Finally, the availability of outside course resources such as Web pages, video links, and social media was also reported as significantly impacting the quality of students' learning experiences.

These findings indicate that while innovative course customization techniques should continue to be explored in PDC development (elements such as video and audio integration, for example), several other recommendations, most based on direct faculty-student interaction, are more likely to result in improved student perceptions of learning:

- Emphasize higher quality and greater frequency of instructor engagement with students via e-mail, phone, Live Classroom sessions, discussion boards, and course announcements. This should be a larger expectation and priority for faculty in their training and professional development in the modification and delivery of PDCs.
- Create faculty professional development training on topics such as creating more effective written responses to assignments, constructing effective discussion board questions and facilitating online discussion, and using personal and class e-mails more effectively as instructional delivery and response tools.
- Ensure continued development of content-rich external instructional resources as well as clearly defined assignments with expectations tied to the course content and learning outcomes.

Student perceptions of learning are not the same as actual student success in achieving learning outcomes. However, student perceptions are important since students with positive perceptions may be able to more effectively engage with course materials. Students who believe they are not receiving adequate feedback, help, or instruction from online faculty, regardless of the actual level of faculty performance, are perhaps more likely to engage course materials and challenge themselves to improve.

RECOMMENDATIONS FOR FURTHER RESEARCH

PDCs and the use of course coordinators to administer and maintain them can be an effective strategy for improving student learning and instructor satisfaction. However, the organizational culture and implementation methods surrounding PDCs must be collaborative for this course template approach to succeed. The risk of the PDC model is that the curriculum is pushed, top-down, to both faculty and students, with little regard for individual preferences, expertise, or simply the human need to have some control over one's professional work. The preliminary results of this study indicate that engaging faculty in the development and ongoing evolution of PDCs is key to faculty engagement and subsequent student perceptions of success.

As Davenport employs a large group of adjunct instructors, the data from this study quite likely reflect a unique point of view in terms of the question of autonomy and creativity. Time constraints for adjuncts in customizing courses are certainly a concern. However, all DU faculty, adjunct or full time, are held to the same expectations in the use and construction of online courses. While a study engaging more full-time DU faculty might yield different results, the heavy general teaching load of full-timers at DU (15 credits per semester) could also quite likely yield the same results as adjuncts in terms of perceptions of creativity and consistency. At other institutions, the level of faculty work load, tenure requirements, and culture of individuality versus collaboration would certainly be variables influencing these results. However, additional research is needed to better understand important differences between different faculty and student populations.

This study was broad-based and primarily focused on instructor actions and perceptions. Additional work on student perceptions of PDCs is needed to better understand the impact of course templates like those used at DU on the student learning experience. Furthermore, a more quantitative comparison of student success in PDC versus non-PDC courses would offer valuable data.

Theoretically, the implementation of PDCs based on a common navigational template minimizes cognitive dissonance and time spent learning how to navigate a course. However, does this navigational consistency translate into improved student success? If not, what potential factors contribute to decreased student performance? Perhaps lack of instructor customization results in courses that are pedagogically sound for a general student population, but that may not reflect the unique needs of students in a specific term/section.

From a faculty development perspective, it would be interesting to examine the ways collaboration on a PDC and the ensuing conversations about teaching a common curriculum shape the community of practice. With the implementation of PDCs at DU, faculty in the Department of English and Communications do have increased opportunities to communicate with each other, have the benefit of a dedicated mentor (via the course coordinator role), and are invited to participate in course development conversations. This study revealed, however, that even with multiple vehicles for collaboration, not all of them are well-utilized, nor do most faculty feel as if their recommended changes are implemented quickly enough in future versions of the PDC. A project comparing relative faculty effectiveness across PDC and non-PDC courses may help to improve understanding of this topic.

Also of interest for further research would be an investigation of the relationship between levels of faculty engagement in the construction of PDCs and success of students in these sections. Specifically, do faculty who are actively engaged in the PDC development process and conversations about the PDC with peers in a community of practice, as well as those who see their suggested changes implemented quickly, demonstrate significantly greater success helping students to learn and achieve course outcomes? Also of research interest would be an investigation of the retention of online faculty using PDCs. Are retention rates for faculty likewise engaged in PDC development, improvement, and maintenance conversations higher than those who opt out of these conversations? As exploration of the implications of using a PDC model continues, institutions dedicated to quality online instruction can better understand how to optimize the use of master-course templates without extinguishing the individual creative talent of instructors essential to faculty retention, professional development, and increased student learning.

APPENDIX A:
Faculty Survey

1. What classes have you taught online for Davenport in a PDC format?

2. To what extent do the following standard elements of the PDC support student learning? (Supports learning significantly, Supports learning somewhat, Supports learning very little, Does not support learning, Element not included in PDCs I have taught)
   - Large group discussion boards
   - Assignment focus areas (speeches, graded papers, reports, etc.)
   - Detailed assignment sheets (the ways assignments are explained)
   - Group assignments
   - Audio lessons/Podcasts
   - Midpoint feedback activity
   - Rubrics
   - Links to outside sites
   - Course link to LInC support tools, online tutoring, etc.
   - PowerPoint presentations on text content
   - PowerPoint lectures/presentations on other content
   - Textbook
   - APA resources
   - Other

3. What kinds of customizations or personalizations do you do typically make during class prep and/or class activity for a PDC class?
   - No customizations during class prep but some modifications during class activities

- No customizations
- Create voice announcement(s)
- Create text announcements in addition to standard welcome message
- Add lectures or other supplemental content resources
- Add supplemental rubrics
- Add more examples of student work
- Create or add podcasts
- Add video or links to videos
- Set up Live Classrooms
- Change discussion questions
- Post additional information or directions on DB posts/threads
- Adding instructor bio either on syllabus tab or in introductions DB
- Add my personal IM information
- Uploading instructor photo(s)
- Uploading other photos
- "Fun" or non–content-related announcements
- Fun links
- Fun DB postings
- Change colors
- Other

4. To what extent do these customizations and personalizations enhance student learning? (Supports learning significantly, Supports learning somewhat, Supports learning very little, Does not support learning, I currently do not customize or personalize in this way)
   - Add voice announcement(s)
   - Create text announcements
   - Add lectures or other supplemental content resources
   - Add supplemental rubrics
   - Add more examples of student work
   - Create or add podcasts
   - Add video or links to videos
   - Chat room/LiveClassroom sessions (online office hours, live "lectures" on key assignments, etc.)
   - Change discussion questions
   - Change agendas
   - Change assignment details
   - Add new DBs or DB threads
   - Interaction via discussion board
   - Adding instructor bio either on syllabus tab or in introductions DB
   - Add link to my personal IM information
   - Add link to my Facebook page
   - Uploading instructor photo(s)

- Uploading other photos
- "Fun" or non–content-related announcements
- Fun links
- Fun DB postings
- Change colors
- Other

5. Why do you make customizations and/or personalizations to the PDC?
   - Student problems with APA
   - Address specific student problem with grammar/mechanics
   - Address student learning need in addition to APA or grammar/mechanics
   - Fix an error in the class
   - Students need additional resources to succeed in class (please list resources you add below)
   - Set an appropriate tone
   - Clarify expectations for student performance
   - Encourage students
   - Give students a sense of instructor personality and teaching style
   - Build community and sense of engagement in students
   - Provide additional examples/samples/models of student work
   - It's fun!
   - Personalization helps students feel more comfortable and get a sense of me as an instructor
   - I want to make the class feel more like "my" class
   - Other

6. If you do NOT make customizations or personalizations to the PDC, why not?

7. To what extent do you believe these modifications to PDCs are acceptable or encouraged by Davenport? (Highly acceptable and encouraged, Somewhat acceptable and encouraged, Minimally acceptable but not encouraged, Unacceptable and not encouraged)
   - Add voice announcement(s)
   - Create text announcements
   - Add lectures or other supplemental content resources
   - Add supplemental rubrics
   - Add more examples of student work
   - Create or add podcasts
   - Add video or links to videos
   - Chat room/Live Classroom sessions (online office hours, live "lectures" on key assignments, etc.)
   - Change discussion questions
   - Change agendas

- Change assignment details
- Add new DBs or DB threads
- Interaction via discussion board
- Other

8. Often increased autonomy in course design and content involves a greater investment in time. Likewise, a predesigned course takes less time to set up and maintain but offers less control. Within this continuum, where do you feel most comfortable?
   - Little to no prep and maintenance time required and little to no autonomy
   - Minimal prep and maintenance time in exchange for some autonomy
   - Increased time investment and increased autonomy
   - Significant time investment and significant autonomy
   - Additional comments or explanation?

9. Which of the following aspects of PDCs do you consider to be advantages, disadvantages or both? (Advantage of PDC approach, Disadvantage of PDC approach, Not affected by PDC approach)
   - Course prep and maintenance time
   - Alignment between sections
   - Quality of instruction
   - Collaboration/community of practice among colleagues
   - Navigation
   - Instructor autonomy
   - Teaching class designed by others
   - Student plagiarism
   - Please explain any answers, especially if you selected more than one answer

10. To what extent does the PDC development and maintenance process engage you in effective collaboration with your colleagues, including course coordinators?

APPENDIX B:
Student Survey

1. Rate the extent to which your mastery of the following skills, concepts, or perceptions increased during this course according to the following scale (Significantly, Some, Very little, Not at all):
   - Collaborating in group projects
   - Peer editing
   - Personal editing
   - Technical skills
   - Critical thinking

- Clear communication
- Openness to opinions of others
- Writing negative messages
- Formatting business documents
- Documenting with APA
- Details of your chosen profession
- Persuasive writing
- Grammar
- Sentence structure
- Paragraph organization
- Research techniques
- Please indicate other skills, concepts, or perceptions not mentioned that you learned or were exposed to in this course.

2. To what extent did the following resources help you improve your learning? My learning was affected (Significantly, Some, Very little, Not at all, Was not used in class):
   - Large group discussion boards
   - Group pages
   - Chats
   - Live Classroom
   - Audio lessons/podcasts
   - Video lesson
   - Individual help
   - Surveys
   - Rubrics
   - Links to outside sites
   - LInC support tools, online tutoring, etc.
   - PowerPoint presentations
   - Textbook
   - Text lectures
   - APA resources
   - Detailed assignment sheets

3. Do you feel like you got a sense of your instructor's personality through the course?
   - Yes
   - No

4. Has your instructor used any innovative teaching technique(s) that is not part of a standard online course?
   - Yes
   - No

REFERENCES

Allen, E., & Seaman, J. (2010). *Learning on demand: Online education in the United States, 2009.* Needham, MA: Sloan Consortium.

Bonk, J. (2001). Online teaching in an online world. *USDLA Journal,16*(2), 1–80.

Gerber S., & Scott, L. (2007). Designing a learning curriculum and technology's role in it. *Educational Technology Research and Development, 55*(5), 461–478.

Hathaway, D. M. (2009). *Assessing quality dimensions and elements of online learning enacted in a higher education setting.* Unpublished doctoral dissertation, George Mason University, Fairfax VA.

Herrington, A., Herrington, J., Oliver, R., Stoney, S., & Willis, J. (2001). Quality guidelines for online courses: The development of an instrument to audit online units. In G. Kennedy, M. Keppell, C. McNaught, & T. Petrovic (Eds.), *Meeting at the crossroads: Proceedings of ASCILITE 2001* (pp. 263–270). Melbourne, Australia: The University of Melbourne.

Kearsley, H. J., & Poitras, G. I. (2007, August 8–10). Achieving CCQ: Consistency, creativity, and quality in the online classroom. *Proceedings of the 23rd Annual Conference on Distance Teaching and Learning, University of Wisconsin, Milwaukee.*

Liaw, S. S. (2004). Considerations for developing constructivist Web-based learning. *International Journal for Instructional Media, 31*(3), 309–321.

Oblinger, D., & Hawkins, B. (2006). The myth about online course development: A faculty member can individually develop and deliver an effective online course. *EDUCAUSE Review, 41*(1), 14–15.

Stamatis, D., Kefalas, P., & Tsadiras, A. (2006, April 10–12). Networked academic societies in collaborative development of e-learning courses. *Proceedings of the 5th Networked Learning Conference, Lancaster, England.*

Stewart, C., Bachman, C., & Babb, S. (2009). Replacing professor monologues with online dialogues: A constructivist approach to online course template design. *MERLOT Journal of Online Learning and Teaching, 5*(3). Retrieved from http://jolt.merlot.org/vol5no3/stewart_0909.htm

Young, A., & Norgard, C. (2006). Assessing the quality of online courses from the students' perspective. *Internet and Higher Education, 9*(2), 107–115.

http://dx.doi.org/10.2190/OE2C4

CHAPTER 4

Communities of Practice Approach: A New Model for Online Course Development and Sustainability

Lisa Meloncon and Lora Arduser

Online courses are quickly being woven into the fabric of "traditional" education because of student demand, institutional demand, and research that suggests students in online classes learn as well as or better than they do in face-to-face classes. Students continue to seek out online educational opportunities because of the flexibility in scheduling, the time-saving features, and the ability to attend to family responsibilities while taking courses (Leh, 2002; Shea, Swan, Fredericksen, & Pickett, 2002; Young, 2006). Colleges and universities, in turn, have felt an increasing demand to offer online courses. According to the National Center for Education Statistics, 61% of 2-year and 4-year institutions reported offering online courses, and an estimated 12.2 million enrollments (or registrations) in college-level credit-granting distance education courses (Parsed & Lewis, 2008). The 2010 Sloan Survey of Online Learning also reports that enrollment in online courses rose by more than 17% from a year earlier (Allen & Seaman, 2010). During times of economic downturn, administrators are also quick to believe that online courses can help solve budgetary problems. Ironically, these economic circumstances create an environment in which resources for course development are scarce. Finally, a meta-analysis by a team from the Center for Technology in Learning of the U.S. Department of Education (Means, Toyama, Murphy, Bakia, & Jones, 2009) claimed that "on average, students in online learning conditions performed better than those receiving face-to-face instruction" (p. ix).

Because online courses are likely to play an increasing role in our work as educators, technical communication instructors need to develop strategies to design and deliver sustainable online courses with limited resources. One way to do this is through collaborative partnerships. These partnerships can help mitigate institutional limitations and expectations while providing a quality learning experience for students. In this chapter, we reflect on one partnership in which we participate: a community of practice (CoP)—a group of people who share a concern for something they do and learn how to do it better as they interact regularly. CoPs are particularly useful for online course development because they provide ongoing support that can alleviate many of the curricular and institutional challenges online instructors face.

We found that the conversations within our CoP helped overcome the social and intellectual isolation often associated with online teaching. We are certain that conversations about face-to-face teaching practices from the teacher perspective take place—in offices, in hallways, in impromptu discussions wherever and whenever instructors gather—even if they are not represented in print. We are less certain as to whether similar conversations are taking place with regard to online teaching and why these kinds of conversations have not been formalized in the literature and scholarship.

By formalizing these conversations about online teaching in a CoP, we are also, in effect, enacting our own form of knowledge management, a term not unfamiliar to technical communicators. Seeing CoPs as a form of knowledge management also helps to legitimize the process from an institutional level. If business organizations worldwide are spending considerable amounts of money in trying to manage, maintain, and retain the collective knowledge of their employees, then why shouldn't online technical communication instructors do the same thing? Each instructor of technical communication brings unique knowledge to a CoP that can contribute more globally to improving teaching practices:

> The needs and opportunities for knowledge management in teaching are analogous to those in business organizations. Every individual teacher develops material resources, classroom activities, pedagogical techniques, and practical insight into learning, development, and human relations. These are knowledge assets that are potentially sharable and reusable. (Carroll et al., 2003, p. 46)

Effective knowledge management systems lead to long-term sustainability because knowledge capital is available to be deployed in multiple situations.

While the formation of our CoP was a progressive, organic process, we argue that forming a CoP early in the process of online course or program development or redesign will not only save time but also lead to ongoing cooperative knowledge creation and sustainability. Therefore we outline the CoP approach we took to online course development and provide heuristics to help other instructors develop a successful CoP.

SETTING THE STAGE: THE NEED FOR BETTER STRATEGIES TO DEVELOP ONLINE COURSES

Many technical communication instructors regularly teach a version of a service course. By "service course," we mean an introductory course for non-majors delivered primarily as a service to other departments and programs on campus. These service courses are designed to better prepare students for the writing they will do on the job, and they usually take on one or both of these roles: the business writing course or the technical writing course. The business writing course focuses on the types and kinds of writing done in business organizations, such as memos and reports. Technical writing incorporates a greater emphasis on the practical knowledge or subject matter in a technical or scientific field (e.g., engineering) and the kinds of writing done in more technical workplaces, such as specifications and technical descriptions. A growing number of these courses are being offered online. In fall 2009, based on a sample of 96 schools, 21% of sections of service courses were being offered online or as a hybrid format (Meloncon, 2009).

We found ourselves in the position of needing to develop an online version of our business writing service course. At the University of Cincinnati, as in many locales, Writing for Business takes on the close relationship of good communication, good management, and successful business practices, as well as issues of ethics, information design, and multiculturalism. It is a required course for a variety of majors, and Writing for Business annually enrolls around 700 students. Approximately 85% of these students are from the College of Business, and they literally walk uphill to go to this class. The students' journey up the hill metaphorically represents the challenges we face as instructors. Because this is a required course, the motivation levels of the students vary tremendously. For the most part, these are not motivated students eager to embrace the course content. Irritated that they have to walk uphill, many enter the class not seeing its necessity and even more nonplussed by the fact that they are expected to work hard. One of the problems is that these students see the course as "other," not a direct part of the business curriculum. Service courses can be notoriously hard to teach because of the amount of content that must be covered in a single term; adding in low student motivation, the multiple issues that come with transferring an existing course to an online format, and limited institutional resources, we found ourselves facing our own uphill journey.

But, like Dick Powell, the professor-turned-screenwriter in the 1953 movie *The Bad and the Beautiful*, we started to work. We began our new course development like many people. We researched, and we were surprised by the limited amount of scholarship available to technical communication instructors.

To date, only a handful of resources about online teaching are available specific to technical communication (special issues of *Technical Communication Quarterly*, 1999, 8.1 and 2007, 16.1; special issues of *Computers and Composition*, 2001, 18.4 and 2006, 23.1; Cargile Cook & Grant-Davie, 2005). While these resources provided important viewpoints and advice, we still felt they left us underprepared for the task at hand. For example, we wanted a list of best practices, something that told us which delivery method works best or what type of assignment is most effective in an online environment.

We performed our own "cross-sectional reading" to fully understand the "electronic landscapes" at work for us, initially focusing our attention on the pedagogical and technical landscapes. When we were unable to find many published resources specific to our needs, however, we began to investigate the institutional landscape and to seek out faculty development opportunities on campus (Meloncon, 2007, pp. 42–43). Through our university's Center for the Enhancement of Teaching and Learning, we attended workshops on different technologies and seminars on online teaching, but we quickly became frustrated on two fronts. First, many of the workshops and seminars were meant for departments or programs launching full degree or certificate programs online, and those in this position had the resources to hire an instructional technologist or e-learning specialist to help with the hands-on course construction.

Second, our background in technical communication meant that we were more technologically advanced than other faculty considering converting a single course to online delivery. Technologically, for example, we knew that the content management platform hosted and supported by the university would limit and constrain our course, so the emphasis on this technology in the majority of the workshops was unhelpful. Moreover, many of the additional topics at technology workshops moved little beyond adding PowerPoints with audio or uploading podcasts to replace face-to-face lectures. The workshop leaders talked in abstract terms of engagement and using various media, but rarely moved to actual successful examples. The ongoing workshop discussions also focused almost exclusively on engaging majors and never addressed how to engage our student population or how to create and integrate the various media we felt would be necessary to engage our students. Finally, our background in Web development meant we already knew more effective ways to include multiple versions of content that students could quickly identify with and select from for assignments. Feeling slightly overwhelmed by the task before us and slightly underwhelmed by the available resources, we realized we were on our own.

While on the surface this may seem to be a negative, this realization was actually an important turning point in moving the development of the online course forward. With our new realization that it was up to us, something else began to happen, and it happened at the gym. We had been workout partners for a while when we realized that many of our informal conversations at the gym often centered on and around pedagogical issues. Increasingly these conversations began to revolve around the design of the online course. For example, Lora was struggling with making peer review work better in her class. After 20-minutes of cardio and discussion, she had the "aha moment": reverse the process and give the students feedback *before* having them revise. In another treadmill session, we decided to integrate a problem-based learning case that was situated within a fictional company but contained realistic workplace scenarios. To develop the cases, we realized we had to draw from our personal experience and interests for these companies. Lisa is a sports nut, so we are working on a sports management agency, and Lora has worked in the textbook publishing field and restaurants, so we currently have companies developed for these two industries.

These conversations also helped to release the frustration of a class that didn't seem to work and a teaching situation that leaves an instructor feeling isolated. It put into perspective what could work better and helped to work through questions with practices, procedures, and assignments. It also helped us to celebrate when assignments or discussions went well, to rejoice when a student "got it," and to improve our overall attitudes about teaching. In short, all these conversations at the gym about the continuous tweaking, adding, changing, and expanding of the curriculum and procedures for the online Writing for Business course marked a major milestone in how we thought about course development: an engaged, happy teacher who can rely on another engaged, happy teacher contributes to a more enjoyable teaching experience that leads to more engaged students.

According to the foundational work of Brookfield (1995), we had proceeded down a well-worn path toward reflective, and in his view, successful teaching: "When teachers start to think about how to deal with the problems that plague them, their instinctive turn is to consultants, experts, texts, or faculty development specialists . . . a useful starting point for dealing with teachers' problems is teachers' own experiences" (p. 160). By talking to one another, we began to believe and to trust our own experiences both in the classroom and in our use of technology. With that realization, we had become a CoP. Forming a CoP for online course development can offer technical communication instructors the resources and support network necessary to develop and to teach the service courses. CoPs have the ability to allay many of the questions and concerns about instructor readiness and preparedness to teach online, and maybe even more importantly, they have the ability to sustain the development and delivery of online courses.

COMMUNITIES OF PRACTICE

The concept of CoP evolved from the theories of learning espoused by Jean Lave and Etienne Wenger in the late 1980s and early 1990s. While other researchers and practitioners have extended Lave and Wenger's concept of a CoP, their original work is still relevant. Wanting to focus on "reconceiving" learning, learners, and educational institutions in terms of social practice, Lave (1993), a social anthropologist, argued that it is clear that "learning is ubiquitous in ongoing activity, though often unrecognized as such" (p. 5). In other words, "people learn from observing other people. By definition, such observations take place in a social setting" (Merriam & Caffarella, 1991, p. 134) and can be described thusly:

> Communities of practice are formed by people who engage in a process of collective learning in a shared domain of human endeavor: a tribe learning to survive, a band of artists seeking new forms of expression, a group of engineers working on similar problems, a clique of pupils defining their identity in the school, a network of surgeons exploring novel techniques, a gathering of first-time managers helping each other cope. In a nutshell: Communities of practice are groups of people who share a concern or a passion for something they do and learn how to do it better as they interact regularly. (Wenger, 2006, para. 1)

This description and definition of a CoP helped us realize that we have been participating in our own CoP. From the conversations at the gym, to the sharing of assignments and classroom exercises, to the affective results of not feeling as though we were teaching alone, the CoP named our activities as a worthwhile pedagogical and intellectual structure.

So how is a CoP different from other collaborative formations? Table 1 is an adaptation of "distinctions between communities of practice and other structures" (Wenger, McDermott, & Snyder, 2002, p. 42), and it illustrates the differences between types of collaborations. CoPs were traditionally concerned with workplace practices, which do not easily transfer to teaching practices, so the questions in Table 1 are important for thinking through how CoPs can benefit teaching practices.

Pedagogical examples for each collaborative structure follow:

- Informal network: "water cooler talk," discussions with colleagues in the hallway or impromptu talks in offices
- Short-term group: workshop, seminar, or conference focused on a topic related to teaching (e.g., specific technology or approach); usual length is half-day, a day, or no more than a couple of days
- Semistructured: similar in approach to the short-term group but is more focused and longer in length, e.g., a week-long institute or year-long course
- Formal department: those involved in curriculum decisions but on a pro- grammatic level

As our brief narrative history highlights, we had participated in each of the collaborative structures outlined. However, our own experience echoed the

Table 1. Distinctions between Communities of Practice and Other Structures

	What is the purpose?	Who belongs?	What holds it together?	How long does it last?
Informal networks	To receive and pass on information, to know who is who	Colleagues and friends	Mutual needs and relationships	Never really starts or ends
Short-term group	To receive information on a specific topic	Those who enrolled or signed up	Common short-term goal	Length of seminar or class, usually 1-3 days
Semi-structured group	To receive information on a specific topic or technique	Those who enrolled or signed up	Common short/ mid-term goal	Length of institute or seminar, usually several weeks or as long as a year
Formal department	To deliver a product or service	Everyone who belongs to the department	Job requirement	Intended to be permanent (or until next reorganization)
Community of practice	To create, expand knowledge, and to develop individual capabilities	Self-selection based on expertise AND passion	Passion, commitment, and identification with the group	Evolve and end organically; last as long as there is relevance and interest

research in education that suggests mechanisms are needed that go beyond the initial workshop or training to sustain and continue learning (Langley, O'Connor, & Welkener, 2004; Pittas, 2000; Ziegenfuss & Lawler, 2008), which is the primary goal of the CoP. Moving past task-based objectives or placing the emphasis on relationships or networks, the defining aspect of a CoP is the emphasis on sharing knowledge and creating collaborative knowledge as a result of the CoP.

FORMALIZING OUR AGREEMENT: OUR COMMUNITY OF PRACTICE

From a pedagogical perspective, the concept of collaboration is not new in technical communication. From the landmark works such as Ede and Lunsford's *Singular Texts/Plural Authors* (1990) and Debs's concept of the corporate author (1993), it is obvious that technical communicators have long been concerned with the collaborative process, which we define as a dynamic and fluid relationship consistent with moving toward a common goal. In technical communication, specifically, instructors also know that students will be embarking on writing projects as social projects with many people writing pieces of a document that does not include or require a byline or identified author. Therefore, technical communication instructors, including us, have incorporated task-based collaborative activities into the classroom where peers collaborate "to produce a jointly authored or created product" (Hewett & Ehmann, 2004, p. 37).

And yet, when it comes to our own teaching, we do not always collaborate as well. Hew and Hara (2007, p. 574) go as far as asking the question, "Why would practicing teachers share knowledge to help others?" Aside from brief flirtations with team teaching in higher education, courses generally are taught solo, and most teachers feel a kind of ownership of their courses and course material. The humanities in general seem to emphasize and prize such a solo mindset over collaboration, still embracing a subjective epistemology of the lone "genius" (e.g., Darling-Hammond & Ball, 1998). In spite of a culture that does not support active collaboration, particularly in teaching and course development, we are both invested in collaboration and in previous industry jobs, we both worked collaboratively extensively. In light of our shared predisposition to collaborate, we quickly agreed that two heads were better than one, and so we placed our two heads into a CoP.

A CoP has three distinguishing characteristics: "a *domain* of knowledge, which defines a set of issues; a *community* of people who care about this domain; and the shared *practice* that they are developing to be effective in their domain" (Wenger et al., 2002, p. 27). Following are examples of how these concepts shifted to teaching online for us.

Domain

Participants are both engaged in teaching effectiveness to improve student learning in online environments. In doing so, a "common ground and a sense of common identity" (Wenger et al., 2002, p. 27) is created that enables the instructor to feel engaged in a legitimate and worthwhile enterprise. The domain is the framework of commitment to topic. Our domain played out in the simplest of ways: it made us realize we were not facing an insurmountable challenge in teaching online because we were facing the task together. Within a few conversations, we also realized that we did share the same problems, same challenges, and usually the same successes. For example, even though Lora's class contained a synchronous section and Lisa's did not, we both still faced the same issue with students "disappearing" only to reappear at the end of the term to turn in all their work for the entire class.

Community

As a community, we also shared the same identity as online writing teachers, a rarely seen breed of teachers in our department. Community is focused on a single goal, although goals can change throughout the lifetime of the CoP. Our community is focused on the development and launch of the online Writing for Business course. As the "social fabric of learning," we "share ideas, expose one's ignorance, ask difficult questions, and listen carefully" (Wenger et al., 2002, p. 28). In more practical terms, we delegated and split tasks. As we started to build the course, Lisa had more experience with open-source technologies, so she explored those platforms while Lora focused on building the companies upon which the assignments are based. We also divided researching existing practices in the scholarly literature and staying abreast of ongoing changes and innovations in online teaching.

Practice

"Whereas the domain denotes the topic the community focuses on, the practice is specific knowledge the community shares, maintains, and develops" (Wenger et al., 2002, p. 29). We built a shared practice by contributing our resources and making them available to one another as well as continuously keeping an eye out for additional resources and materials to be added. We shared ways to make online presentations effective and keep an eye open to new technologies that may facilitate this process better, such as the use of Skype and Wiggio, an online group environment that allows for conference calls and file and calendar sharing. We responded to each other as teachers who each have valuable knowledge and experience to share and problems to solve. We engaged one another through the solicitation of advice, sharing of assignments and exercises, and discussions of best practices for assessment. A quick look at our courses reveals the shared practice, such as common language in course policies, but at the same time recognizes our unique teaching styles. Lisa's syllabus contains a "Teaching Manifesto" and a reference to the Kentucky Fried Chicken's secret herbs and spices, for example, whereas Lora's syllabus contains references to not being regarded as a student's "personal Google tool" and "We the Robots" cartoons. These examples show our expectations for student interactions and work in the class while incorporating our individual senses of humor.

KEEPING UP THE MOMENTUM: SUSTAINABILITY AS A LONG-TERM GOAL

While our process was more organic than planned, we argue that an intentional community of practice for online course development improves the online course and can lead to sustainability. It moves us past simply sharing and managing knowledge toward creating new, collaborative knowledge about best practices in online course development, delivery, and sustainability. Some rhetoric and composition scholars have begun to use the word "sustainable" in discussions of technology and writing (see DeVoss, McKee, & Selfe, 2009; Grabill, 2006; Johnson, 2004; Selfe, 2005), but none attempt to use sustainability to frame the development and delivery of online courses. We argue that CoPs offer technical communication instructors the opportunity to sustain online course development as technologies, pedagogical practices, and content continue to shift over time. In the context of online course development and delivery, we take sustainability to mean the process of maintaining and reworking an online course without additional resources for an indefinite period of time. Much like Johnson (2004) argued, "to be sustainable suggests maintenance *and* reflection are part and parcel of any movement we may be contemplating or actually practicing" (p. 102). This view of sustainability intersects with the primary tenets of CoPs.

In our minds, a CoP ensures sustainability because it helps to erase the barriers and challenges faced by technical communication instructors. We see this type of community as specifically mitigating the challenges of time, economics, culture, and increasing workloads. General studies about online education show developing an online course takes considerably more time than a face-to-face course development (Allen & Seaman, 2010; Seaman, 2009). The collectivism, reciprocity, personal gain, and altruism associated with CoPs are motivators that can move past such barriers (see Hew & Hara, 2007). More specific to technical communication instructors are the findings that reported the results of a 2-semester study. Worley and Tesdell (2009) found they "spent more time per student in the online classes—approximately 20% more" (p. 143). Incorporating a CoP approach and drawing on the resources of that community can reduce the time of development. When Lisa developed her course after Lora's pilot course, it did not take as much time to develop content. She was able to use the problem-based learning case and several assignments that had been created collaboratively for Lora's course. Another time-saving example is that we were able to give a structure to a "debrief" document that provides an overview of common problems, explanations as to why the situation could have been addressed more effectively, and examples of how to improve the problem. The "debrief" document, combined with limited specific comments on individual papers, saves time in commenting and from initial results, improves student writing. Finally, our CoP helped us to share strategies to reduce the amount of time we spent with each online student.

Economics is tied directly to whether an instructor chooses the institution's content management system (CMS), chooses open-source delivery, or opts for another delivery mechanism (e.g., an instructor-supplied and financed Web site). Each of these options comes with its own set of pros and cons. Choosing to work within the institution's CMS will provide CoP members with a level of technological support that does not come with an open-source or instructor-funded option. On the other hand, using multimedia content with many of these systems can be challenging. Because most institutions are heavily invested in their CMS, they provide little technological support for other systems. Other systems may be more flexible for online course content needs, but that means the onus falls completely on the instructor to research and test other options. To maintain a sustainable course means instructors have to decide how to deliver the course within the confines of such economic considerations. We discussed at great length the pros and cons of CMS versus other types of delivery. Over the course of a year, we tested and piloted a variety of tools to deliver the online course, including Blackboard, various wikis, and personal Web sites. The CoP allowed us to divide the testing of possible tools and then share the results. Had each of us been faced with attempting this sort of comparative analysis on our own, it's likely we would each still be using the CMS provided by the university.

Culture is also important when using CoPs to sustain course development and delivery. Many technical communication instructors work within departments that only offer technical communication service courses—the main focus of the department curriculum lies elsewhere. For these instructors, as well as many others, the departmental culture may be unconcerned, uninterested, or ambivalent toward the development and delivery needs of a technical communication online course even while insisting on the need for such a course. At the institutional level, there may be an interest in online course and program development without any funding. These cultural considerations make CoPs even more important for sustainability since the CoP may be the only resource for people to turn to as they discuss course (or program) development and then implement the initiatives. The scenario outlined in this paragraph is similar to our local situation in that our departmental culture is ambivalent toward online courses. A CoP requires an epistemological shift from an acquisition metaphor to one of participation (Jonassen & Land, 2000). In other words, rather than seeing knowledge like a package that teachers acquire, potential participants in a CoP need to see knowledge of a new subject area or a technology as a socially constructed activity.

Work is the final challenge embedded within the issue of sustainability. Work in this sense means the actual labor involved in developing and delivering an online course in the context of the labor involved with the rest of instructor workloads. Instructors at all ranks and at all institution types are doing a full range of teaching, service, and research. While the literature suggests that in the best-case scenario, instructors would be granted a course release to design an online course, this is rarely the case. Therefore the work of online course development must be completed at the same time instructors are trying to teach two or three face-to-face courses, maintain progress on their research, and continue their service obligations. Like many other technical communication instructors, these were the same work challenges we experienced. Neither of us was granted release time to develop the online course so we had to fit into already overloaded schedules all the training sessions and research we completed. However we did find that our CoP helped to mitigate this barrier and has been vital to sustaining the course without increasing our workloads. We have imported the idea of single-sourcing by using and reusing pieces of text that we have written. For example, we have a growing set of assignments and related information and explanation for those assignments that we can use and reuse to keep the course fresh and updated. We created an assignment that asks students to research current technologies (e.g., social networks, online video conferencing tools, alternatives to PowerPoint, open-source tools). This general idea has been repurposed in several ways. In a recent term, for example, Lora's students wrote informational reports, while Lisa's students prepared a presentation and handout.

Beyond helping to overcome barriers associated with developing and delivering online courses, a CoP provides specific additional benefits that can positively affect sustainability:

- Providing a community instructors can rely on for all issues, large and small
- Encouraging instructor professional development and course enhancement
- Embodying a social constructivism theory of teaching that encourages sharing knowledge and experience
- Organizing this social body of knowledge and experience into one place, which mimics the knowledge management of corporate organizations
- Validating teaching as an intellectual endeavor

These benefits mean that those involved in a CoP continue to focus on pedagogical sustainability and innovation at the course, curricular, and departmental levels. Our own experience as university teachers and our own experiences with a CoP has confirmed that teachers can make "small-scale changes to their practices without pushing against the structural boundaries marked by time-tables, workloads, program structures, institutional assessment arrangements, colleagues' priorities and so on" (Knight, 2002, p. 196). We can do little to change institutional structures, especially during a particularly trying term. We can, and should, make small-scale changes to our practices that can help us positively affect student learning outcomes because "the depth of knowledge that results compensates for the boundaries that inevitably arise. Communities can be instruments of agility in the face of change" (Wenger et al., 2002, p. 159).

The relationship between a single course to the program and/or departmental goals also can be realized through the visibility of the CoP as a site for professional and programmatic identities. "Communities of practice create value by connecting personal development and professional identities of practitioners to the strategy of the organization" (Wenger et al., p. 17). If faculty members are connected personally and professionally in a CoP that has as its primary aim to ensure the success of programs and curricula, the time spent to develop such a community is well worth the investment. Online courses, and even face-to-face courses, will continue to be impacted by changes in technology and changes in staff at the departmental and institutional level. Placing sustainability as the primary objective, these fluid factors are lessened because of the programmatic structures, including CoPs, that are already in place. Wenger et al. (2002) offer seven principles for CoPs. We feel that three of these principles are key to sustaining a community of practice devoted to teaching online: invite different levels of participation, open a dialogue, and focus on value (pp. 53–63).

Invite Different Levels of Participation

New members of the community have to invest in "legitimate peripheral participation" (Lave & Wenger, 1991, p. 29) and the goals of the community. Legitimate peripheral participation "provides a way to speak about the relations between newcomers and old-timers, and about activities, identities, artifacts, and communities of knowledge and practice" (Lave & Wenger, 1991, p. 29). As this quotation suggests however, the emphasis is not so much on the acquisition of a particular kind of knowledge; it is more about the members participating in "the *practices* of social communities and constructing *identities* in relation to these communities" (Wenger, 1999, p. 4). In our case, for example, for the initial development of the online course, Lisa was "assigned" the role of tenure-track faculty advisor and Lora was assigned the task of developing the course when she was hired. Initially Lisa participated from the margins and Lora took the lead in development, but throughout the process, we have each continued to move from center to periphery and back again, creating a situation of co-participation (Wenger, 1999). Working in the CoP put us both on the same level because we were both learning the same material from the periphery of online teaching practice.

Open a Dialogue

CoPs can be vital for professional development and the development of collaborative work partnerships. The reflective professional "critically reflects on multiple and diverse discourses, on practice within broader contexts and critical frameworks of his or her professional situation, however situated, constituted or clustered: teaching-research-administration; discipline-department-institution; ethical-social-economic-political; local-national-international" (Light, Cox, & Calkins, 2009, p. 14). The open dialogue of a CoP enables technical communication instructors to follow this advice much easier, and the open dialogue allows both agreement and disagreement. For example, we still have an ongoing discussion (and disagreement) about whether the online course should be asynchronous or have a synchronous component. We have found that our constant communication, even when we disagree, has been a key feature of our process in online course development.

Focus on Value

"Frequently early value mostly comes from focusing on current problems. . . . As the community grows, developing a systematic body of knowledge that can be easily accessed becomes more important" (Wenger et al., 2002, p. 59). An ongoing concern of value is the issue of technology and the accessibility of the community's resources as the community grows. One of the primary ways we focus on value is to keep the student-learning objectives at the forefront of our discussions so that our innovation does not veer off course. We also work hard at trying to develop assignments, readings, exercises, and such that can be scaled and/or reused. For example, the final assignment, "Communication Strategy," asks student to address a particular issue and deliver information about this issue to multiple audiences in different formats. While the topic changes to stay relevant to current trends in business, the basic premise and much of the background of the scenario can be used and reused. Thus we focused on the value of building a framework that could be adapted and implemented based on our own teaching strategies and strengths. The tangible and intangible benefits derived from the CoP ensure that it continues to provide value to our teaching practice.

LOOKING TO THE FUTURE: IMPLICATIONS FOR TECHNICAL COMMUNICATION INSTRUCTORS

According to the Sloane Consortium annual survey of online education in the United States (Allen & Seaman, 2010), 19% of all institutions provided no training for their faculty teaching online. Of the institutions that do provide training, the most common approach, 65%, is training courses (Allen & Seaman, 2010, p. 11). Furthermore, writing faculty "have not distinguished well among types of writing courses or stressed the importance of innovation in teaching writing" (Sullivan, 2007, p. 250). Because of this, the nuances and complexities of teaching writing, especially an upper-level technical communication service course, are often lost on administrators or program coordinators who encourage (or are forced to encourage) the development of an online writing course. Unlike didactic courses with low interaction and the option of multiple-choice tests to assess student learning, writing courses take much more time to develop, much more time to deliver, and much more effort to sustain.

A CoP focuses on using all available resources, including human capital, to provide a collaborative, dynamic framework for knowledge management. By sharing and managing the knowledge of community members, the CoP becomes a valuable resource that technical communication instructors can leverage over time. The CoP provides a support network, serves as a repository of information (e.g., assignments or classroom exercises) that can be accessed at any time for any need, and facilitates the creation of new knowledge and teaching practices. Having a community to turn to that understands and shares a common concern increases the likelihood of sustaining courses at a high level and mitigating factors of time economics, culture, and workload, all which can lead to instructor burnout. A CoP can provide a structure that enables sustainable online course development. More importantly however, the CoP demonstrates the "importance of collaboration in the ongoing process of perpetual redesign" (Salvo, Ren, Brizee, & Conard-Salvo, 2009, p. 109), particularly since a "collaborative conversation-based course design process" can be more successful than more structured course design processes (Ziegenfuss & Lawler, 2008, p. 154). The CoP survives because the members draw on the community to support their engagement with the teaching process and reflective practice necessary for effective teaching. The CoP also survives and ensures sustainability because while the community shares a common goal, members do not have to share a singular vision. For example, while our courses have much in common, we incorporate different assignments to achieve the course goals, and we incorporate different delivery mechanisms. But each version and variation of the assignment was developed through our CoP.

While we've focused on our experience with one course, implementing a CoP can lead to sustaining a variety of courses, as well as sustaining programs. What makes a CoP work is the commitment to a formal dialogue about issues involved in creating and delivering a course, a set of courses, or a program. This same commitment to dialogue and continuous reflective engagement can only make technical communication programs stronger. The formalization of pedagogical knowledge structures is the most important cause and effect of a CoP. As technical communication instructors, each one of us carries implicit and explicit knowledge about creating courses, crafting assignments, managing the classroom, facilitating classroom discussion and activities, as well as a wider knowledge of how courses should integrate toward programmatic goals and objectives. But what instructors rarely do is formalize this knowledge in a way that can be shared viably, reducing workloads through distribution of tasks, and ultimately, this sharing and formal interaction leads to improved practices.

While not a direct implication of teaching online, we feel that formalizing how we constructed pedagogical knowledge for this course has enabled us to better reflect on all our teaching practices. Connected to this reflection are the insights that technical communication instructors need to do a better job of sharing information about teaching. Increasing the knowledge flow about teaching practices has the potential to alleviate issues with teaching online as well as improving teaching practices in all courses, thus leading to sustainable pedagogical practices that will enhance programs and curricula.

REFERENCES

Allen, I. E., & Seaman, J. (2010). *Learning on demand: Online education in the United States, 2009.* Babson Park, MA: Babson Survey Research Group.

Brookfield, S. D. (1995). *Becoming a critically reflective teacher.* San Francisco, CA: Jossey-Bass.

Carroll, J. M., Choo, C. W., Dunlap, D. R., Isenhour, P. L., Kerr, S. T., MacLean, A., et al. (2003). Knowledge management support for teachers. *Educational Technology Research and Development, 51*(4), 42–64.

Cargile Cook, K., & Grant-Davie, K. (Eds.). (2005). *Online education: Global questions, local answers.* Amityville, NY: Baywood.

Darling-Hammond, L., & Ball, D. L. (1998). *Teaching for high standards: What policy-makers need to know and be able to do.* Philadelphia: Consortium for Policy Research in Education, University of Pennsylvania.

Debs, M. B. (1993). Corporate authority sponsoring rhetorical practice. In R. Spilka, (Ed.), *Writing in the workplace: New research perspectives* (pp. 158–170). Carbondale: Southern Illinois University Press.

DeVoss, D. N., McKee, H. A., & Selfe, R. (Eds.). (2009). Technological ecologies and sustainability. Logan: Computers and Composition Digital Press/Utah State University Press. Retrieved October 23, 2009, from http://ccdigitalpress.org/ebooks-and-projects/tes

Ede, L., & Lunsford, A. (1990). *Singular texts/plural authors: Perspectives on collaborative writing.* Carbondale: Southern Illinois University Press.

Grabill, J. (2006). Sustaining community-based work: Community-based research and community building. In P. Takayoshi & P. Sullivan (Eds.), *Labor, writing technologies, and the shaping of composition in the academy* (pp. 325–339). Cresskill, NJ: Hampton.

Hew, K. F., & Hara, N. (2007). Empirical study of motivators and barriers of teacher online knowledge sharing. *Educational Technology Research and Development, 55,* 573–595.

Hewett, B. L., & Ehmann, C. (2004). *Preparing educators for online writing instruction: Principles and processes.* Urbana, IL: National Council of Teachers of English.

Johnson, R. (2004). (Deeply) sustainable programs, sustainable cultures, sustainable selves: Essaying growth in technical communication. In T. Hunt & G. Savage (Eds.),

Power and legitimacy in technical communication Volume 2: Strategies for professional status (pp. 101–119). Amityville, NY: Baywood.

Jonassen, D. H., & Land, S. M. (2000). Preface. In D. H. Jonassen & S. M. Land (Eds.), *Theoretical foundations of learning environments* (pp. 3–9). Hillsdale, NJ: Lawrence Erlbaum.

Knight, P. (2002). *Being a teacher in higher education.* Buckingham, England: The Society for Research in Higher Education and Open University Press.

Langley, D., O'Connor, T. W., & Welkener, M. M. (2004). A transformative model for designing professional development activities. In C. M. Wehlburg & S. Chadwick-Blossey (Eds.), *To improve the academy Vol. 22* (pp. 145–155). Bolton, MA: Anker.

Lave, J. (1993). The practice of learning. In S. Chaiklin & J. Lave (Eds.), *Understanding practice: Perspectives on activity and context* (pp. 3–32). New York: Cambridge University Press.

Lave, J., & Wenger, E. (1991). *Situated learning: Legitimate peripheral participation.* Cambridge, MA: Cambridge University Press.

Lay, M. (Ed.). (1999). Technical communication, distance learning, and the World Wide Web [Special issue]. *Technical Communication Quarterly, 8*(1).

Leh, A. (2002). Action research on hybrid courses and their online communities. *Education Media International, 39,* 31–39.

Light, G., Cox, R., & Calkins, S. (2009). *Learning and teaching in higher education: The reflective professional* (2nd ed.). London, England: Sage.

Means, B., Toyama, Y., Murphy, R., Bakia, M., & Jones, K. (2009). Online learning: A meta-analysis and review of online learning studies. Washington, DC: U.S. Department of Education Office of Planning, Evaluation, and Policy Development Policy and Program Studies Service. Prepared by Center for Technology in Learning.

Meloncon, L. (2007). Exploring the electronic landscape: Technical communication, online learning, and instructor preparedness. *Technical Communication Quarterly, 16*(1), 31–53.

Meloncon, L. (2009). [Programmatic information in technical communication]. Unpublished raw data.

Merriam, S. B., & Caffarella, R. S. (1991). *Learning in adulthood: A comprehensive guide.* San Francisco, CA: Jossey-Bass.

Parsad, B., & Lewis, L. (2008). *Distance education at degree-granting postsecondary institutions: 2006–07* (NCES 2009–044). Washington, DC: U.S. Department of Education, National Center for Education Statistics, Institute of Education Sciences.

Pittas, P. A. (2000). A model program from the perspective of faculty development. *Innovative Higher Education, 25*(2), 97–110.

Salvo, M. J., Ren, J., Brizee, H. A., & Conard-Salvo, T. S. (2009). Usability research in the writing lab: Sustaining discourse and pedagogy. *Computers and Composition, 26,* 107–121.

Seaman, J. (2009). *Online learning as a strategic asset, Volume 2: The paradox of faculty voices: Views and experiences with online learning results of a national faculty survey, part of the online education benchmarking study.* Washington, DC: Association of Public and Land Grant Universities and Sloan National Commission on Online Learning.

Selfe, C., & Hawisher, G. (Eds.). (2001). Distance education: Promises and perils of teaching online [Special issue]. *Computers and Composition, 18*(4).

Selfe, C., & Hawisher, G., (Eds.). (2006). Distance learning: Evolving perspectives [Special issue]. *Computers and Composition, 23*(1).

Selfe, R. (2005). *Sustainable computer environments: Cultures of support for teachers of English and language arts.* Cresskill, NJ: Hampton.

Shea, P. J., Swan, K., Fredericksen, E. E., & Pickett, A. M. (2002). Student satisfaction and reported learning in the SUNY Learning Network. In J. Bourne & J. C. Moore (Eds.), *Elements of quality online education* (pp. 145–155). Needham, MA: Sloan Consortium.

Sullivan, P. (2007). Literacy work in e-learning factories: How stories in popular business imagine our future. In P. Takayoshi & P. Sullivan (Eds.), *Labor, writing technologies, and the shaping of composition in the academy* (pp. 229–260). Cresskill, NJ: Hampton.

Wenger, E. (1999). *Communities of practice: Learning, meaning and identity.* Cambridge, MA: Cambridge University Press.

Wenger, E., McDermott, R., & Snyder, W. M. (2002). *Cultivating communities of practice: A guide to managing knowledge.* Boston, MA: Harvard Business School Press.

Wenger, E. (2006). *Communities of practice: A brief introduction.* Retrieved October 23, 2009, from http://www.ewenger.com/theory/

Worley, W. L., & Tesdell, L. S. (2009). Instructor time and effort in online and face-to-face teaching: Lessons learned. *IEEE PCS, 52*(2), 138–151.

Young, S. (2006). Student views of effective online teaching in higher education. *The American Journal of Distance Education, 20*(2), 65–77.

Zachary, M. (Ed.). (2007). Online teaching and learning: Preparation, development, and organizational communication [Special issue]. *Technical Communication Quarterly, 16*(1).

Ziegenfuss, D. H., & Lawler, P. (2008). Collaborative course design: Changing the process, acknowledging the context, and implications for academic development. *International Journal for Academic Development, 13*(3), 151–160.

http://dx.doi.org/10.2190/OE2C5

CHAPTER 5

Training Faculty for Online Instruction: Applying Technical Communication Theory to the Design of a Mentoring Program

Janie Jaramillo-Santoy and
Gina Cano-Monreal

Over the past decade, program administrators have witnessed the exploding enrollment of students in online courses and have felt the pressure to transition their course offerings online. The Instructional Technology Council (ITC) and the Sloan National Commission on Online learning report a 20%–22% increase in distance learning enrollments at colleges, versus overall campus enrollments, which averaged a less than 2% increase in the 2008–2009 academic year (ITC, 2010; McCarthy & Samors, 2009). Trends indicate enrollment growth in distance learning courses will continue at 2- and 4-year colleges (ITC, 2010).

However, as program enrollments grow, administrators find themselves rethinking program strategies in order to meet the competing demands of developing and teaching online courses with tight and oftentimes shrinking budgets. One major challenge colleges face is recruitment of trained faculty who can offer the number of online sections required to meet student demand (ITC, 2010). Recruitment can be even more difficult; 85% of faculty with experience teaching and/or developing online courses have reported that it takes more effort and different skills to develop an online course in comparison to a face-to-face course (Seaman, 2009).

These challenges of reduced funding, increased demand, and changing skill requirements provide opportunities for technical communicators to extend their expertise beyond their own programmatic boundaries. To meet recruiting and training needs, growing programs that lack funds for specialized training can utilize in-house talent and expertise, via a mentoring program, to train faculty new to, and sometimes hesitant to attempt, online education. Technical communicators can use their knowledge and skills to serve an instrumental role in helping institutions and programs face the pressures to increase online course offerings by developing and implementing innovative methods for training faculty new to online instructional design and delivery.

TECHNICAL COMMUNICATION AND FACULTY TRAINING

More than 5 years ago, in her article "Applying Technical Communication Theory to the Design of Online Education," Marjorie Davis (2005) argued that technical communicators are ideally situated to use their theoretical knowledge to help in the design of online education programs. Davis lists the knowledge domains and explains how each can be used to develop such programs. She asserts that "the theoretical application demonstrates that technical communicators are not only qualified to develop online education within their own specialties, but, through this knowledge, are also capable of leading and assisting others as they develop online learning programs" (p. 16). Although Davis emphasizes program development, in this chapter we argue that the knowledge and skills she outlines—mastery of "the important concepts of audience, purpose, persona, and usability; . . . the knowledge of the technology for online delivery; . . . a strong collaborative work ethic and experience in project management; and . . . strength in instructional design" (p. 16)—can also be applied to develop training programs focused on preparing faculty for online course development and delivery. Our experience has taught us that this type of training is an essential component for the long-term success of any online education program. In the rest of this chapter, we expand on Davis's argument and explain how we applied the domains she outlines to our particular institutional training needs in order to demonstrate how, as technical communicators, we were able to employ our theoretical knowledge to develop, direct, and participate in a training-mentoring program designed to help faculty transition from teaching face-to-face to teaching online and, at the same time, help faculty build a community that would sustain quality improvement practices.

Background

Our own experience in developing an online education training program comes from having designed the training to meet the expanding needs created by the exponential increase of student enrollment in online education at our institution,

Texas State Technical College (TSTC) in Harlingen, Texas. TSTC is a 2-year technical college with an enrollment of approximately 6,000 students. Enrollment in online learning courses at TSTC Harlingen increased 448% (171 to 938) from the fall of 2007 to the summer of 2010. To meet this demand, program administrators increased the number of courses offered by 333% (6 to 26 courses) from the fall of 2007 to the summer of 2010. (To meet demand, multiple sections of certain courses are offered.) Similar to many institutions around the country, our program administrators, seeking to develop online courses, originally turned to individuals who demonstrated one of the knowledge domains outlined by Davis: "Familiarity with a broad range of tool technologies, along with a willingness to experiment and learn more" (2005, p. 17). These faculty, though, were unable to keep up with the demand. Administrators then turned to recruiting adjunct faculty and full-time faculty who were hesitant to enter a teaching arena in which they lacked expertise.

Meeting the demand brought several training challenges. Faculty members new to online instruction, Cargile Cook (2007) asserts, usually expect that training for online teaching will focus on the technical tools that can be used to deliver the course online. We have learned that faculty development professionals, especially those with limited knowledge of online teaching, can also hold this misconception. Initially, the only formal training provided to our faculty for online instruction focused on how to use the learning management system (LMS) and selected software. Our college, like many others across the nation, has a limited number of faculty development professionals. They were able to design and deliver several formal sessions focused on the LMS. These workshops, though, were not sufficient to provide the intensive training and support faculty members needed to develop and deliver an online course. They provided individualized instruction, but the low numbers of personnel limited the number of faculty they could train.

Similar to Powell's recommendation that faculty use a "checklist of 25 course design principles . . . to critique or evaluate their online course sites prior to launch" (Powell, 2001, p. 43), our distance learning program established criteria for course design based on best practices in published research about online pedagogy, especially those practices endorsed by Quality Matters, "a nationally recognized, faculty-centered, peer review process designed to certify the quality of online courses and online components"(Quality Matters, n.d.). The Quality Matters organization has designated eight general standards with which online courses can be evaluated to gauge quality design. These include (a) Course Overview and Introduction, (b) Learning Objectives (Competencies), (c) Assessment and Measurement, (d) Instructional Materials, (e) Learner Interaction and Engagement, (f) Course Technology, (g) Learner Support, and (h) Accessibility. (More information about best practices for online course instruction endorsed by Quality Matters can be found on their Web site: http://www.qmprogram.org)

Because of the scope of this chapter, we cannot delve into all the best practices for online teaching. We can say, though, that those practices fall into two general areas that are relevant to our training model: online instructional design and course delivery via the Internet. Although our staff development office recognized the importance of these best practices, they had few resources to offer formal faculty training in online learning pedagogy or instructional design. Many times faculty had to find ways to learn these valuable and essential skills on their own. To accomplish these goals, they often turned to self-teaching or informal mentoring by other knowledgeable instructors. Despite their efforts, the heavy teaching load (5-5-5) of our full-time faculty and the limited time our adjunct faculty spent on campus afforded little time for them to experiment and explore on their own and, at the same time, design a course that would meet our institutional requirement that it be 100% ready for delivery and that it meet rigorous design standards before the first day of class.

Out of this context, we (two faculty members with administrative duties at a small 2-year technical college) developed a mentoring program to help faculty design online courses that were fully developed by the first class day and to support those faculty during their first semester of teaching online. We used Leidman's definition of mentoring to mean a "mutually supportive culture which encourages sharing of ideas and norms allowing experienced personnel to lead and openly and unjudgmentally create interpersonal communications resulting in a faster and more constructive/progressive start-up" for a faculty member entering a new assignment (Leidman, 2006, p. 1). Informal mentoring relationships, according to Hezlett (2005), have less structure than formal ones but serve many of the same functions. Hezlett's study identified eight commonalities in informal and formal mentoring:

> (1) coaching and advising in three areas (specific problems related to mentees' current roles, longer-term skill development, and career decisions), (2) providing information in three ways (providing a new perspective on situations, sharing information, and mentors' disclosure of their own experiences), and (3) intervening on the mentee's behalf, either to solve problems or create opportunities. . . . (4) providing feedback, (5) managing the mentoring relationship, (6) facilitating the mentees' self-exploration, (7) offering encouragement, and (8) protecting mentees from office gossip. (pp. 455–456)

We considered these functions as we developed our informal mentoring-training program, which was also guided by institutional requirements and guidelines. We call our program Mentor2Mentor (M2M).

As we faced this new training situation and conceived of M2M, we considered many of the same questions Marjorie Davis (2005) addressed: What audiences are served by the training process? How can the training meet the needs of each audience? What is the purpose of the mentoring program? What are the different types of mentoring? What purpose does each serve? How can the mentoring program purpose align with the purpose of the online education program? In what ways can the mentor assist with course development and testing? How can the mentoring process effectively introduce digital tools that can be used for the design and eventual delivery of the course? Such questions, outlined by Davis, led us to consider the negotiations technical communicators must make when using their theoretical knowledge for an application in a context complicated by many challenges. We describe how we answered these questions in developing the M2M Training Model that we have now instituted at TSTC-Harlingen.

COMPONENTS OF THE MENTOR2MENTOR TRAINING MODEL

We designed the M2M program to utilize the expertise of faculty with experience teaching online. These faculty help develop the skills of those new to online instructional design and/or online course delivery by providing different types of support individual faculty need as they transition from face-to-face to online instruction (Katz, 2003). This process is outlined in Figure 1: The Mentor2Mentor Training Model. As Davis recommends, the first phase in the M2M training is a form of audience analysis conducted by the program directors. In this initial audience analysis, we assess the mentee's knowledge regarding online pedagogy, digital tools, and institutional requirements for online teaching; this information is then used to match the mentee with a mentor who can provide extensive guidance in needed areas or support the knowledge the mentee already possesses. Depending on the mentee's needs, the pair then collaborates by reviewing institutional and accreditation guidelines; designing, delivering, reviewing, and assessing the course; and finally assessing the M2M process.

Mentor2Mentor (M2M) Training Model

In developing the M2M Training Model, we were able to follow many of the steps Davis (2005) outlines but not always in the chronological order she suggests. For example, Figure 1 does not include two key considerations that preceded model development: our commitment to collaboration and articulation of program goals. More clearly identified, however, are steps such as audience analysis and instructional design. Our discussion of the M2M program, for these reasons, does not replicate Davis' recommended steps exactly, but it does illustrate how these recommendations came into play in actual practice as we utilized our mentoring program.

We begin our discussion with the importance of collaboration, explain how we arrived at our purpose statement, and detail how audience analysis is critical to the process. Further, we explain the development and testing of our course prototype, discuss how tools are evaluated and selected, explain how we offer

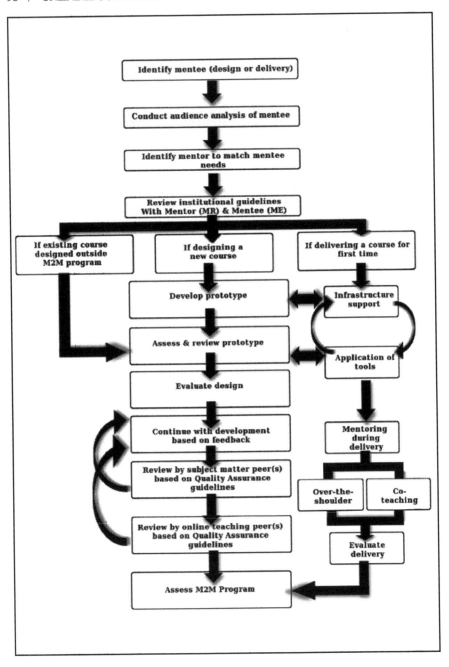

Figure 1. Mentor2Mentor (M2M) Training Model indicates the progression for each of the three mentoring processes.

support for course delivery and evaluation, and finally discuss the training program assessment.

Collaboration

Davis (2005) asserts that successful development of an online program requires the formation of collaborative relationships between faculty, technicians, support staff, faculty outside of the institution, or with anyone with pertinent expertise to achieve the program's goals (p. 24). These relationships are also fundamental in the development of a successful training program and online teaching experience; in fact, we have found that collaborative relationships are the seeds from which the entire process grows.

The course development process, the testing of the course at various stages, and continual course improvement all depend on collaborations, which the M2M program supports and sometimes even creates. Faculty who are new to online instruction collaborate with faculty members (internal or external) experienced in online course development and delivery. These experienced faculty members provide important information about strategies or tools that have or have not worked in their courses. The collaborative relationship that develops between the mentor and the mentee is the first and most crucial in the training, which includes both course development and approval process. The mentor assists in the collaboration between the mentee and support staff, faculty members, and others who will be valuable resources. The relationships built during the course development and testing phases are essential to promote the continual improvement of developed courses. Similar to Davis's experience at Mercer (2005, p. 24), we have courses that are developed by a single author but shared among faculty and other courses that are co-authored. These situations foster collaborative relationships among faculty who are experts in the same content area, because they share experiences and methodologies specific to the online delivery, and sometimes redesign, of the shared content.

Purpose

Growing from an awareness of our collaborative relationships, we have articulated the purpose of the M2M program. To design the purpose statement, we used questions similar to the ones Davis poses:

- Why does the department or institution want to engage in a mentoring program?
- What will the program attempt to accomplish?
- Why is the program needed?
- What benefits will the program offer mentors, mentees, departments, and colleges?

These questions have helped us, as technical communicators, to craft a purpose statement for the program that, ideally, explains the benefits to the mentee, the mentor, the online program, and the institution. These details have allowed us to build collaboration and support from both faculty and administrators. The statement also clarifies to those participating that a mentoring relationship is different from one between a content expert who provides the course content and an instructional designer whose sole purpose is to publish the content online. The purpose statement emphasizes that the goal of the program is not solely for cost-saving benefits.

Using the questions and the answers generated from them, we developed the following mission statement for the TSTC-Harlingen M2M program:

> The Mentor2Mentor program prepares and supports faculty new to online learning course design and/or delivery by assessing the needs of the individual and providing personalized instruction. The network of faculty who have successfully completed the program create a professional learning community which can sustain the increased demand for online instruction despite limited budgets.

The mission statement, as we have articulated it, serves as a touchstone throughout the online course development process. It characterizes the goal of the mentoring relationship as a collaborative effort to move the mentee in the mentoring continuum from "support" to "expert" so that mentees become independent of the mentor and can be given the opportunity to become mentors. The support provided by the mentor minimizes the design and teaching anxiety of the first-time online teaching experience by providing someone to guide them through the process and to point out where they can focus their energies at different points in the development or delivery process. During the mentoring relationship, the mentor shares best practices gathered from online pedagogy and online course design research and assists new faculty in navigating the institutional process of online course evaluation. The mentoring program has also benefited faculty teaching online by allowing them to extend and expand their expertise by serving as a mentor—to help guide, to share their experience, to have someone with whom to share and test ideas. With this shared mission, those who work within the mentoring program create and sustain a community and network of faculty committed to professional growth. In addition, the program has helped us meet the increased demand for online learning.

Audience Analysis

Understanding the audiences involved in the mentoring relationship has been crucial for the success of the training program; equally important is knowledge of the audiences who can support and sometimes constrain the process of online course development. M2M is designed for both types of audience analysis. Davis argues that "audience analysis is one of the strengths of skilled technical communicators, and this strength provides a solid foundation for planning education or training programs" (2005, p. 17). She identifies six types of audiences: local audiences, distance audiences, employers, competitors, accrediting agencies, and peers in the appropriate community. In identifying, as Davis suggests, even those audiences who are on the periphery (p. 18), we translated the audience dimensions to the training program using a series of questions:

- What audiences are served or affected by the training program and process?
- What are the needs and function of each audience?

The audiences that Davis outlines map well to those that we considered when designing a training program. We list and define each briefly below; following this list, we describe how and when each of these audiences comes into play in the M2M process:

- Target audience: mentor/mentee faculty or staff who want to participate in the programs;
- Supervisors: department chairs or deans who approve participation of faculty as mentor or mentee, authorize faculty release time or compensation, and evaluate the benefits of the knowledge gained;
- Peers: individuals who assess the product quality and may teach designed courses;
- Local audiences: department, college, and institutional committees who approve the online course designed;
- Accrediting agencies: organizations that evaluate the course designed and certify online courses/programs;
- Competitors: entities offering online course design and delivery training or other mentoring programs on campus.

We have found that analysis of these audiences often takes place at different stages of the mentoring process: early in the mentoring process to pair mentees and mentors; midprocess to establish institutional and accreditation audience requirements for online courses; and late-process to understand and prepare for peer, administrative, and outside quality assurance.

Early Analysis: Matching Mentees and Mentors

According to Davis, the audience for which the program is specifically designed is the target audience—in our case, the mentees and mentors who are paired—and this audience forms the most important and earliest audience analysis component of the training program. The target audience is analyzed to evaluate the needs and capabilities of each individual, the mentor and mentee, before they are paired. This analysis reveals the technical skills and confidence level of the participants as well as recognizes the limits of the exploration capacity of each during the design or delivery phase of the course. Even though Davis argues technical communicators are keen to experiment and learn (2005, p. 17), recognizing the limits of the exploration capacity of each individual during the design or delivery phase of the course is critical. The correct match with an experienced mentor has been critical in our program because the sharing alleviates anxiety experienced by faculty new to online teaching.

Faculty entering the mentoring program have ranged from those who have never taught online and consider themselves novices to those who have designed and taught online courses at other institutions and may consider their skill levels as "expert" and therefore need less support from the mentor. To represent the mentee/mentor relationship visually, we created a set of continua that reflect the mentee's level of knowledge in three domains addressed by our mentoring program:

- Knowledge of **Pedagogy** for Online Course Design or Delivery
- Knowledge of **Tools** for Online Course Design or Delivery
- Knowledge of **Department and Institutional Requirements** for Online Learning

We will illustrate with the example of a faculty member who, during the mentee interview, reveals he has no experience in fully online course design or delivery. Figure 2 shows how this mentee (M^E) would be mapped on the first continuum, which represents Knowledge of Pedagogy for Online Course Design or Delivery, and matched with a mentor (M^R) who can offer the extra training in online course design and delivery that this faculty member needs.

While this faculty mentee has little knowledge of the *pedagogy* involved in online course design and delivery, the interview revealed that he has some limited

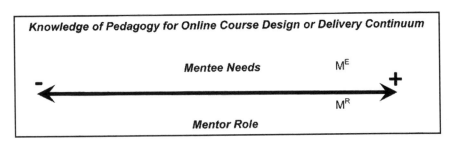

Figure 2. Mentee (M^E) with little knowledge of online pedagogy is placed at the "needs +" end of the continuum and matched with a mentor (M^R) who will provide a correspondingly high level of support.

experience using the discussion board feature of a learning management system (LMS) in his face-to-face (F2F) course. Therefore, on the second continuum, which represents knowledge of *tools* for online course design or delivery, the mentee would be placed as in Figure 3—toward the "needs +" end of the continuum but not as far over as on the Pedagogy continuum. This placement reflects that he still requires substantial training, not only regarding the LMS tools available but also regarding additional digital tools that he can utilize in the design and delivery of their course. As on all the continua, the mentor's role would be enlarged or reduced to mirror the mentee's level of knowledge and experience.

The position of mentees on the continua is based on their level of experience and expertise, which we determine after a brief interview. The exception applies to the third continuum, which represents Knowledge of Department and Institutional Requirements. All mentees, whether they are entirely new to online course design and delivery or have designed and taught online courses at other institutions, are placed on the "needs +" end and paired with mentors who know both types of requirements. Our expectation is that everyone new to online course design and delivery at our campus will need to learn how to meet our institution's online learning requirements.

After the mentee's skills and online course development needs are mapped, we choose a mentor who can provide the right combination of skills to support the mentee's work. The results of the audience analysis reveal which mentor/mentee pair will be compatible with regard to knowledge and skills. As important is that the training program directors match the pair according to temperament. Once matched, the newly formed team, mentoring pair, is ready to begin its collaboration.

Mid-Process Audience Analysis: Working Within Institutional and Accreditation Requirements

Their first activity is yet another form of audience analysis: reviewing and understanding institutional and accreditation guidelines for course development. To begin this work, mentee and mentor explore what Davis (2005) calls "local

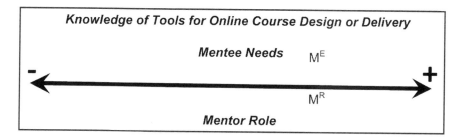

Figure 3. Mentee (ME) has limited knowledge of online tools. Mentor (MR) provides matching level of support.

audiences." Local audiences refer to those internal audiences that evaluate the worth of the program to the institution. Our mentoring program was designed to align with the local audiences as well as take into account the different types of internal evaluation and approval to which an online course will be subject. These evaluations can be part of the department, the college or division, and the institution. Because in our institution, as in many others, an online course is evaluated before it is offered and then again after it has been delivered, it was imperative that the training program work within the guidelines established by the institution. One of the main objectives of the mentoring program is to help the new faculty member navigate the departmental, programmatic, and institutional requirements for the course while the course is being planned, designed, and delivered. A review of departmental, programmatic, and institutional requirements before beginning course development familiarizes the mentee with these requirements and alleviates frustration from learning that design does not match required components in the evaluation.

Our M2M program is designed so that the mentor will lead the mentee through two levels of required evaluation: the departmental evaluation and the Distance Learning Committee online course evaluation. The curricular evaluation, occurring at the departmental level, by subject matter peers, guarantees that the course meets the content scope and learning objectives of the course, while the online course review and approval by online teaching peers verifies that the course design meets the recommended standards of "Best Practice" as established by the institution which, in our case, mirror those provided by Quality Matters. The training program director or mentor works with the local audience responsible for the evaluation of the course, in our case the department chair and the Distance Learning Committee respectively, so that these individuals understand their role in the process.

Knowledge of the role of accrediting agencies is another aspect of audience analysis that comes into play prior to course design and development. Accrediting agencies function as audiences that directly or indirectly guide the development and evaluation of online courses. Some have strict requirements that must be part of the course design, while others only provide recommendations for providing a quality course. Regional accrediting agencies, like Southern Association of Colleges and Schools (SACS), provide recommendations for online course design. When more than 50% of the courses toward program completion can be taken online, the program must be approved by the agency. To gain this approval, most recommendations identified by the agency as best practices must be implemented. Although SACS only provides recommendations, our institution's online course approval requirements parallel the recommendations. Some courses at TSTC, such as Medical Terminology, are subject to more prescriptive programmatic certification requirements for course design by its certification agency (American Health Information Management Association). A third type of certification agency can be interinstitutional. For example, Quality

Matters is an external "peer review process designed to certify the quality of online courses and online components" (Quality Matters, n.d.). Mentors do not have to become experts in all agency requirements, but they communicate with the mentee about such possible requirements and suggest that they speak with their program director for more specific information. Awareness of these agencies as audiences provides useful information, as direct evaluation or recommended guidelines, which is utilized during online course design.

Late-Process Audience Analysis: Preparing for Review and Evaluation Audiences

After the mid-process audience analysis is complete, one final set of audience analyses is required. The work of this audience comes into play after the course has been designed and again after delivery, but we have found that it is worthwhile to keep them in mind as course development begins. These audiences are composed of peers and administrators. According to Davis (2005), individuals who belong to the same discipline would be considered peers. The mentoring program contends with two types of peer audiences: the subject matter peers and the online teaching peers. Both types are involved in the evaluation of the product. The subject matter peers assist with evaluation of the course content and learning objectives, while the online teaching peers provide feedback about the design of the course and the use of computer technology tools. For our program, individuals who make up the Distance Learning Committee and evaluate the developed course are faculty members experienced in online course development and delivery; thus, they classify as online teaching peers. The Distance Learning Committee members may not be content experts in the subject area in which a particular course is developed; therefore, the Department chair and respective faculty members are more suited as this audience. They are the most knowledgeable audience for the course's content, even if they are not currently involved in online course instruction.

Administrators, such as department chairs and deans, who approve participation of faculty as mentors or mentees, are integral to the success of the training program. Supervisors knowledgeable of the process and the quality of the program can better support the needs of the faculty. Training program directors, mentors, and mentees communicate periodically with these administrators about the progress of the mentoring process. This communication is crucial especially with the department chairs or those individuals who will be responsible for evaluating the course designed during the final phase of the design mentoring relationship. Administrators are also able to provide support by developing recognition and/or incentives for the valuable service of those who participate in the program. We return to the roles of these audiences later in the chapter when we discuss prototype and course review and assessment.

Instructional Design, Course Development, and Delivery

A vital component in the development of an online course is the preliminary instructional design process and testing of the course prototype. During this component of the faculty training program, the mentee develops skills used to design the course and receives feedback to improve and ready the course for delivery to the student audience (see Figure 1). Davis proposes a 5-step preliminary design model be followed in the development process (2005, p. 22). We used a variation of this 5-step model to think through the training process needed so faculty can acquire the skills to be successful in the online teaching environment.

As we discussed in the previous section, the boundaries for course design and approval may be outlined by the department, program, or institution. Ideally these guidelines (borrowing from our accrediting agency, we use the term "quality assurance") can also align with the requirements of external accreditation agencies. For example, at our institution, this document is called *Quality Assurance for Online Learning*. The college's Distance Learning Committee developed it to ensure that all distance learning courses developed and approved for delivery by the college adhere to the Quality Matters best practices for online education.

If possible, the quality assurance document should be composed of two sections, each addressing a different set of course guidelines. One section provides guidelines for correlating the content to be delivered in the online course with its counterpart face-to-face course. These guidelines address course learning objectives, assessments, and assignments to ensure that the depth of the knowledge to be delivered and assessed aligns with the face-to-face course. Another section of the document details guidelines to meet online instruction best practices with regard to overall course design, tool selection, the presence of materials and assessments appropriate to the online environment and learner and instructor interaction. In our case, both the Department Chair and the Distance Learning Committee use the best practices detailed in the quality assurance document to review the developed course. Both sections provide faculty the needed "guidance . . . to identify which practices or processes should be planned or improved" in an online course (Neuhauser, 2004, p. 2).

Orientation of the mentee to the best practices serves as a fast-track on the Online Course Design Maturity Model developed by Neuhauser (2004, p. 2). Neuhauser's Online Course Design Maturity Model contains five distinct levels: Level 1 Initial, uses mostly text, minimal use of CMS, and no assessments are conducted online; Level 2 Exploring, consists of use of a blended course with notes and some assignments collected online; Level 3 Awakening, contains lectures with links and student participation in discussion, use of CMS to deliver tests, and collect papers from students; Level 4 Strategizing, includes use of multimedia, collaborative tools, structured content, student-generated content;

and Level 5 Integrating Best Practices. For more details on the Model, see Neuhauser's "A Maturity Model: Does It Provide a Path for Online Course Design?" Instead of waiting for faculty to advance by identifying and implementing best practices on their own, the mentoring process provides direct support and guidance for the faculty to implement required strategies that may be too advanced for their level. As we noted earlier, the mentor discusses the quality assurance document with the mentee before the course development process begins, and the mentor and mentee are encouraged to use the document as a reference throughout the development process. Once the above guidelines are discussed, the design of the course can begin.

As course development begins, the mentor and mentee together plan the instructional design, including learning objectives, materials, and methods for instruction, interaction, and assessment. The quality assurance document guides this step of the process so that the learning objectives provided in the online course are understandable and address measurable outcomes, content mastery, and critical thinking. Since the learning objectives are set by departmental guidelines, this step in the development of a new course can be centered on planning how the design will effectively address the course objectives. For mentees who have developed an external online course, an evaluation of their course will indicate changes that will need to be made to meet departmental guidelines. The mentees are subject matter experts; therefore, they have a clear knowledge of the course learning objectives. The mentor's responsibility is to assist the mentee to select one module or unit of the face-to-face course and analyze how the content can be effectively delivered. This analysis directs the appropriate selection of the materials, instructional methodologies, and technology tools to deliver the content in the online environment. Through development of this module, mentees typically realize that although the environment (online or on-site) in which they will be delivering their course will change, their course objectives must not change dramatically.

When the first course content module has been designed, the mentor and mentee discuss different delivery methods, including the advantages and disadvantages of various technology tools. The audience analysis reflects the mentee's technical experience and comfort level with various delivery methods specific to the online environment. At this stage, the mentor informs the mentee of the available media that may be constrained by institutional choices. The constraint of institutional choices of technology tools may require additional changes. If the mentee in this situation is not familiar with the tools provided by the institution, the audience analysis places them closer to the "needs +" end of the Mentor Relationship Continuum, reflecting a need for training in the use of the new tools to deliver their developed content. Depending on the mentee's technical experience, the mentor provides individualized training or identifies appropriate support staff to provide training on the use of various technology tools. Importantly, consideration must be given as to whether the tools are pedagogically sound. The mentor and other distance learning faculty serve as valuable resources by sharing their experiences with the use of tools supported by the institution as well as affordable alternatives that may be more appropriate for the delivery of the content in a particular course.

With at least one course module and tools in place, the mentor then prepares the mentee for future evaluation and accreditation issues regarding the course design, the design for testing and evaluating the student's achievement of learning objectives, and the instructors' delivery of educational services. Standards set by the institution and/or its accreditation agency regarding online course design and evaluation are in place in anticipation of accreditation issues. The mentor helps the mentee ensure that the design of the course meets these standards regardless of whether the course is developed at the college or developed externally.

When the mentoring pair has completed these steps, the prototype is ready for review and testing. Review and testing of the course by local and peer audiences also has a significant role in verifying that the course adheres to set standards.

Prototype Review and Assessment

Testing provides crucial feedback to the mentee so appropriate improvements can be made prior to delivery to the student audience. Davis (2005) advises that a paper prototype of the course be evaluated before course tools are selected and actual course development begins (p. 22). To meet the constraints of a shorter course development timeline, our prototype is defined as one completed online module or unit of the course. Davis also suggests that user and task analyses described by Hackos and Redish and Rubin (as cited in Davis, 2005, p. 23) be used to ensure that the product is usable and practical. In this type of analysis, the product is evaluated to determine its ease-of-use, effectiveness, learnability, and likeability. The findings from the analysis then dictate the changes that need to be made prior to delivery to the students. Proper testing of the online course can include evaluation criteria found in a user and task analysis. Although our testing process does not include actual student users, the standards within our institution's *Quality Assurance for Online Learning* document serve this purpose.

When possible, evaluations should be done more than once during the development process, with the first test preferably done early in the development process. The mentor's preliminary evaluation of the prototype prevents the mentee from designing a course using methods that may be detrimental to student learning. This initial evaluation guides the remainder of the course development and ensures that major overhauls of the course design are not necessary. After the mentor's preliminary evaluation and feedback, the mentee completes course development. At this point, the online teaching peer audience, made up of faculty members who have experience developing and/or delivering distance learning courses at TSTC, evaluates the course. Both the preliminary and final evaluations utilize the quality assurance for online learning document. The feedback provided to the mentee following each evaluation is essential to the production of a quality end-product that will be approved for delivery to the student audience.

Tool Evaluation and Selection

After prototype development and evaluation, mentees are ready to identify the best delivery of instruction based on the prototype design. The technical communication theory presented by Davis suggests that online education tools be selected after prototype development (2005, p. 23). This concept of pedagogy driving the selection of the delivery technology, not vice versa, is also suggested by Cargile Cook (2005) and Ascough (2002). A challenge to our faculty members is that while we agree that "the learning goals must drive the selection of the delivery technology" (Davis, 2005, p. 23), our institution, as well as many other colleges and universities, have adopted technology tools that faculty are urged, if not forced, to use. Therefore, the mentor must be able to guide the mentee concerning the available choices that will best fit their pedagogical goals.

At our institution, the faculty must use the provided learning management system (LMS) to deliver their course. However, the mentor can guide the faculty member as to the selection of the available LMS tools best-suited to meet their course objectives. In addition to the tools provided in the LMS and other technology tools provided by the institution, the mentor can direct the mentee to open-source or low-cost alternatives that may be more pedagogically appropriate to achieve their course goals. One of the goals of our courses is to design for interaction between students and faculty. Many technology tools promote inter-action within the LMS, while numerous open-source options function outside the LMS. In a case like this, other factors can be considered, such as ease-of-use by the instructor and the student. Whereas our evaluation and selection of tech-nological tools is pedagogically driven, in agreement with the technical com-munication theory, faculty within institutions that demand use of their pre-determined tools possibly face a more limited pool of technological tools from which to choose.

Given these constraints, the mentor and mentee discuss different delivery methods, including the advantages and disadvantages of various technology tools. The continua maps reflect the mentee's technical experience and comfort level with various delivery methods specific to the online environment. At this stage, the mentor informs the mentee of the available media that may be con-strained by institutional choices. The constraint of institutional choices of tech-nology tools may require additional change. Depending on the mentee's technical experience, the mentor provides individualized training or identifies appropriate support staff to provide training on the use of various technology tools. Impor-tantly, consideration is given as to whether the tools are pedagogically sound. The mentor and other distance learning faculty serve as valuable resources by sharing their experiences with the use of tools supported by the institution as well as affordable alternatives that may be more appropriate for the delivery of the content in a particular course.

Finally, before the course is delivered, the mentor explains the infrastructure of support available to the mentee, including instructional media or support staff. Regardless of whether the mentee is entirely new to online course design and delivery or if they have designed and taught online courses at other institutions, the mentor acts as the primary support contact for technology training and faculty development training. The mentor also serves as a liaison to identify and contact appropriate support staff at the institution or an outside entity. This relationship facilitates the course development process in a situation in which time constraints are an issue. The mentor confirms that the mentee is familiar and comfortable with seeking assistance from instructional technologists, network services, and faculty training offices once the training program is completed. Additionally, standards set by the institution and/or its accreditation agency regarding online course design typically require that the online course provide the student with contact information for all college academic services, student support services, and technical support services.

Course Delivery and Evaluation

Once the course is approved for delivery, a second mentoring relationship is established to guide the mentee. We have found it preferable to have the same mentor, if at all possible, shadow the mentee during the first semester that the mentee delivers an online course. This practice provides an accessible resource to the mentee and eases their transition into online course delivery.

At this point, the relationship takes one of two forms: what we call "over the shoulder" or "co-teaching." In the over-the-shoulder method, the mentor continues to provide general guidance and answer questions as they arise. We used this method with faculty who are already comfortable with the technology because of their considerable experience teaching hybrid courses. Alternatively, the mentor provides more direct instruction in the "co-teaching" approach. The mentor, in coordination with the mentee, establishes the parameters of the co-teaching relationship to determine what responsibilities each will have during the delivery of the course. For example, we have had mentoring relationships in which both mentor and mentee served as instructor of record for several sections, and both had contact with the same students. In this instance, the mentor verified that the mentee had a variety of experiences and gained enough knowledge to independently teach the course in subsequent semesters. A variation of this relationship involves both mentor and mentee teaching different sections using the same designed course. In this variation, the mentee observes the mentor and attempts to duplicate the same instruction, but the mentee has much more independence and responsibility.

Because the mentor is present as a resource and to protect the relationship between the individuals, we recommend that the mentor does not participate in direct evaluation of the mentee. Evaluation of the instructor's delivery of the online courses may be assessed formatively by a peer or supervisor and summatively by students in an end-of-course evaluation administered by the online program. In addition, data that demonstrates student learning can be collected and analyzed. These evaluations provide data to indicate course success and areas for continual course improvement. If the faculty evaluator is not an expert in online course delivery, he may contact the mentor to discuss possibilities for assistance with course improvement. Evaluation is best conducted by someone outside the mentoring relationship. We recommend the mentor not participate in evaluation of the mentee so that the mentoring relationship can remain intact.

Once mentees have completed the M2M training program and delivered an online course successfully for one semester, they "graduate" to certified mentor status. A mentee's successful completion of the M2M program and graduation to a certified mentor can be dependent on various evaluation measures:

1. Approval of the designed course by subject matter peers and online teaching peers;
2. Positive reviews from the mentor in interviews carried out through the course design and delivery phases; and
3. Student evaluation of the course and its delivery during the first semester the course is offered online.

Throughout this process, appropriate feedback is provided to the mentee from the mentor and communicated to supervisors. In addition, the course and its delivery is continually reviewed by student and peer evaluators. The experience and expertise the mentee receives through this process enables the mentee to become a valuable mentor for other faculty new to online course design and delivery.

Although the evaluation and "graduation" marks the end of the formal mentoring process, an informal collaborative and supportive relationship between the mentor and the mentee in the program often continues.

MENTOR2MENTOR ASSESSMENT AND COMMUNITY BUILDING

We have developed formative, as well as summative, evaluation to facilitate continual quality improvement of the M2M training program. Formative evaluation allows the mentor to determine if the strategies and methods being used are effective and provide feedback to the program director about how to help the mentor provide better service. On the other hand, summative evaluation allows both mentor and mentee to provide feedback about how to improve the process for future mentoring relationships. Mentees and mentors are interviewed at the beginning, middle, and end of the M2M training program. Answers to interview questions provide information to the program director about program expectations that the mentee and mentor have and whether or not these expectations are being met. Throughout the mentoring process, the mentor and mentee document their interactions using a short questionnaire. This allows for the collection of ongoing documentation that provides information and suggestions that can be used improve the mentoring program.

Assessment allows our program to address its weaknesses and nurture its strengths, which in turn builds its reputation and ability to recruit. We agree with Davis, though, that "the best advertising is by word of mouth" from current participants, especially to recruit mentors (2005, p. 25). Even when the mentoring program is mandatory for new faculty, it can be difficult to recruit faculty experienced in online instruction, many of whom have developed their expertise by working on their own, to be mentors if the program is not marketed correctly or is perceived as taking advantage of faculty or not providing the type of support it promises. Recruitment of mentors is facilitated by providing clear and institutionalized benefits to the mentor for participation in the program. Creating a community of sharing and support and collecting testimonials helps with word-of-mouth marketing.

Another crucial component of the program management further supports faculty and staff who participate in M2M. This component includes certification, recognition, and compensation for distance learning faculty and program administrators. As Davis suggests for online programs, training programs "define and gain acceptance on workload issues for faculty and administrators, . . . commit to providing total learner support online, and . . . secure budgetary commitments to keep technology current" (2005, p. 26). Enough compensation opportunities are designed into the program so that mentors and other possible participants do not feel exploited. Mentoring takes a considerable amount of time and energy, and a successful program must compensate mentors in ways that align with institutional expectations of faculty. The program is developed so that each faculty member receives institutional certification and recognition for their participation in the mentoring program. For example, at our institution we were able to secure stipends for our mentors. Also, participation in the program is applied to meet yearly professional development requirements. We are currently developing a certification system to recognize the skills faculty have acquired and applied through their mentoring relationships. We will use a two-tiered system to acknowledge the number of individuals mentors have guided through the mentoring program. Other institutions that have access to a large adjunct and teaching assistant pool may be able to offer release time or partial-release time for faculty who serve as mentors. Additionally, faculty may be more willing to participate if they are able to include such participation as part of their tenure and promotion materials. Program administrators can work to guarantee that the institution acknowledges the mentoring as teaching and training of other faculty rather than service, if service is weighed lightly compared to teaching or scholarship. Finally, program administrators can create scholarship opportunities for or support research by those participating in the mentoring process.

CONCLUSION

In 2005, Davis challenged technical communicators to participate in online program development at their institutions. Developing a strong program must include a faculty training component that builds the expertise needed for sustainability; however, decreasing budgets create challenges to providing the appropriate training to faculty who lack the required skills to teach online. Few external training programs exist that provide personalized guidance through the complex course design and delivery process. We answered Davis's call for active participation by applying the technical communication theory she outlined to design an in-house training program that utilizes experienced faculty to mentor those new to online instruction.

The challenge in applying the theory in a specific context is the negotiation required between the ideal application of the theory, the needs of the individuals, and context created by the institution. We found that one type of negotiation arose from the time constraints imposed by the increasing, and at times urgent, demand for certain courses. For example, creating and testing a course prototype according to Davis's recommendations was time-prohibitive. A second type of negotiation was due to cost issues. Although instructors would have liked to use certain tools in our course design, we were limited by those provided and supported by the institution.

Despite the limitations, we were able to use the technical communication theory to create a strong training program. Our skills as technical communicators allowed us to take a leadership role to identify acceptable alternatives when faced with certain challenges. Additionally, we became advocates for faculty needs that we identified as the training program developed. Most importantly, our focus on mentoring highlights the skills of faculty leaders from different disciplines to create a larger network of leaders who are able to sustain quality online education.

REFERENCES

Ascough, R. S. (2002). Designing for online distance education: Putting pedagogy before technology. *Teaching Theology and Religion, 5*(1), 17–29.

Cargile Cook, K. (2005). An argument for pedagogy-driven online education. In K. Cargile Cook & K. Grant-Davie (Eds.) *Online education: Global questions, local answers* (pp. 49–66). Amityville, NY: Baywood.

Cargile Cook, K. (2007). Immersion in a digital pool: Training prospective online instructors in online environments. *Technical Communication Quarterly, 16*(1), 55.

Davis, M. (2005). Applying technical communication theory to the design of online education. In K. Cargile Cook & K. Grant-Davie (Eds.), *Online education: Global questions, local answers* (pp. 15–29). Amityville, NY: Baywood.

Hezlett, S. A. (2005). How do formal mentors assist their proteges? A study of mentors assigned to cooperative education students and interns. *Online Submission*. Retrieved from http://www.eric.ed.gov/ERICWebPortal/contentdelivery/servlet/ERICServlet?accno=ED492458

Instructional Technology Council (ITC). (2010). *Distance Education Survey results. Trends in elearning: Tracking the impact of eLearning at community colleges.* Washington, DC: Instructional Technology Council. Retrieved from http://www.itcnetwork.org/file.php?file=%2F1%2FITCAnnualSurvey2009Results.pdf

Katz, R. N. (2003). Balancing technology and tradition: The example of course management systems. *EDUCAUSE Review, 38*(4), 48–54, 56–59.

Leidman, M. B. (2006). Utilizing role theory and mentoring to minimize stress for new faculty. *Online Submission*. Retrieved from http://www.eric.ed.gov/ERICWebPortal/contentdelivery/servlet/ERICServlet?accno=ED502287

McCarthy, S. A., & Samors, R. J. (2009). *Online learning as a strategic asset volume I: A resource for campus leaders. A report on the Online Education Benchmarking study conducted by the APLU Sloan National Commission on Online Learning.* Washington, DC: Office of Public Affairs, Association of Public and Land-Grant Universities. Retrieved from http://www.aplu.org/NetCommunity/Document.Doc?id=1877

Neuhauser, C. (2004). A maturity model: Does it provide a path for online course design? *The Journal of Interactive Online Learning, 3*(1). Retrieved January 10, 2006, from www.ncolr.org/jiol/issues/PDF/3.1.3.pdf

Powell, G. (2001). The ABCs of online course design. *Educational Technology, 41*(4), 43–47.

Quality Matters. (n.d.). Retrieved June 26, 2010, from http://www.qmprogram.org

Seaman, J. (2009). *Online learning as a strategic asset volume II: The paradox of faculty voices: Views and experiences with online learning. Results of a National Faculty Survey, Part of the Online Education Benchmarking study conducted by the APLU Sloan National Commission on Online Learning.* Washington, DC: Office of Public Affairs, Association of Public and Land-Grant Universities. Retrieved from http://www.aplu.org/NetCommunity/Document.Doc?id=1879

http://dx.doi.org/10.2190/OE2C6

Section II: Adapting to Changing Student Needs and Abilities

CHAPTER 6

Teaching Technical Communication to a Global Online Student Audience

Emily A. Thrush and Susan L. Popham

For at least the last 17 years, an active dialogue has been taking place in technical communication journals, at conferences, and on e-mail lists, about the importance of preparing students for a globalized workplace. We have talked about raising awareness of cultural differences in communication strategies and preferences, increasing the students' ability to write for diverse audiences, and using materials that reflect the realities of international and intercultural communication. Now it's time to practice what we preach and internationalize our classes.

Online delivery of certificate and degree programs in technical communication is expanding the possibilities for participation by students around the globe. Many universities see online programs as a way of reaching new populations, while students overseas see online classes as a way to obtain a U.S. degree without the expensive and difficult process of getting a visa, relocating, and finding financial support adequate for studying and living in the United States. Having students who represent various cultures offers advantages to instructors who want to incorporate an international perspective in their courses, but it also poses new opportunities and challenges. We have to be prepared to answer the following:

- How can assignments take advantage of the skills and knowledge of the participants from different countries and cultures?

- How can students learn from each other about communication practices in other places?
- How do syllabi, materials, and assignments need to be globalized?
- What are the expectations for documents such as résumés and cover letters?
- How do document design preferences vary from culture to culture?
- What persuasive strategies are most effective?
- What adjustments in guidelines for writing style need to be made? Are the Plain English guidelines effective for speakers of English as a second language?
- Are there specific ways of writing for translation into other languages?
- What are the implications of having international students who are not in English-speaking settings in online courses? What kinds of support need to be offered to these students to support language development along with instruction in technical communication?
- Most importantly, does the instructor of a technical communication class need to be an expert in all these issues, or are materials available to help guide teachers through these questions?

We cannot offer definitive answers to all these questions at this time. What we hope to do is to open a dialogue on these issues by discussing the need to make changes in what we teach and how we teach it. We will look at the state of English usage around the world and approaches to education internationally that have gone beyond the often limited perspective of the U.S. academy. We will also suggest some approaches to dealing with the challenges of educating a truly multicultural and multilinguistic student body.

It should be noted that we are not specifically writing about joint programs between U.S. and foreign universities, or what Starke-Meyerring and Wilson (2008) call Globally Networked Learning Environments (GNLEs). Their excellent book on GNLEs covers many issues, including the negotiating process between institutions and examples of activities that link students in the cooperating schools. Much of what we suggest in this chapter might apply to those situations as well, but we are primarily writing to the teacher who suddenly finds students enrolled in an online course from any non-English-speaking country.

For those new to the issue of online, global teaching, a few standard definitions may be helpful. According to Hoft (1995), localization refers to the communication practice of developing documents or other texts for a highly specific, local community. A memo designed to circulate among only the workers in a single office may be said to be localized: the diction, purpose, style, format, and other communicative elements are likely to be known and familiar to everyone in the office. Internationalization refers to the communicative practice of developing a text or document from one country for use in another specified country. Thus, a document or other text would need only two countries, an originating country and a receiving country, to be considered international. Likewise, an online course might have students from only two countries, or possibly just one student from a different country, to be considered international. Globalization refers to the practice of preparing documents for use in multiple countries by multiply diverse audiences. Thus, a Web site is certainly a document that could be used around the world, as is a memo circulated to employees in several different branches of a global company. Similarly, an online course, in which students from several different countries are enrolled, could be perceived as global. In this sense, globally oriented describes the practice of emphasizing global issues and globally diverse audiences. Thus, a class that is globally oriented would do more than teach students from several different countries; it would try to focus on, highlight, and make integral to the course elements from several different cultures, and it would pay attention to the differences that the students bring to the course culture and course assignments. For the purposes of this chapter, we will try to adhere to these definitions about local, international, and global audiences.

Like the messy definitions that often accompany thinking beyond the borders of one's own country, so too does the term "English" seem complex and often without definition. Within our own department, for example, English can be the name of our department, something our students study, the language of England, the literature of England, the literature of English-speaking nations, the supposed Standard Academic English that some of us try to enforce in student writing, and so on. We argue all the time about what "English" means. And for the most part, we labor these argumentative efforts without even acknowledging the complexity of addressing World Englishes, International English, Business English, Global English, Globish, and English as the de facto Lingua Franca (it has not escaped our notice that this term uses two other languages, Latin and Italian, to describe English). Even the term "online," another messy issue, implies the Internet, the World Wide Web, Web 2.0 technologies, asynchronicity, synchronicity, distance, piracy, privacy, security, and open source. When teachers begin to think about the online teaching of English to a global audience, the archaeological layers that we must unearth may often seem overwhelming. We will try to cut through those complexities to deal with the issues most critical to teaching and learning: who the students are, what the content of the course is, why we teach professional communication, which English we should be teaching, and how we deliver the content.

CHANGES IN WHO WE TEACH

Online degree programs often encourage international and global student participation. Our own university's online degree programs allow nonresident students, including both out-of-state students and international students, to pay the same tuition rate for the online classes as the state resident students. And our online degree programs are being strongly marketed on our university's

Web site, in the local and regional newspaper (including the online newspaper presences), and in databases of educational programs. Because our online programs are relatively new—at this time, just three semesters—it is difficult to know how many international students are enrolled in those online classes. However, the number of international students enrolled in our university has risen 6% over the past two years: in the fall of 2007, of those students who declared nationality, 839 total students were categorized as "foreign." In the fall of 2009, the number had risen to 889. While we cannot state with certainty that these students were all enrolled in online courses, it seems probable that the advent of online degree programs during that time may have had an impact on our university's enrollment of international students. Another university, well-known for its online degree programs, Texas Tech University, hosts 33 online or video-interface degree and certificate programs; from 2007 to 2008, this university experienced a 16% increase in nonresident alien student enrollment (Texas Tech University Historical Fact Book, 2008). Again, while the increase in international student enrollment does not specify online degree enrollment, it is important to note that these increases occurred during the time the university was increasing its online degree presence. Better tracking of international student enrollment figures would help faculty and university administrators prepare for teaching online global student audiences. Significantly, however, the increase in international student enrollment shows the growing interest that students in other countries have for U.S. degrees. Better marketing of the online degree programs available in the United States may prompt greater enrollment of international students, including those who find themselves unable to leave their homelands. More and better targeted marketing of our online degrees in technical communication would certainly help to increase the number of globally based students in our courses as the need for strong English communication skills increases globally.

Extending our programs to students globally does more than enhance the bottom-line financial prospects of our universities. Globally oriented learning can offer all students better skills for participating in international workplaces and for learning about the complex process that we call Technical Communication. Noted by Herrington and Tretyakov (2005), online global teaching "helps to make our students aware of the complexity of the processes of communication and teaches them how to deal with at least some of its elements in action" (p. 280). For U.S. students, learning with students from other countries offers them a way to learn from firsthand accounts about other cultures and other styles of communicating. As we strengthen the global presence in our online technical communication courses, our own local students learn to expand their own cultural and language boundaries. One can only hope that they can learn to be less insular and bound to national or local value systems as they encounter students from other cultures in their courses. At our own university, 75% of our student enrollment comes from the county in which our university is located, with another 10% coming from neighboring counties. Moreover, many of these students are financially unable to venture much beyond the county boundaries. For these students, their sense of the world, of people, of cultures, and of English communicative practices is only known through their highly localized view. Being able to perceive how other cultures use communicative practices and English to function in workplaces, without having to bankrupt their college endeavors can often mean the difference between finding a job in an international company or not finding a job at all. Herrington (2008) points out that contact with students from other countries in a class can "provide them with a forum for learning how to develop a critical cross-cultural literacy through negotiating multiple perspectives" (p. 39).

CHANGES IN WHY WE TEACH

As experienced teachers of fully online courses whose students often participate from across the nation and from around the world, we work with the assumption that globally oriented teaching is a benefit for us, for our universities, and for all our students. This assumption is not unexamined, as we fully realize that we are participating in what many would perceive as only financially motivated, and hence impure in some way. Nor does it escape our recognition that by participating in such endeavors, we may be helping to "colonize" the international world to U.S. standards, thus making our work somehow tainted by the stink of imperialism and cultural domination. Nevertheless, we believe that such global teaching is primarily an enhancement to us and to our students, and that when we participate in such endeavors while being critically aware, we can help to further improve the future of global online teaching.

Despite the recent economic recession, more and more corporations, those based both in and outside the United States, are increasing their international/ global business. Because these employers and customers are likely to value high-quality, global, and international communication skills, we teach in online global environments so that all our students, both international and local, are more adept and skilled in entering such workplaces. For example, one of our technical communication students worked as an intern in an anthropology lab in which she was required to prepare reports and newsletters for funding agencies. She told us that every researcher and employee of that lab was international and that she found herself at a cultural disadvantage because everyone else was already so familiar with global and international communication patterns. Not only did she have to learn how to communicate within the discipline of anthropology, and then to communicate that knowledge about anthropological knowledge to nondisciplinary specialists, she also had to learn how to understand and write in a globally oriented environment, a skill that she carried into her next job. Such language expertise as knowing when to drop the article before a noun, very common in scientific disciplines and in international communication, is an essential skill that our local students may never encounter without prompting from a globally oriented online class. Students who enter technical communication, usually with the hope of securing a career as a technical communicator, are well-served when we help to prepare them for a global workplace: they learn to prepare for local jobs that are increasingly focused on international markets, they learn to communicate internationally, they learn to analyze and negotiate cultural contexts, and they are better prepared for jobs around the world.

We also do global online teaching because it enhances our own pedagogical skills. As teachers, when we learn to stretch and expand our own horizons, when we learn to analyze cultural contexts in which we teach, when we learn to appreciate new and different ways of communicating, we thus learn to be better teachers. And quite frankly, it makes our academic lives more interesting. We all know colleagues who dust off their decades-old notes from their own graduate school days and reteach the same old tired course semester after semester. But teaching online global classes helps to renew and refresh our interest in teaching, in meeting the ever-changing needs of our students and of workplaces. Further, when we emphasize global contexts and issues in our online classes, we do so in hope that we make our own workplaces, our academic disciplines and departments, more welcoming to international colleagues.

CHANGES IN WHAT WE TEACH

When we teach an online globally contextualized class, we must be ready to change the content of our writing-instruction classes to better meet the needs of international students. One of the challenges in offering writing-intensive classes to international students is that they frequently have no prior formal instruction in any type of writing, either in their native languages or English. In some cases, this is because only members of the cultural elite in other countries attend universities, and they all speak the same variety of the native language. Writing instruction in the United States became a focus of undergraduate education with the expansion of colleges and universities to regions with dialects that varied from the "standard" English encoded in the textbooks and when the G.I. Bill made postsecondary education more affordable for a wider range of students. In countries where that has not happened, there has been no push for universal writing instruction. Crabtree and Sapp (2004) reported that Brazilian students themselves recognized that their reading and writing skills were not as advanced as their speaking and listening skills, and that "most students in Brazil also do not receive instruction in academic writing and research skills—even in their native language—until late in their undergraduate education or, more likely, until graduate school" (p. 112). The first author of this chapter found the same situation in a leading university in Mexico, where students in a degree program in teaching English as a second language had to first take a course on writing in Spanish and then one on writing in English, because they had no previous explicit instruction in writing. This lack of experience with writing instruction is going to affect the students' knowledge of how to approach writing assignments, how to analyze writing tasks, and how to revise and edit their written work. Building that background knowledge of how writing courses work is going to take more effort on the part of instructors. To use a common term from education, students will need more scaffolding or in plainer terms, more virtual "hand-holding."

Another challenge for teachers is the recognition that introductory technical communication classes in the United States are often organized around genres—types of documents typically produced in work environments, such as letters, memos, proposals, recommendation reports, and such. These typical writing tasks may be irrelevant for international students. As Brewer (2010) reports, many of these genres are either not widely used or take quite a different form in other cultures. For example, much of what is done in U.S. business through memos, e-mail, and letters occurs orally in other cultures. In multicultural organizations, there may be serious communication problems among people with different expectations about the mode, numbers, and level of detail of correspondence. Years ago, on a tour of the Sharp manufacturing plant, a U.S. engineer discussed the adjustments he had had to make to work in a Japanese-owned company. He pointed out the long glass wall behind the assembly line and told us that all the managers and engineers had desks there, not separate offices. He had discovered after a few incidents of miscommunication that he was supposed to be keeping his ears open while working at his desk, to hear others talk about the need for a meeting and when they would get together. There were no memos announcing meetings or e-mail reminders. In a high-context culture, oral communication is more important than written, and written communication is less detailed (Thrush, 1993). When our university had an internship program for students to teach in high schools in China, the contract was worked out only after we had taken the first group of students over, and only at the insistence of the American lawyers. The Chinese officials considered the oral agreement with us binding and had been assiduous about observing the details of it. They did not understand the need for a written document. These global examples show that we teachers cannot take for granted that all of our students will immediately understand the exigency of producing a résumé like most of our local students will. It will be challenging for the instructor to keep the course objectives and materials relevant for international students while still meeting the needs of students in the United States.

Wherever our students come from, they may be able to inform us of how jobs are obtained and what communication skills they may need for the search process. In a writing class for students in Russia, Bowen, Sapp, and Sargsyn (2006) discovered that résumés are either seen as not needed or take on a very different role in the hiring process, partly because jobs were (and still are, to a great extent) gotten by contacts rather than an application process. Also, students were frequently unable to produce résumés that differentiated themselves from others because in the Russian educational system, the curriculum is standardized, so everyone in, for example, an engineering degree program, took all the same courses. In Russia, as in many other parts of the world, it is unusual for students to work while in high school or university, so the students tend not to have any work experience or volunteer experience to record on their résumés. They also found the cover letter even more difficult to write than U.S. students typically do, because it is even more culturally inappropriate to "brag" about one's own abilities. Meanwhile, the job-hiring process in the United States is undergoing significant changes that are not yet reflected in the writing textbooks. Web sites such as Monster.com and Jobsearch.com ask applicants to post a generic résumé rather than the customized ones we usually advocate, because companies run searches for specific words in the résumés of applicants to identify qualified individuals. Applications posted on these sites may need to look quite different from the traditional résumé, including, perhaps, the use of icons to visually represent job skills (Jobsearch.com, n.d.). Thus, the hiring process is changing, both to meet international demands and technical advances.

With the growth of multinational companies, the hiring process is changing in many countries, and more documentation of skills and experience may soon be required, but the American model of the résumé may not be the most appropriate or effective. In some cultures, there is less separation of work and personal life than there is in the United States. The first author of this chapter taught a writing class for employees of a Canadian insurance company years ago. In an exercise in which the students applied for an "employee of the year" award, many of the students wrote as much about their home lives, their children, their church or volunteer work, and their good character as they did about their performance on the job. These aspects of their lives were all seen as testaments to their value to the company, and indeed, residents of some communities might be more likely to buy insurance from companies who employ workers of exemplary character and personal integrity. Some of the legal restrictions on gathering personal information about prospective employees in the United States do not apply in other contexts, so the job application might be required to contain information that we advise students not to reveal. But our perception of work life as separate from personal life may be changing as well. Melissa Cidade from the Center for Applied Research in the Apostolate at Georgetown University commented that when she found that a prospective employer had looked her up on the Internet,

> Maybe it's OK to be Googleable. Maybe it's okay for the workplace to have a fuller picture of me as a person rather than just as a worker. And I think that's in keeping with some of the data that we've seen about Millennials in the workplace, which is that they want better work-life balance, they want more satisfaction, they want to be seen as a person and not just a worker. So maybe it's more of that reflective technology going on. (Pew Research Center, 2010)

The variations in job-search processes across the globe highlight the need for teachers of technical communication to be attuned to these variations as they develop course assignments.

Given that job-search processes and the genres traditionally used for those processes are changing, it may be time to consider changing the way introductory technical communication courses are organized. Rather than an approach that focuses on workplace genres, such as résumés, letters, memos, documentation manuals, and the like, an approach that asks students to analyze the communicative exigency and the cultural context before beginning to write might be more effective for an online global student population. This might work better for domestic students as well. For global technical communication courses, an overemphasis on U.S. genres may not be helpful to international students or for local students who hope to work in international workplaces. Instead, global technical courses might find it more effective to emphasize communicative and analytic skills, such as analyzing the audiences and their cultural expectations for a document; learning to work effectively on collaborative documents using Web 2.0 media, like Google docs; learning to analyze the purposes and exigencies of various existing genres and potential genres; and finally, learning to recognize one's own cultural expectations that shape one's view of successful communicative practices. Maylath, Vandepitte, and Mouston (2008) relate their experiences with students who recognized the need to adapt their communication in documents, but failed to do so in e-mail negotiations about completing a joint project (p. 57). They cite an incident in which two students used "irony and sarcasm" to communicate about a disagreement—neither of which work well in e-mail or translate across cultures. More instruction and intervention is needed to help students develop appropriate negotiation strategies, especially in a globally focused online course.

Other forms of workplace communication are changing rapidly as well. We might find that we need to structure our classes around newer virtual genres, such as blogs, wikis, text messages, tweets, Web pages, social bookmarking sites, Google docs, and social networking sites instead of the old genres. Given the current generation's technological skills for cell phones, computers, and social networking, international students are more likely to share the same newer technological skills with their localized counterparts than either group is likely to find in common with the previous generation or even with the generation of their teachers (Accenture, 2010). One student in a graduate class recently reported that one of her job assignments had her working under a supervisor who wanted all communication to take place through text messaging, a communication medium in which she had no training. Technical communication textbooks offer very little advice on texting, but an analysis of the audience, purpose, and rhetorical strategies appropriate for this communication situation would have been helpful for this student.

For teachers wondering how to know which communication scenarios are likely in international environments, it would be worthwhile to have students investigate local organizations of the type they might one day work for. For example, in a course that used video conferencing to connect students from the United States and Hong Kong, Du-Babcock and Varner (2008) assigned the students to find out about the communication practices in a local McDonald's. The students were to assume "the role of management consultants advising McDonald's top management on how to adapt business and organizational practices from the United States to Hong Kong, or vice versa" (p. 157). While the researchers in this case were primarily interested in looking at the interactions among the students, an assignment such as this could lead to a better understanding of the needs of students from other countries.

Which English to Teach?

Changes in what we teach—job-search processes, genres, and style—may not be the only challenge for teachers of online global technical communication courses. These teachers must also consider the global complexity of requiring the "English" language. Several phrases are used to describe the varieties of English used among nonnative speakers, including World Englishes, Global English, and English as a Lingua Franca. These terms are used in different ways, often with political implication. English as a Lingua Franca is the most limited concept, describing the English that might be used by members of a particular profession or trade and consisting of the vocabulary specific to that field of endeavor along with general English structures needed to construct sentences and questions. Global English, as used by Crystal (1997), Graddol (2000) and the Oxford Dictionary refers to more general usage. Sources advocating Global English, such as the BBC, the English Company Ltd. (which produces a newsletter called "Global English"), and others see it as a standardized form based on British and American English, with some allowance for local dialects around the world. "World Englishes" was coined by Braj Kachru (1992) to refer to the varieties of English that were emerging naturally from the interactions of nonnative speakers. The English used by some speakers of Asian languages, for example, will often lack articles and plural endings, while most speakers of English as a second language have trouble with the idiomatic use of prepositions in expressions such as "based on" and "search for" (Thrush, 2001).

While the use of these terms is sometimes controversial, the main point that instructors of online global courses need to recognize is that communicators in international settings do not need the idiomatic features of the American, British, Indian or Australian dialects of English. Many of the surface-level errors that make the writings of nonnative speakers look different from native speaker writing do not interfere with communication and are unlikely to be noticed by other nonnative speakers. For example, speakers of World English are more likely to use the sense verbs (see, hear, taste, etc.) in the progressive form than are speakers of American or British English. One software developer posted a question on a forum that said, "Sometimes, I am seeing yellow triangle symbol with 'I' symbol" (http://forums.adobe.com/thread/881370?tstart=0). In addition to using "am seeing" instead of the simple present "see" for a repeated action, this writer demonstrated the typical omission of articles before "yellow triangle" and "'I' symbol." However, neither of these "errors" interferes with communication. Furthermore, it will become increasingly important for native speakers to be able to comprehend and communicate with nonnative speakers, a skill they can develop in globally oriented courses. Kennon (2008) reported on the problems that arose in a multicountry course because the U.S. students were unaware of the colloquial and idiomatic nature of the English they were using (p. 122). Learning about these differences in a course with other students is far preferable to learning it on the job, when important negotiations are involved, or when there is greater urgency about getting a message across accurately. Thus, it's a mistaken concept to assume that because our students "know English," that they will all know the same English; teachers must be ready to address cultural differences in the English language. This implies that teachers themselves must improve their awareness of the emerging varieties of English and of how English is used among nonnative speakers.

Changes in How We Teach

Along with adaptations in what content and what language we teach, we may also need to change the way we teach if our student population becomes more diverse. The culture of learning and teaching differs widely from country to country. Crabtree and Sapp (2004) write about an on-site class offered by U.S. university faculty in Brazil. Some of the issues they discuss (differences in amount of physical contact and concepts of personal space) do not apply to an online class. However, many of the cultural differences could have a profound effect on teaching in an online environment, such as the varying perspectives on time and deadlines. While North Americans tend to treat schedules as fixed and unchangeable, Brazilians see deadlines as negotiable, depending on the circumstances and needs of the individuals (p. 114). This practice is echoed in Venezuelan business arrangements in which each branch manager expected exceptions and accommodations to fit each office's situation. The second author also found these same cultural expectations about loose scheduling and deadlines in a recent visit to India. Thus, teachers may need to reconsider their requirements for strict adherence to deadlines and due dates. This flexibility poses an additional burden for the teacher, who will have to confront the expectations of the American students that any degree of flexibility is somehow "unfair."

Another cultural difference concerns the expected relationship between the student and the teacher. Crabtree and Sapp (2004) found that the professional distance usually kept by postsecondary teachers in the United States, no matter how concerned they are with their students' learning, was found to be inappropriate in Brazil. When the American teacher of the intercultural communication course became more open to revealing her life and hearing about her students' lives, it had a powerful affect on her ability to reach the students with the course content. Brewer (2010) reports on her own experience teaching Business English in Taiwan, where many of the students were more responsive and much more interested in her cultural experiences at Appalachian State University than they were in the class sessions on language rules. The classes in which she and another student showed pictures of her campus and region were some of the classes in which the Taiwanese students showed the most interest and excitement. From Brewer's perspective, the students needed less instruction in correct English and more knowledge about cultural differences and how those differences may affect the use of English. Teachers need to be ready to adapt their traditional pedagogical strategies to those that more appropriately address the diverse needs of a global student audience.

Different expectations of the presentation of course material is another challenge that Crabtree and Sapp (2004) observed. They comment that the Brazilian students "sought to contextualize abstract theories, personalize concepts, and connect the topics of the course to the cultural and political realities of their lives. . . . They interjected personal examples and related course issues to contemporary political concerns" (p. 118). While many of us already incorporate in our classes and assignments applications that relate to student experiences and goals, we may not be prepared for some of the issues students raise. For Brazilian students in the communication class, "the course content was inextricable from the interethnic and class conflicts in their country . . . or their own efforts to overcome personal adversity for education's sake" (p. 118). Fortunately, the discussion boards in most courseware for managing online classes allows for the kinds of discussions that students may need to feel connected to the course content.

Teaching the global class requires us to be more aware of the cultural assumptions underlying our pedagogical practices in order to help our local students learn to appreciate cultural differences, to tolerate differences in language use, and to see that their own language use is highly marked by local standards and expectations. For example, our local students are very familiar with a conversational pattern of point and counterpoint, and a conversational pattern that would be very comfortable with highlighting areas for improvement when collaborating with another student. Many of our native students cannot imagine someone being hesitant to point out someone else's flaws. However, as reported in Bosley's (1993) study of cross-cultural collaboration, international students may be very unwilling to critique another student's writing, something that they perceive as insulting. Online teaching, by its very distance, may make collaboration very difficult for international students. Yet online education also makes this kind of cross-cultural exchange more likely to happen and easier to resolve. For our local students, seeing that their familiar classroom and conversational patterns could be perceived very differently, perhaps as insulting, is an essential piece of knowledge that they can carry with them to other classes and to other workplaces. Learning that language use is determined "acceptable" more by its cultural context than by its strict adherence to rules and learning how to gauge the cultural context are admirable skills. Our international students learn these skills as well. For those international students who have been well-drilled with the rules of English, learning that such rules are helpful insomuch as they lead one to acknowledge the cultural context of a piece of writing, a context that can change with the internationalization or globalization of the document, or even the discipline of the document, is quite a revelation.

SUPPORTING LANGUAGE DEVELOPMENT

One of the most controversial issues involved in having international students in technical communication courses is how much support for the development of language skills the technical communication teacher should be asked to provide. In a recent e-mail exchange among members of the ATTW listserv who are interested in international issues, one person commented that his institution was heavily recruiting international students, and the English Department faculty were expressing a very strong feeling that they did not want to become ESL teachers. While they certainly had a point—their training and expertise are in other areas—the fact is that few of our students come to us with all the language skills we would like them to have. Whether we are dealing with native speakers of English who do not know the difference between a restrictive and nonrestrictive relative clause or the nonnative speaker who has not yet mastered the very complex use of the article "the," we are just as responsible for teaching them those general language skills as we are for teaching theories of document design or rhetorical strategies for proposal writing.

Another problem may be that students may have studied a different variety of English and now have to learn American English. If they spell words with a "u" as in "honour" or "colour," we usually recognize that as British spelling. But if they use a phrase such as "at the weekend" or "he's in hospital," we think of those as examples of a second-language learner making a very basic mistake rather than an example of another variety of English. Few Americans know that collective nouns take a plural verb in British English rather than the singular verb preferred in American English, as in this example from the Web page of the Scientific Committee on Antarctica (n.d.): "*The group propose* a timeline with production of data, a scientific publication and a report to SCAR to be completed by July 2010."

(http://www.scar.org/researchgroups/physicalscience/pact/). Teachers must be amenable to working with international students and realizing that one's own language rules may be nothing more than familiar preferences.

Why is it unreasonable to expect perfect fluency in English? Because language skills take years to develop. Collier's research (1989) found that children immersed in English in K–12 schools with daily ESL instruction took 5–7 years to develop the skills to do academic work. Even very proficient users of their second language, who regularly work, read, research, and write in that language, still do not have native-like control of all structures. Many of the renowned experts in science, math, and other disciplines at your university may need help with editing their written work to make it acceptable to native speakers of American English. If they have become highly successful in their fields without perfect fluency in English, is it reasonable to expect more from students?

BEYOND THE U.S. MODEL

Teachers of international global student audiences must be ready to perceive language learning beyond that of our own tongue, as evidenced by the European Union framework for language education called Content and Language Integrated Learning (CLIL). This framework is now also being used in Australia, New Zealand, and areas of Asia. A report prepared for the EU on CLIL states that "The importance of linguistic diversity in education and training in making Europe the most competitive and knowledge-based economy in the world means that existing language barriers need to be lifted" (Marsh, 2003, p. 9). For that reason, the EU has adopted an M+2 goal (mother tongue plus two other languages) for all students.

While there is not a single model for CLIL instruction, Coyle (2002, 2007) laid out the four key principles of CLIL in a report for the European Commission, and later in articles and a book:

1. **Content**: The language of a specific content area is typically taught with the content itself, so that the student is learning, for example, the vocabulary of engineering in the engineering class, and the format and grammatical choices appropriate for a lab report in the lab. This curriculum contrasts with the traditional approach which separates the language class from content classes.

2. **Context**: Language is a tool that only has meaning in contexts that are meaningful for the students. That is, when certain aspects of English are learned in the technical communication class, they will be learned better because they are in a context that gives them meaning, rather than in a decontextualized language class.

3. **Cognition**: Integrating language with content poses more cognitive challenges for the students, which helps to develop thinking skills along with language skills and content area knowledge.
4. **Culture**: Learning a content area through a foreign language provides opportunities for students to learn about the culture of that language. This will help students gain a different perspective on their own culture, and perhaps become more tolerant and more skilled in cross-cultural communication.

These four principles make a compelling case for the benefits of integrating technical communication, online teaching, and global student audiences because these principles are often implemented in the process of such integration. An online technical communication class could easily ask students to complete a group project by working with online students from another country; for example, one such assignment might ask students to write a manual on how to manage diabetes in India and in the southern portion of the United States. In this project, students would need to communicate with peers in India, easily accomplished online, and would ensure that students understand the context, the culture, and the content while developing their cognition in language skills, for many native Indian students, second-language skills. These kinds of online global assignments help students develop skills in CLIL. One of the aspects that distinguishes CLIL from bilingual education or the Content Based Language Learning used in U.S. K–12 schools is that not just any subject is chosen for study in a target language. Subjects are taught using a language in which the learner might actually use in that domain; so, for example, topics related to EU law might be taught in languages that could be used in international discussions of those laws (Coyle, 2007, p. 77). Technical communication, then, is a perfect discipline for nonnative speakers to learn in English, since that is the language often used in technology and frequently used in addition to the native language in product documentation, correspondence within and between multinational companies, and communication with mass media outlets. Teachers of technical communication in a globally focused online course would serve their students well if they incorporated the CLIL communication-learning qualities of content, context, cognition, and culture.

WAYS TO SUPPORT LANGUAGE DEVELOPMENT IN TECHNICAL COMMUNICATION CLASSES

The most effective teachers with nonnative speakers of English in their classes will have a certain degree of awareness of language development. Although we may have taken foreign language classes in which we were expected to memorize grammar rules and vocabulary and then put them together into sentences, that is not really the way languages are mastered (as evidenced by how few who study languages that way can actually speak them). Learning to speak a language is not like memorizing the capitals of the states or other sets of knowledge that we learned in school. It is a skill that involves instant and unconscious processing by the brain and muscular habits of the tongue, teeth, and lips in pronunciation. We often liken teaching a language to teaching someone how to ride a bicycle. You can demonstrate how to pedal and tell them how to work the brakes and the gears, but there's no way to transfer knowledge about how to stay balanced on the bike. The learner has to practice repeatedly so that the brain learns how to send the right signals to the muscles. In the process of that practice, the learner is likely to fall down a few times. Language learners also need opportunities to practice until production of the new language becomes effortless. They are also going to "fall down"—to make errors and learn from them.

The stages of acquiring mastery of a second language are similar to those of children learning English as their native language. Many of us have observed our children learning to communicate about past events, in which they first tend to overgeneralize the most obvious form and attach the syllabic ending of "waited" and "needed" to other verbs. When they tell us "I eated it all up," we don't usually explain the rules for past tense endings to them, and make them do practice drills with the past tense verbs. We understand that they will, if exposed to the correct forms, gain a good grasp of both regular and irregular past tense verbs. We may not know enough about language acquisition to be excited when a 3-year-old says, "I drink-ed the milk," but we should be. That "error" shows learning. It shows that the child has noticed one way of indicating past time and is applying it. It is a major step forward from the child who says, "I drink it yesterday." Similarly, the second-language learner who writes, "the process which they developed it" has learned to use adjectival clauses but is still using the syntax of the native language, in which the pronoun "which" does not replace the noun. If we can now think of our students' errors as part of the developmental process, we can provide appropriate input and prompting to move the learner along in the acquisition of accurate forms.

That error in using an adjective clause is an example of an "interlanguage" error; one that results from the grammar rules of the native language being used with English vocabulary. These are also called "transfer errors" and are a common source of errors in English learners. If you studied Spanish, you may remember learning the rule that states that most adjectives go after the noun, as in "casa blanca" for "white house." You may also remember that when you tried to produce Spanish sentences, you would often translate from English and put the adjective before the noun. If your teacher gave you a chance to self-correct or modeled the right form back to you ("Es un grande perro." "Oh, un perro grande?" "Si, un perro grande."), you eventually started putting the adjective after the noun *most* of the time. You were moving from putting Spanish words into English syntax to using both Spanish vocabulary and syntax.

Another type of error is the "intralanguage" error. These result from the complexities of English itself. The use of the definite article "the" often produces this kind of error. It's hard for us to explain—and harder for the learner to understand—why it's "The company has high standards" but "*The* standards clearly communicate the expectations to employees." Or "Life is beautiful" but "*The* life of a teacher is a hard one." Or "The headquarters is in China" but "a branch office is in *the* Philippines." We've learned the usage of "the" from years of hearing and reading it in many contexts. There are rules, but most native speakers can't tell you what they are, and most English learners have not been taught the usages with enough chances to practice. Many other aspects of English are similarly complex and defy simple explanation. Even after students have tested at a high level on one of the standardized tests used for college admission, they still need all the stages of the writing process to get feedback, edit their own work, and gain automaticity in the use of the structures of English.

Perhaps the best way to assist English learners in gaining this automaticity is to choose materials that will model the vocabulary and structures needed to complete the writing/speaking tasks. Considerable research shows that reading is the most effective way to acquire language structures and improve writing skills (Krashen, 2004). A study by Hudson (1991) of chemical engineering students found that intensive reading in their subject area was the most effective way to improve their writing skills. From reading, students acquire not only the vocabulary of their fields but a variety of sentence structures, knowledge of how paragraphs are constructed, and models of design and organization. While we typically have students look at samples of the kinds of documents they are writing, they may need more focus on close reading of those samples and analysis of the language used and the strategies employed.

Finally, professional writing teachers may need to be willing to assess the students on their knowledge and application of the concepts of the technical communication class and their improvement in English skills rather than on the surface features of their writing or their ability to produce native-like usage of American English. This is going to require a major shift in thinking for some teachers, who find it easier to mark surface-level errors than to identify more, shall we say, "global" errors?

CONCLUDING THOUGHTS

It can be safely assumed that online teaching and international students will likely increase, and that these two dimensions will intersect with greater frequency as our field adapts to changing workplaces and economies. Here we have opened up and described many of the challenges and questions that teachers will encounter as they enter this arena. These pedagogical challenges arise from the complexities of teaching in online environs, teaching to a technologically savvy and increasingly more international and global student body, understanding the ever-changing language that we teach, and addressing the changing expectations of the field of technical communication. We have refrained from stipulating strong guidelines for teaching technical communication to a global audience, mostly because this issue is still relatively new in our country and in our universities. Much more research will have to be conducted before any strongly occurring themes can be recognized and shaped into prescriptions for effective teaching styles and pedagogical strategies. However, we have offered suggestions for addressing these challenges, suggestions arising out of other fields such as Second Language Teaching, linguistics, content learning, and educational research. As they put into practice some of these pedagogical suggestions, we hope that technical communication teachers face these challenges with interest and vigor.

REFERENCES

Accenture. (2010). *Accenture global research on millennials' use of technology: Jumping the boundaries of corporate IT.* Retrieved March 10, 2010, from http://www.accenture.com/Global/Research_and_Insights/By_Role/HighPerformance_IT/CIORe search/Jumping-Boundaries.htm

Bosley, D. (1993). Cross-cultural collaboration. *Technical Communication Quarterly, 2*(1), 51–62.

Bowen, B., Sapp, D. A., & Sargsyn, N. (2006). Résumé writing in Russia and the newly independent states. *Business Communication Quarterly, 69*(20), 128–143.

Brewer, P. (2010, March 17). *Researching and teaching technical communication in Taiwan.* Presentation at the 13th Annual Conference of the Association of Teachers of Technical Writing, Louisville, KY.

Collier, V. P. (1989). How long? A synthesis of research on academic achievement in second language. *TESOL Quarterly, 23,* 509–531.

Coyle, D. (2002). Relevance of CLIL to the European Commission's language learning objectives. In D. Marsh (Ed.), CLIL/EMILE—The European dimension: Actions, trends and foresight potential. European Commission.

Coyle, D. (2007). Content and language integrated learning: Towards a connected research agenda for CLIL pedagogies. *International Journal of Bilingual Education and Bilingualism, 10*(5), 543–562.

Crabtree, R. D., & Sapp, D. A. (2004). Your culture, my classroom, whose pedagogy?: Negotiating effective teaching and learning in Brazil. *Journal of Studies in International Education, 8*(1), 105–132.

Crystal, D. (1997). *English as a global language.* Cambridge, MA: Cambridge University Press.

Du-Babcock, B., & Varner, I. (2008). Intercultural business communication in action: Analysis of an international videoconference. In D. Starke-Meyerring & M. Wilson (Eds.), *Designing globally networked learning environments: Visionary partnerships, policies, and pedagogies* (pp. 156–169). Rotterdam, The Netherlands: Sense.

Graddol, D. (2000). The future of English. *The British Council.* Retrieved December 28, 2010, from www.officiallanguages.gc.ca/docs/f/Future_of_English.pdf

Herrington, T. (2008). The global classroom project: Multiple relationships in global partnering. In D. Starke-Meyerring & M. Wilson (Eds.), *Designing globally neworked learning environments: Visionary partnerships, policies, and pedagogies* (pp. 37-51). Rotterdam, The Netherlands: Sense.

Herrington, T., & Tretyakov, T. (2005). The global classroom project: Troublemaking and troubleshooting. In K. Cargile Cook & K. Grant-Davie (Eds.), *Online education: Global questions, local answers* (pp. 267–283). Amityville, NY: Baywood.

Hoft, N. (1995). *International technical communication: How to export information about high technology*. New York: John Wiley and Sons.

Hudson, T. (1991). A content comprehension approach to reading English for science and technology. *TESOL Quarterly, 25*(1), 77–104.

Jobsearch.com. (n.d.). *Enhancing your résumé*. Retrieved July 3, 2010, from http://www.careerbuilder.com/JobSeeker/Résumés/RésuméIconify/ResIconDescription.aspx?cblid=scpripr001&lr=cbc_jsdc

Kachru, B. B. (1992). Meaning in deviation. In B. B. Kachru (Ed.), *The other tongue*. Urbana: University of Illinois Press.

Kennon, J. (2008). International collaboration and cross-cultural communication. In D. Starke-Meyerring & M. Wilson (Eds.), *Designing globally networked learning environments: Visionary partnerships, policies, and pedagogies* (pp. 114–128). Rotterdam: The Netherlands: Sense.

Krashen, S. D. (2004). *The power of reading: Insights from research*. Westport, CT: Libraries Unlimited.

Marsh, D. (2003). *CLIL/EMILE—The European dimension: Actions, trends and foresight potential*. Retrieved January 21, 2010, from http://ec.europa.eu/education/languages/pdf/doc491_en.pdf

Maylath, B., Vandepitte, S., & Mouston, B. (2008). Growing grassroots partnerships. In D. Starke-Meyerring & M. Wilson (Eds.), *Designing globally networked learning environments: Visionary partnerships, policies, and pedagogies* (pp. 53–66). Rotterdam, The Netherlands: Sense.

Pew Research Center. (2010). *Millennials, media and information*. Retrieved March 22, 2010, from http://pewresearch.org/pubs/1516/millennials-panel-two-millennials-media-information

Starke-Meyerring, D., & Wilson, M. (Eds.). (2008). *Designing globally networked learning environments: Visionary partnerships, policies, and pedagogies*. Rotterdam, The Netherlands: Sense.

Scientific Committee on Antarctica Research. (n.d.). *Polar Atmospheric Chemistry at the Tropopause (PACT) Action Group*. Retrieved July 10, 2010, from http://www.scar.org/researchgroups/physicalscience/pact

Texas Tech University Historical Fact Book. (2008). Fall to fall one-year comparison, enrollment by ethnicity. Retrieved July 3, 2010, from http://www.irim.ttu.edu/NEWFACTBOOK/Comparison/Fall2007-08EnrollmentComparison.pdf

Thrush, E. A. (1993). Bridging the gaps: Technical communication in an international and multicultural society. *Technical Communication Quarterly, 2*, 271–285.

Thrush, E. A. (2001). Plain English? A study of plain English vocabulary and international audiences. *Technical Communication, 48*(3), 289–296.

http://dx.doi.org/10.2190/OE2C7

CHAPTER 7

Students in the Online Technical Communication Classroom: The Next Decade

Angela Eaton

Knowing about our students—their demographics, likes, dislikes—is useful in any teaching situation. What are online students like? What do they enjoy about online instruction, and what do they dread? How can I reach them when I am advertising my program? Pertinent student information can help us preview pitfalls, advertise our programs, and provide a useful benchmark to compare with our own student populations. In Chapter 2 of *Online Education: Global Questions, Local Answers*, I reported the results of a survey investigating attributes of students in technical communication online distance courses. This chapter is a replication of that study. Replicating any study in which time might change the results is necessary; with online education becoming more common and more accepted nationwide, as students become more comfortable in the process, and as Internet use increases in every age group, our results might change. Add in the explosion in online technical communication programs, which multiplies the geographic range, the number of schools, and the student populations they draw from, not to mention the growth in online technical communication PhD programs, and we have an exigence for updating the data.

The data for the original chapter were collected from March 4 to April 20, 2002; these new data were collected from July 10 to August 24, 2010. For the replication study, data was collected by sending an e-mail survey invitation to chairs or directors of technical communication distance programs identified in an article on applying to graduate school in technical communication (Eaton, 2009);

the e-mail included a request to forward it to their online technical communication students. Many graciously helped by sending on the invitation and a reminder; the forwarding added a level of privacy for students, because their e-mail addresses were not shared outside their department, but it did preclude collecting the possible number of respondents so that response rates could be calculated. Some schools' directors did not respond to the invitation or reminder; some programs did not have an electronic mailing list for distance students only, one program outside the United States required a second human subjects review, and one program had discontinued its distance efforts. Overall, 12 schools are represented in the data from 17 invited (71%).

Of the six schools originally represented in the 2002 data, four reappeared in 2010—Mercer University, Southern Polytechnic State University, Texas Tech University, and Utah State University (Rensselaer Polytechnic Institute and Indiana University Purdue University at Indianapolis no longer have distance programs). The eight new schools included University of Central Florida, East Carolina University, Minnesota State University Mankato, New Jersey Institute of Technology, Old Dominion University, Sheffield Hallam University, SUNY Institute of Technology, and Texas State University. These schools generally offer Master's of Arts or Science. Students pursuing PhD programs came from Texas Tech University, Old Dominion University, and East Carolina University. The sampling frame was made up of graduate programs, so the data is primarily from graduate students.

In addition to the increase in programs participating, there was a 311% increase from the 37 respondents from 2002. In total, 12 respondents in 2010 stopped answering before the fourth question and were dropped from the dataset, and 152 participants completed the survey. Respondents were asked about demographic information, including gender, age, workload, degree pursued, courseload and mode, and workload perception; reasons for pursuing distance education; features they like and dislike in online education; advice they would offer instructors; and research methods they used to locate and investigate their program.

WHAT TYPES OF STUDENTS CAN INSTRUCTORS EXPECT TO TEACH IN ONLINE TECHNICAL COMMUNICATION PROGRAMS?

Respondents were asked about gender, age, workload, degree sought, and courses taken.

Gender: In this sample, 70% of respondents were female, 28% were male, and 2% preferred not to answer. Even though the 2002 and 2010 samples differed greatly in size ($N = 37$ vs. $N = 152$, respectively), the gender ratios in the 2002 data were only 1% different—70% female, 27% male, and 3% preferred not to answer.

Age: The respondents from 2010 were slightly older, on average, and also had more respondents in the older age groups (see Table 1 and Figure 1).

Workload: Knowing the workload of our students is helpful in getting to know our demographic. In the 2010 survey, I asked respondents to report the time they spent each week on paid and, in a separate question, on unpaid work (defined as "childcare, elder care, housework, carpooling, yard work, car maintenance, etc."). Some 92% of respondents in 2010 worked for pay every week, and they did so for an average of 35 hours per week (SD = 15). Respondents performed unpaid duties an average of 20 hours per week (SD = 17).

Table 1. Average Age of Respondents

Respondents	2002 data	2010 data
Total responses	36	149
Mean age	36.0	40.6
SD	8.8	10.6

Note: The total responses were lower than all respondents for the year because some chose to skip the question.

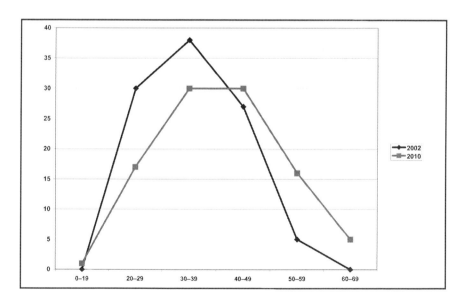

Figure 1. Grouped ages of respondents for 2002 and 2010, in percentages of respondents.

To compare responses across data collections, Table 2 shows the 2010 paid and unpaid hours added together along with the 2002 data. As the table shows, most respondents in the 2002 survey reported working in the range of 31–50 hours per week, whereas the 2010 respondents reported working more hours per week—in the range of 41–60. This greater number may be due to the separate question about unpaid work in 2010, prompting respondents to evaluate their overall workload more accurately, or respondents may have been working more in 2010.

Overall, our distance students continue to have very challenging schedules. There are 168 hours in a week; remove 56 for sleeping 8 hours a night, the 55 average hours respondents work for pay or at home, and we're left with 57 remaining—8 hours a day for commuting, meals, leisure, family time, and

Table 2. Hours Respondents Worked, 2002 and 2010

Hours per week	2010 unpaid	2010 paid	2002 paid and unpaid together	2010 paid and unpaid together[a]
0	3	8	3	0
1-10	41	3	0	3
11-20	28	9	0	3
21-30	5	5	3	5
31-40	13	44	34	7
41-50	3	25	54	26
51-60	1	3	9[b]	25
61-70	1	1	n/a[c]	14
71-80	2	0	n/a[c]	11
81+	0	0	n/a[c]	5
Mean	19.9	35.3	n/a[c]	55.2
Standard Deviation	16.5	15.3	n/a[c]	19.9

Note: Hours respondents worked in percentage of respondents. $N = 37$ for 2002, $N = 152$ for 2010.

[a]Respondents' answers were added by respondent, so the paid and unpaid numbers were not added across columns. (In other words, while 3% of respondents worked 0 hours of unpaid work per week, not one respondent worked 0 hours in both categories, so 0% appears in the column for paid and unpaid together).

[b]In the 2002 survey, the highest number of hours respondents could choose was "More than 51 hours a week, excluding coursework."

[c]The 2002 survey asked respondents to choose a range (ex: 41-50), so mean and standard deviation could not be calculated.

classes. The 16% of respondents who worked 70+ hours per week had only 6 hours a day for all of those tasks. It might seem like a lot of time, but if you remove 3 hours for getting ready, commuting to and from work, and eating dinner, weeknights only have 3 hours for these students to attend class, work on homework, and spend any time with family or friends. One can imagine the pressure a schedule like this might put on students and how that pressure might influence their patience.

Degree sought: Degrees pursued changed dramatically between 2002 and 2010. In 2002, only one student pursued a PhD while jointly pursuing an MA in Natural Science. In 2010, a total of 30% of the respondents pursued a PhD online (see Table 3).

Courseload and mode: Respondents reported how many semesters they had taken distance education. Students were asked if they take traditional classes along with distance courses (see Table 4).

As for the number of courses students took each semester, 68% of respondents took one course per semester, 24% varied between one and two courses, and 9% took two courses each semester in 2002. In 2010, I asked for the total number of semesters and the total number of courses for each respondent and calculated the mean; the average number of courses was 1.46 per semester.

Perception of workload: In the 2002 data, I noticed students mentioning excessive workloads when they gave advice to teachers, and I noticed that they (understandably) resented others thinking their degrees were easier because they were earned via distance. To clarify whether they thought their workloads were too much or too little, in 2010 I asked them their perceptions of the difficulty of the coursework. Of the 151 respondents who answered this question, 37% responded that their distance courses were more work than traditional courses, 38% said they were equal, 5% said they were less work, and 20% couldn't compare or didn't know.

Table 3. Degree Sought by Respondents

Degree pursued	2002 data	2010 data
Non-degree certificate	0	7
BS/BA	5	3
Master of Science	54	28
Master of Arts	38	33
PhD	1	30

Note: Degree pursued by respondents is represented in percentage of respondents. $N = 37$ for 2002, $N = 152$ for 2010.

Table 4. Semesters in Distance Education
and Course Delivery Method

Semesters in DE	2002	2010
1-2 semesters	31	23
3-4 semesters	28	29
5-6 semesters	17	21
7-8 semesters	25	12
9+ semesters	0	15
Delivery Method		
Only online	86	70
Online and traditional occasionally	14	22
Traditional every semester	n/a	9

Note: In percentage of respondents. N = 36 for 2002, N = 150 for 2010.

To summarize this demographic data, online technical communication students are twice as likely to be female and are most likely in their 30s or 40s (60% of respondents were in these age groups). They almost certainly work outside of the home (92% of respondents do), and they do an additional average of 20 hours of work at home. They are twice as likely to pursue a Master's than a PhD. They are a more experienced group; 15% have had nine or more semesters, compared to no one having more than eight semesters in 2002, and that difference is almost certainly due to the longer PhD programs 30% of respondents are participating in. They are twice as likely to be online only than to mix in traditional courses. Approximately one-third perceive their coursework to be harder than traditional courses, one-third think that it is equal, and approximately 20% can't compare.

REASONS FOR CHOOSING DISTANCE EDUCATION

In 2002, reasons students pursued distance education were taken from the literature, and respondents were asked to check all the answers that described their personal reasons for choosing distance education, a simple yes or no answer. In 2010, rather than asking for a simple checkmark, respondents were asked to rate how important each reason was for their personal decision to attend distance courses on a 7-point scale. Table 5 shows the percentages of 2002 respondents who checked yes for each reason. For the 2010 column, the percentage represents

Table 5. Percentage of Respondents Choosing Each Reason

Reasons for choosing distance education	2002 data	2010 data
Distance education courses fit into my schedule better than traditional courses.	95	90
I want to improve my skills.	78	85
I can participate in a program that is not available locally.	82	82
These courses will improve my chances at retaining my job *or gaining a new one.**	19	81
I save commuting time.	64	73
I prefer to work from my home or office.	61	65
I have access to better faculty.	11	39
My classmates are more diverse than in a traditional classroom.	19	31
My employer pays for this program.	33	29

Note: In percentage of respondents. N = 37 for 2002, N = 146-151 (respondents occasionally skipped a question) for 2010 data.
*Indicates slightly altered response for 2010, the addition of "or gaining a new one."

every respondent who ranked the answer above the neutral midpoint of 4 on the 7-point scale. The table is organized from most to least popular reason for 2010. Four reasons were chosen by 80% or more of respondents—"distance education fitting schedules," "improving skills," "participating in a program not available locally," and "improving chances at retaining or gaining a job."

Four responses were rated within 5% between 2002 and 2010—"distance education fitting schedules better," "the employer paying for the program," "participating in a program not available locally," and "preferring to work from home or office." "Improving skills," "saving commuting time," and "having diverse classmates" became slightly more popular, a 7%–12% increase over 2002 respondents' answers.

Two reasons grew substantially in support compared to 2002. "Access to better faculty" grew from only 11% to 50% of respondents, and "the courses improving chances at retaining or gaining a new job" grew from 19% to 81%. The 2010 survey added "or gaining a new one" to the retaining a job option, which is likely responsible for some of the large change for that answer.

However, it is very interesting to note that both "access to better faculty" and "improving chances at gaining or retaining a job" increased more than 200%. The latter can probably be explained by the economy plus the change in the question. The former, however, we can only speculate. As the number of distance programs increases, are students more cognizant of the choices they have in faculty? If they were simply more eager to access a better program, the "participate in a program not available locally" percentage should have increased over the 2002 number, but it was exactly the same. Only further research can tell us definitively.

Table 6 shows the percentage of respondents who chose each rating in 2010, and the right column provides the average rating on a 7-point scale. Those looking for advertising messages for their programs should pay careful attention here to the reasons currently enrolled students found distance education to be the correct choice for them.

The 18 "other" reasons for pursuing distance education in 2010 were revealing. Along with a few unique answers, such as "distance education providing access to better libraries" or "the state providing free distance education to seniors," three themes appeared: "distance education was the only way for respondents to take a specific course" (four responses—two of whom mentioned that they prefer traditional courses), "to participate in a specific program" (two responses), or "to receive any education or to receive education that fits with their current job requirements" (six responses).

Respondents were also asked what was their *primary* reason for choosing distance education (as opposed to rating all possible reasons; see Table 7). The top two reasons, each gaining a third of responses or more, were "participating in a program not available locally" and "distance education fitting into schedules." Five reasons had very similar scores in both data collections—"diverse classmates," "employer paying," "better faculty," "distance courses fitting into schedules," and "working at home or office." "Improving skills" increased 9%, and "saving commuting time" decreased 9%. "Participating in a non-local program" decreased in importance (49% to 37%), and "improving chances at retaining or gaining a job" changed dramatically, from being no one's primary reason in 2002 to being the primary reason for 19% of respondents in 2010 (again, adding "or gaining a new job" to the answer is likely responsible for part of this change).

Respondents were also asked what features they liked about distance education. In 2002, respondents were asked to check every feature that they liked. In 2010, rather than asking for a simple checkmark, respondents were asked to rate how much they liked each feature on a 7-point scale. Table 8 shows the percentages of 2002 respondents who checked yes for each reason; the 2010 column represents the percentage of respondents who ranked the answer above the neutral midpoint of 4 on the 7-point scale.

Four reasons showed hardly any change between 2002 and 2010: "the lack of commute," "the privacy," "the flexible schedule," and "the ability to prepare

Table 6. Reasons for Choosing Distance Education (2010 Data)

Reasons for choosing distance education	Extremely unimportant (1)	2	3	4	5	6	Extremely important (7)	Average rating on 1-7 scale
Distance education courses fit into my schedule better than traditional courses.	2	0	0	8	8	18	64	6.30
I can participate in a program that is not available locally.	4	1	2	11	7	9	66	6.06
I want to improve my skills.	2	0	3	11	10	21	54	6.05
These courses will improve my chances at retaining my job or gaining a new one.	4	3	1	10	11	21	49	5.83
I save commuting time.	3	2	5	17	18	23	32	5.40
I prefer to work from my home or office.	4	7	6	18	18	20	27	5.08
I have access to better faculty.	4	4	2	39	10	28	12	4.81
My classmates are more diverse than in a traditional classroom.	16	9	5	38	14	11	6	3.83
My employer pays for this program.	32	4	2	33	10	7	12	3.52

Note: Center columns provide the percentage of 2010 respondents for each rating; shaded boxes indicate the highest percentage for the answer. The last column, Average Rating, provides the average rating on a scale of 1 to 7 for 2010 respondents (N = 146-151 due to a few skipped questions).

Table 7. Primary Reason for Choosing Distance Education

Reasons for choosing distance education	2002 data	2010 data
I can participate in a program that is not available locally.	49	37
Distance education courses fit into my schedule better than traditional courses.	27	30
It will improve my chances at retaining my job *or gaining a new one.* *	0	19
I want to improve my skills.	3	12
I prefer to work from my home or office.	5	2
I save commuting time.	11	2
I have access to better faculty.	5	1
My employer pays for this program.	0	1
My classmates are more diverse than in a traditional classroom	0	0

Note: Primary reason for choosing distance education is expressed in percentages of respondents. $N = 37$ for 2002, $N = 145$ for 2010 data.
*Indicates slightly altered response for 2010, the addition of "or gaining a new one."

answers" were approximately as popular in each data collection. "The varied student body" decreased in popularity. Two other reasons increased: "the convenience of working from home/office" was selected by 90% of 2010 respondents (compared to 68% in 2002), and "the personal communication with the instructor" doubled in popularity, being selected by 59% of 2010 respondents.

Only seven respondents included comments in the "other" entry. Four comments did not have to do with features of distance education. Two mentioned it allows them to keep working while taking courses, and another noted it suited her/his learning style better.

Respondents were also asked for their rating of different features of distance education (see Table 9) plus their *most liked* feature of distance education (only one selection allowed; see Table 10). Most of the change between datasets occurs in the top three features liked by respondents: "the flexible schedule" was the favorite feature of 27% in 2002, but is favored by 49% in 2010. "The convenience of working from home or work" was more popular in 2002,

Table 8. Liked Features of the Distance Education Classroom

Feature	2002 data	2010 data
Flexible schedule	87	93
Convenience of working from home or work	68	90
Lack of commute	79	79
Personal communication with the instructor	32	59
Ability to prepare answers before answering in discussions/chat rooms/bulletin boards	57	55
Varied student body (having classmates from all over the world)	62	46
Privacy	28	33

Note: Column labeled "2002 data" provides the percentage of respondents from 2002 who liked that feature (multiple answers possible). The 2010 percentages were calculated from any respondent who chose 5-7 on the scale, all the choices above the neutral midpoint. $N = 37$ for 2002 data, $N = 150\text{-}152$ for 2010 data.

from 35% to 26% in 2010. Finally, "the lack of commute" was favored by 19% in 2002 but only 11% in 2010. The five other features changed only 0%–2% between the data collections.

Disliked Features of Distance Education

Respondents were asked their opinion of features often described negatively in the literature (see Tables 11 and 12). The most noticeable attribute of these disliked features is that they aren't rated as strongly as the positive features. Notice the overall lower ratings compared to the liked items; the highest rating is 4.64, slightly above the neutral point, whereas the liked items had four items with higher average scores. No score exceeds 5, which means that as a group, the respondents don't dislike these features (if the group disliked them, the group average would be 5 or higher).

Between 2002 and 2010, all but two of the features stayed within 10 percentage points. Only "not having a classroom to go to" was seen more negatively in 2010. And "others thinking my program isn't rigorous because it is distance"

Table 9. Features Respondents Like in Distance Education (2010 Data)

Feature	Extremely unimportant (1)	2	3	4	5	6	Extremely important (7)	Average rating on 1-7 scale
Flexible schedule	1	2	1	3	9	29	55	6.23
Convenience of working from home or work	1	4	1	6	15	33	42	5.94
Lack of commute	1	5	4	11	20	30	29	5.50
Personal communication with the instructor	2	5	6	28	16	32	11	4.91
Ability to prepare answers before answering in discussions/chat rooms/bulletin boards	3	11	9	23	29	17	9	4.48
Varied student body (having classmates from all over the world)	9	11	5	30	23	18	5	4.17
Privacy	13	19	6	30	14	12	7	3.74

Note: Center columns provide the percentage of 2010 respondents who chose each rating; the shaded boxes contain the highest percentage for that answer. The last column, Average Rating, provides the average rating on a scale of 1 to 7 for 2010 respondents (N = 150-152).

Table 10. Most Liked Feature of Distance Education

Feature	2002 data	2010 data
Flexible schedule	27	49
Convenience of working from home or work	35	26
Lack of commute	19	11
Ability to prepare answers before answering	5	5
Personal communication with the instructor	5	4
Varied student body—having classmates from all over the world	3	3
Privacy	3	1
Other	3	1

Note: In percentage of respondents. $N = 37$ for 2002, $N = 152$ for 2010 data.

moved from being mentioned in the "other" section by two people in 2002 to being noted by 53% of 2010 respondents when it was introduced as an option.

A total of 18 other responses were provided. Seven respondents noted that the importance scale was difficult to apply to disliked features (the scale was used for liked features and liking distance education, and it was kept for disliked features for consistency). The remaining responses were unique; they included "not having enough professor interaction," "feeling isolated after finishing PhD coursework," "technology failing," "infrequent feedback," and "difficulty of forming relationships with faculty members."

In 2010, respondents were also asked about the feature of distance education they dislike the most (see Table 13). The least liked feature was "others thinking the program isn't rigorous because it is distance," followed by "not being able to interact with the instructor face-to-face." Another 12 "other" responses were provided; two both stated that none of the listed features apply. The remaining 10 "other" items had no common themes.

ADVICE FOR INSTRUCTORS

Respondents were asked to give advice to instructors who are designing or who are considering designing distance technical communication courses. Overall,

Table 11. Disliked Features of Distance Education

Feature	2002 data	2010 data
Not being able to interact with my instructor face-to-face	66	61
Not being able to interact with my classmates face-to-face	60	55
Others thinking my program isn't rigorous because it is distance*	5	53
Communicating online taking longer than communicating face-to-face**	n/a	39
Having to learn new software or technology to complete course requirements	19	24
Having to interact with technology during class	16	21
Not having a campus or classroom to go to	4	17
Not having a set class time (if your class is asynchronous)	4	10

Note: Column labeled "2002 data" provides the percentage of respondents from 2002 who disliked that feature (multiple answers possible). Percentages in 2010 column were calculated from any respondent who chose 5-7 on the scale, all the choices above the neutral midpoint. $N = 37$ for 2002 data, $N = 152$ for 2010 data.

*These were "other" answers in the 2002 study, and the reason was included as an option in 2010.

**Indicates a new response option for the 2010 survey.

127 of the 152 respondents provided suggestions (84%). Each suggestion had 0 to 6 suggestions contained within it (respondents had plenty of space to enter their advice), and these answers were coded into 32 categories, which were generated by reviewing the data and creating categories. These categories were split into five main groups: technology, course design and content, communication, personal behaviors of the professor, and unclear answers. Each group had 5–8 possible categories within it, plus an "Other" category.

To determine the stability of the coding scheme, I trained a colleague by providing the scheme and a fresh portion of the data for two rounds of coding. Between rounds, we discussed our assignments, and I tweaked the coding scheme. Then we coded 47 new answers of the 127, or 37%. Technically, some authors say that coding 10% of the data with two coders is enough to determine whether a coding scheme is stable, but we wanted to exceed that minimum

Table 12. Features Respondents Dislike in Distance Education Classrooms (2010 Data)

Feature	Extremely unimportant (1)	2	3	4	5	6	Extremely important (7)	Average rating on 1-7 scale
Not being able to interact with my instructor face-to-face	7	10	11	12	23	23	15	4.64
Others thinking my program isn't rigorous because it is distance	15	7	8	17	20	18	15	4.35
Not being able to interact with my classmates face-to-face	13	9	12	12	28	19	8	4.24
Communicating online taking longer than communicating face-to-face*	18	14	10	20	22	11	5	3.67
Having to learn new software or technology to complete course requirements	34	16	7	18	13	9	3	2.95
Having to interact with technology during class	34	21	5	19	13	7	2	2.83
Not having a set class time (if your class is asynchronous)	34	16	8	33	7	3	1	2.74
Not have a campus or classroom to go to	36	18	9	21	11	2	3	2.72

Note: Center columns provide the percentage of 2010 respondents who chose each rating; the shaded boxes contain the highest percentage for that answer. The last column, Average Rating, provides the average rating on a scale of 1 to 7 for 2010 respondents. For 2010, there were 151-152 respondents.

*Indicates a new response option for the 2010 survey.

Table 13. Most Disliked Feature of Distance Education

Feature	2010 data
Others thinking my program isn't rigorous because it is distance	32
Not being able to interact with my instructor face-to-face	23
Not being able to interact with my classmates face-to-face	15
Communicating online taking longer than communicating face-to-face	12
Other	7
Having to learn new software or technology to complete course requirements	5
Having to interact with technology during class	3
Not having a campus or classroom to go to	2
Not having a set class time (if your class is asynchronous)	1
None of the above	1

Note: Most disliked feature of distance education is expressed in percentages of respondents. $N = 152$ for 2010 data.

substantially because the data corpus is smaller. Finally, we calculated Cohen's kappa and received a 77.6% reliability between coders, which is above the minimum 70% agreement cited by many researchers (for example, see Beach, 1992; Hughes & Hayhoe, 2007). If we were running elaborate statistics on significance, we would have continued with the training to get the agreement number above 80%, but as I am providing descriptive statistics only, 77.6% is quite accurate.

Communication suggestions made up the largest group of answers (27.7%) (see Table 14). What was most interesting about these answers is that every single one could also be given in a face-to-face course. Providing a detailed syllabus is standard educational advice. However, many students mentioned that these issues increased in importance in the distance environment. For example, five students suggested faculty make an extra effort to initiate communication with students; several specifically mentioned that either they personally or the class in general seemed less likely to initiate faculty member contact in the online setting. They also thought their faculty should do more to foster student interaction than they were currently experiencing.

For suggestions about course design and content (27.6% of answers), all but two would apply equally to distance and face-to-face classes, such as accommodating learning styles and providing interesting content. However, naturally only online instructors would be advised to keep their effort, grading, and class times the same as a face-to-face class. The other item that is more important in distance education (but would apply equally to institutions with older adult student populations) is to consider the workload of graduate students outside of the classroom. I was pleased to see that no student actually requested an easy class or a lessening of work, especially since 37% of them mentioned they think their courses are harder than face-to-face courses. Instead, they urged instructors to consider the demands of their assignments in the context of their lives and work, noting that sometimes faculty members didn't realize how much time their assignments took.

Here I can share an aside: this past year I have had all of my graduate students keep track of their time spent on the class and enter it anonymously into an online survey. I pair this time-tracking with a very clear discussion the first week of how much time I expect that they will be spending on my class. I let them know that if the survey shows that as a class they are spending more time than I intend, I will reduce smaller assignments later in the semester. This approach helps me verify if my perception of the time an assignment takes matches students' speeds. It also helps alert students to their effort; they have little grounds for complaint if they see they are entering only 3 or 4 hours a week. Finally, it shows students that I care about course design and their investment and strive to make them match. Do watch for outliers if you try this. Occasionally you will get a student who takes 3 or 4 times as long to do the assignments; if you use an average and don't filter that person out, you'll be cutting the course right and left and shortchanging the other students.

Technology suggestions (24.7%), while you might think would apply more to distance education than face-to-face classes, could also be applied nearly identically. Having a backup plan for when technology doesn't work (four answers) takes on a new exigence in distance education, as does providing tutorials. Other than that, these suggestions could be applied to any of our courses.

I hoped that I would get a clear sense of whether students wanted cutting-edge technology with lots of bells and whistles that are often more likely to malfunction or stripped-down classes that are more often tried and true (I am an "if it isn't broken" instructor who prefers to spend her time on content rather than technology). Unfortunately, the data did not show a clear mandate. Seven responses said to use more technology and means of interaction, while six responses said to lessen them or standardize them across the entire program. Some just wanted newer technology (three responses), but not necessarily more than what they're using now. Other suggestions were surprising to me—three

Table 14. Advice to Distance Education Instructors from Respondents

	Times mentioned	Percent of responses
Communication	**58**	**27.7**
Give detailed/clear instructions or course info or syllabus	17	8.1
Communicate regularly (including promptly)	10	4.8
Foster community among students	10	4.8
Provide feedback	8	3.8
Other communication suggestions (such as e-mail and introduction to class)	7	3.3
Initiate communication connection with students	5	2.4
Ask for student feedback about course	1	0.5
Course Design and Content	**58**	**27.6**
Other course design suggestions (less theory and more practice, include multicultural components, give examples, offer optional FtF seminars, keep classes small, have all materials ready early, etc.)	25	11.9
Consider audience (e.g., survey students about their needs, don't use jargon)	7	3.3
Don't change class time/grading/homework/effort from face-to-face class	5	2.4
Be aware of workload students have in classes and at home/work	5	2.4
Accommodate learning styles	4	1.9
Be interesting/provide interesting content	4	1.9
Provide structure for overall class or parts of class	3	1.4
Group work (anything to do with group work, positive or negative)	3	1.4
Due dates (anything about due dates)	2	1.0

Table 14. (Cont'd.)

	Times mentioned	Percent of responses
Technology	**52**	**24.7**
Use this specific program/don't use this specific program	13	6.2
Other technology comments (including use it effectively)	8	3.8
Use more technology/means of interaction	7	3.3
Use less technology/means of interaction and/or standardize across classes or programs	6	2.9
Make info easy to find (on websites, etc.)	5	2.4
Have a backup plan for when technology doesn't work	4	1.9
Teacher should know technology or make sure technology is working	3	1.4
Use newer technology	3	1.4
Provide tutorials about technology	3	1.4
Personal behaviors	**35**	**16.7**
Be available (for communication, questions)	12	5.7
Other personal behaviors for the teacher (have content expertise, avoid typos in materials)	11	5.2
Get to know/interact with students	5	2.4
Follow syllabus and/or instructions/be consistent	4	1.9
Don't patronize/be condescending/realize students are adults	2	1.0
Be on time	1	0.5
No advice/no clear advice	**7**	**3.3**
Total	**210**	**100**

Note: Advice to prospective distance education teachers expressed in total number of answers plus percentages of responses: 127 respondents provided 210 answers for 2010 data.

students felt that they needed to advise faculty members to know the technology they are using for the course and make sure it is working; one would think an online instructor would have that covered.

Personal behaviors of the instructor (16.7%) had a handful of comments. By far the most popular one was to be available to students (12 responses). Other answers were less popular: get to know/interact with students (5), follow the syllabus/instructions and be consistent (4), and don't patronize or be condescending and realize the students are adults (2).

Table 14 provides the number of answers in each group's category. Here we'll discuss the most popular answers overall. The most popular suggestion, given 17 times, was to provide detailed and clear assignment descriptions, course descriptions, and syllabi. Suggestions about using or not using a specific program (Skype, Blackboard) were next (13 answers), followed by 12 pleas that instructors be available to students for communication and questions. Communicating regularly (10) and fostering community among students (10) were two other popular comments. All other comments had fewer than 10 instances each.

I am of two minds about these answers from students. First, I'm frustrated. Most of their advice, what they feel they should point out as important insights, are very common suggestions that appear in both the regular classroom literature and the distance education literature and have for years. Suggestions for exact requirements and clear goals and creating community (McKeachie & Svinicki, 2006, pp. 16–17), knowing content and interacting with students (Hativa, 2000, pp. 15, 44), giving grades promptly and being accessible (Gross-Davis, 2009, pp. 340, 492), giving feedback (the fifth essential skill in *The Teacher's Craft: The 10 Essential Skills of Effective Teaching*, Chance, 2008, p. ii)—these have been consistently recommended.

I also consulted older distance education texts to see if the students' advice was represented there. Planning ahead (p. 150), interacting with students (p. 153), and having a back-up plan (p. 153) are common recommendations (Simonson, Smaldino, Albright, & Zvacek, 2012). Supporting students (p. 72), providing personal feedback (p. 78), and choosing technology based on objectives have been recommended at least since 1992 (Rowntree, 1992). Even in 1984, choosing media carefully (p. 227) and considering how to foster interaction between faculty and students (p. 224) were discussed, back when the context was personalizing distance cassette courses (Bates, 1984). That students' top tips are tips I feel we ought to know by now is frustrating.

However, there is another way to think about these comments—perhaps, in terms of what the students wish faculty members would do, teaching online isn't all that very much different from teaching face-to-face. That said, this advice should make us think carefully about our current teaching Achilles' heels. We all have one (or more), something we're not terribly good at in teaching, something we're always trying to improve. We can tell from this data that teachers who don't like to or can't communicate frequently with students should not teach online. Period. Instructors who have had students complain in the past about unclear directions or about frequently changing assignments? Skip teaching online or work really, really hard to be clear, consistent, and ahead of schedule. Don't give much feedback and tend to be slow about returning it? Not for you. However, if you look at Table 14 and see a picture of your own best practices, it's likely you will succeed as a distance instructor. Digging up past course evaluations and comparing them to the list might be useful to determine whether past students indicate we are strong in these skills (and double-checking our self-perception is often a fruitful exercise).

LOCATING AND RESEARCHING PROGRAMS

One of the most intriguing questions in distance education is whether a distance program can compete when a local program exists. In 2002, I wanted to know if the respondents knew about local programs. I asked them if traditional courses in technical communication, defined as "courses that take place on a college campus with the instructor and students in the classroom at the same time," were available within commuting distance (see Table 15). The results from 2002 remain relatively stable today: traditional courses are available to approximately 40% of respondents, they are not available to approximately 50%, and approximately 10% don't know if they are available. These stable results indicate that even if a local program exists, a distance program can find students in that geographical area. I found these numbers surprising in both data collections; I anticipated (incorrectly) that students would seek online education only if local face-to-face courses were not available. Neither data collection supports that idea, which is good news for those of us with distance programs.

Respondents were also asked how they first learned of their program's existence (see Table 16). By far, the most frequent method used was electronic marketing, particularly the Web search. Word of mouth, professional organizations, and traditional marketing followed.

Table 15. Availability of Courses

	2002	2010
Traditional courses are available.	43	39
Traditional courses are not available.	46	53
I do not know whether traditional courses are available.	11	8

Note: $N = 37$ for 2002 data; $N = 150$ for 2010 data.

Table 16. How Students First Learned of Their Program's Existence

Method	2002	2010
Electronic marketing	**38**	**52**
Listserv or newsgroup*	8	1
Web search	27	51
Webpage (web search or direct access)	3	0
Word of mouth	**30**	**28**
Employer	5	3
Friend or co-worker	14	10
Professor or advisor	11	11
I am a current student*	0	4
I am a current employee*	0	1
Professional organizations	**22**	**12**
Magazine or journal	3	1
Professional organization	19	9
Conference*	0	2
Traditional marketing	**11**	**8**
Contact with university (phone, catalog, pamphlet in office)	8	0
Newspaper article or advertisement	0	3
Radio*	0	1
Direct mail	3	3
Book or graduate guide*	0	1

Note: How respondents first heard about their programs in 2002 and 2010 is expressed in percentage of respondents. $N = 37$ for 2002 data; $N = 158$ for 2010 data (some respondents gave multiple answers).
*Indicates that answer was coded from "other" in 2010.

In the two data collections, traditional marketing and word of mouth had similar percentages. Professional organizations alerted 22% of respondents to their program in 2002, but only 12% of 2010 respondents learned of their program this way. Electronic marketing, specifically Web searching, became even more popular, representing 52% of respondents finding programs in 2010, up from 38% in 2002.

In 2010, respondents were asked how they researched their program; they could choose multiple answers. One method was used by nearly every respondent (program Web site, 93%), but no other method was used by even half of respondents (see Table 17). I found the responses surprising; considering the effort and expense in gaining a graduate degree, I thought the students would research their programs more thoroughly than simply reading departmental Web pages.

I also analyzed the answers of just the respondents who have a local program to see if their search strategies differed (see the third column in Table 17). Respondents with local programs did differ from all respondents in a few ways. Only two differences seem dramatic—only 12% talk to alumni and 12% talk to current students, compared to 41% of all respondents. I can't think of a compelling reason that explains this difference. It may be due to chance.

RECRUITING AND ADVERTISING
BASED ON THE DATA

The 2002 chapter provided advice about how to recruit students to an online technical communication program. The four marketing messages provided in the 2002 chapter were (a) participate in a unique program not available locally,

Table 17. How Respondents Researched Their Programs (2010 Data)

Method of researching program	Percentage of all respondents	Respondents who have a local program
I looked at the program's website	93	91
I talked to alumni about it	41	12
I talked to current students about it	41	12
I e-mailed a faculty member(s)	35	40
I did a web search on the program (not just their own website)	24	33
I read publications written by the faculty	14	23
I did a web search on faculty members	10	23
I attended an information session	1	2
I called the chair, staff, or faculty	1	2
I spoke to faculty at the other institutions about my program	1	0
I spoke to hiring managers/people in the field	1	0
Other	1	2

Note: $N = 148$ for all respondents, $N = 57$ for respondents who have a local program.

(b) fit your busy schedule, (c) experience the convenience of learning from home or work, and (d) save the commute. These messages are still useful, but they do need to be updated. Based on the 2010 data, marketing messages should be (a) fit your busy schedule, (b) improve your skills, (c) participate in a program not available locally, (d) retain your job or gain a new one, and (e) save the commute. Stressing the flexibility of the program, the convenience, the lack of the commute, and the personal communication from the faculty—echoing the most liked features of distance education—should also be beneficial.

For advertising modes, because the respondents' answers were so similar between 2002 and 2010, that advice still holds: ensure that your program's Web site is excellent, be on the first page of search results, use word of mouth, and recruit through professional organizations. Naturally, the suggestions about improving Web search results are even more important since Web searching nearly doubled as a strategy for discovering programs.

To help prospective applicants research your program, facilitate any of the methods used by more than a third of respondents. Make it easy for prospective students to e-mail or talk to faculty members, current students, and alumni; consider including these contacts on your Web pages because only 41% or less of respondents requested contact information. Make sure the departmental Web pages (the only method used by nearly every respondent) are perfect—they must represent your program at its best.

CONCLUSION

Overall, this data gives us a good snapshot of the online distance education technical communication student, whose attributes and opinions have remained relatively steady over the 8 years between data collections. Respondents are still approximately 70% female and 30% male, working, and busy inside and outside the home. As a group, they have filled out into more age groups, and their ages shifted older—they are now more likely to be in their 30s and 40s than 20s and 30s. They take an average of 1.46 courses per semester, which is slightly more courses per semester than the 2002 respondents took. They have completed more semesters. Some 30% of them mix online and face-to-face classes, some every semester, some occasionally (only 14% mixed modes in 2002).

These students take their work seriously; while 75% perceive their classes to be harder or equal to face-to-face classes, only 5% find them easier (20% cannot compare or don't know). They pursue distance education because it fits their schedule better than traditional courses, it will improve their skills, it allows them to participate in a program that isn't available locally, it will help them retain or gain a job, and it will give them access to nonlocal faculty. Most of these reasons held steady over the past 8 years, but two increased by approximately 200%. Retaining or gaining a job was a reason for 19% of 2002 respondents but 81% in 2010 (note the addition of "or gaining a new job" to the answer in the 2010 survey). Having access to better faculty was important to only 11% of respondents in 2002 but 39% of respondents in 2010.

The features of distance education liked by more than half the respondents are the flexible schedule, the convenience of learning from home or work, the lack of commute, the personal communication with the instructor, and the ability to prepare answers ahead of time. The convenience of working from home or work and personal communication with the instructor grew in popularity, while having a varied student body fell, and all other features stayed relatively constant.

The scores for items respondents disliked weren't as high as the scores for what they liked. Nothing had an average score higher than 4, the neutral point; certainly, some respondents disliked features strongly, but as a group, they did not have a strong reaction. All of the disliked features stayed within 10 points over the 8 years, except for "Others thinking my program isn't rigorous because it is distance." This answer was written in the "other" category by two respondents in 2002, so it was made an official option in 2010; it was chosen by 53% of respondents in 2010.

Although students and their ratings of distance education have stayed relatively steady, competition in online technical communication programs has increased dramatically. The 2010 survey had twice as many schools participating. Three schools were offering PhD classes or degrees entirely online. Four times the number of students responded in 2010 versus 2002. Increasing students and increasing programs make effective advertising and recruiting more important. For students first hearing about their programs, electronic marketing grew in importance, word-of-mouth techniques and traditional marketing held steady, and professional organizations fell. Students researched their programs primarily through the program's Web site (93%); no other method, such as e-mailing faculty or talking to alumni, was used by more than 41% of respondents. Marketing messages based on students' reasons for pursuing distance education should be (a) fits your busy schedule, (b) improves your skills, (c) participate in a program not available locally, (d) retain your job or gain a new one, and (e) save the commute. Using the most liked features of distance education to create selling points will result in stressing the flexibility of the program, the convenience, the lack of the commute, and the personal communication from the faculty.

This data prompts some questions that it can't answer. For example, students' workloads prompt parity questions. How much, if at all, should a course be modified due to the limited time of the students? Where is the line between respectful acknowledgment of adult responsibilities and watering down a class?

The data revealed that students want structured courses with clear instructions, thoughtfully chosen and implemented technology, and prompt feedback and availability from their instructors. These are reasonable expectations. Chapters 1, 2, 3, and 5 can provide useful information on training and supporting new and existing instructors at the departmental and university level. Chapter 4 describes a model for creating a community of practice, which can also provide a network of support.

There are other questions to be answered outside of this book. How do students feel about their online courses, other than their likes and dislikes? Are they passionate about them? Deeply satisfied? Are there any long-term benefits or negatives for being an online student versus an on-campus one, such as tighter or looser professional networks? There is no shortage of future research.

It seems that distance education is becoming more popular. The flexibility and inclusion that we hoped for seems to be coming to fruition as more respondents are incorporating distance with face-to-face classes, earning more types of degrees, and are enrolling from more age groups. The data's steadiness in what attracts students to online education, what features they like, the milder ratings of what they dislike—with only a few options changing in popularity for each topic—could be interpreted that we have a stable educational mode that students will continue to pursue.

REFERENCES

Bates, A. W. (1984). *The role of technology in distance education.* London, England: St. Martin's.

Beach, R. (1992). Experimental and descriptive research methods in composition. In G. Kirsch & P. A. Sullivan (Eds.), *Methods and methodology in composition research.* Carbondale: Southern Illinois University Press.

Chance, P. (2008). *The teacher's craft: The 10 essential skills of effective teaching.* Long Grove, IL: Waveland.

Eaton, A. (2009). Applying to graduate school in technical communication. *Technical Communication, 56*(2), 149–172.

Gross-Davis, B. (2009). *Tools for teaching* (2nd ed.). San Francisco, CA: Jossey-Bass.

Hativa, N. (2000). *Teaching for effective learning in higher education.* Dordrecht, The Netherlands: Kluwer Academic.

Hughes, M. A., & Hayhoe, G. F. (2007). *A research primer for technical communication: Methods, exemplars, and analyses.* London, England: Routledge.

McKeachie, W. J., & Svinicki, M. (2006). *McKeachie's teaching tips: Strategies, research, and theory for college and university teachers* (12th ed.). Boston, MA: Houghton Mifflin.

Rowntree, D. (1992). *Exploring open and distance learning.* London, England: Routledge.

Simonson, M., Smaldino, S., Albright, M., & Zvacek, S. (2012). *Teaching and learning at a distance: Foundations of distance education* (5th ed.). Boston, MA: Pearson.

http://dx.doi.org/10.2190/OE2C8

CHAPTER 8

From Gamers to Grammarians: How Online Gaming is Changing the Nature of Digital Discourse in the Classroom

Virginia Tucker

In 2004, while teaching a technical writing class, I was looking through student peer reviews when I found the word "noob" scribbled on a student's paper by his peer reviewer. Already familiar with the term's meaning in gaming discourse, I was prompted to write a cautionary note to the offending student. I have discovered since then that discourse common to virtual communities has gradually affected online discussions in my hybrid technical writing courses. Over the years, my students have engaged in more passionate arguments in virtual chats than I have yet to witness in an on-site classroom, and student-created discussion threads possess increasingly clever and intriguing titles, while traditional essays written by on-site students are still clumsily titled "Essay 1." I wondered to what extent students' growing participation in virtual communities was affecting online class activities; and more specifically, the term "noob" called into question the relationship between collaborative learning practices and the popularity of online gaming.

When online classroom chats began to out-participate and out-think the in-class discussions, it seemed to me that online gaming discourse was responsible for pioneering a positive change in the way college students engage in knowledge-making discourse. With an increased proficiency in digital communication, students can now be expected to make greater strides in virtual classroom

159

discussions and use the class time more productively than was the case a decade ago. Such competency in virtual collaboration may also hasten students' immersion into the classroom discourse community, thereby improving the outcomes of discussion and collaboration in the classroom. While this could in part be attributed to the growing popularity of social networking, sharing character-limited messages with friends and family does little to engage goal-driven groups the way online gaming does. Certainly, online gaming influences how incoming students communicate and associate with their friends, how they obtain information, and how they view and share media. But what effect has online gaming had on how students engage in knowledge-making activities in a classroom?

Gaming discourse resembles collaborative practices in the writing class, meant to show students how to discover and construct knowledge in social settings, such as the workplace (Howard, 2001, p. 57). To test this theory, I turned to Kirkpatrick's 2001 conversation analysis of his 300-level Research Methods class. Kirkpatrick (2005) found that his students did not take the virtual classroom meetings seriously, wasting much of the class time on non–work-related conversation. Certain that, 8 years later, students are now better suited for online learning environments due to their frequent participation in virtual discourse communities, I attempted to replicate Kirkpatrick's study by analyzing Blackboard virtual classroom chat recordings for three sections of English 131: Technical and Scientific Writing at Old Dominion University. The results of this conversation analysis show notable improvements from those of Kirkpatrick's performed in 2001, indicating a change in the way students engage in social construction practices online. Comparing the exchange of conversation to that of gaming discourse samples, I discovered that similar conversation threads exist across the two communities, which suggests that student writers are affected by grammar and rule-making discourses that take place within their game communities. Grammar and rhetoric are critical to gamers entrenched in game-related argument and theory, and for gamer-students this provides a knowledge community engaged in writing outside of the classroom. Students participating in gaming communities develop proficiency in virtual forms of goal-driven, high-stakes collaboration that aid in the social construction of knowledge, and my findings suggest that they apply these virtual behaviors when they enter online classroom discussions.

VIRTUAL CLASSROOMS IN 2001

Replicating the 2001 case study, I examined students' use of synchronous online classroom environments using Kirkpatrick's (2005) framework. The study, published 4 years later, found that students were reluctant to participate in the academic chat, either by ignoring Kirkpatrick's efforts to stimulate discussion or by simply logging out (p. 151). He determined that the time spent in the virtual classroom could be divided into four categories: (a) 45% was time spent *working* and discussing course content, (b) 27% was time devoted to *self-conscious* activities such as explaining the assignment or how to perform functions in the virtual classroom, (c) 25% was time used to merely greet and acclimate students to the environment, and (d) 3% of the time spent in the chat room was used up on *irrelevant* discussion (Kirkpatrick, 2005, p. 153). Aware that his students found the session "trivial," Kirkpatrick concluded his study by reflecting on the causes of students' desire to engage in nonacademic discourse in the virtual classroom:

> Students talk nonsense with greater confidence than usual. This seems to be a function of the novel environment of the VC, in which the physical proximity and mutual visibility of the classroom situation are overturned. Students may have been familiar with such environments from other, more flippant contexts, and have internalized an association between chat-rooms and a trivializing attitude. (p. 157)

My first experience using virtual synchronous discussions 9 years ago were, like Kirkpatrick's, discouraging. Students complained that they couldn't keep up with the conversations taking place and couldn't type fast enough to share their thoughts before someone else expressed a like idea—a symptom of our dependency on conversational principles like turn-taking and direct responses (Sacks, Schegloff, & Jefferson, 1978). But I became certain that, if in 2001 most virtual environments were little more than chat rooms encumbered by frivolous topics devoted to small talk, then surely by 2011, as we observe the popularity of continuous online game worlds, participants of digital discourse see less novelty and more purpose in their exchanges.

VIRTUAL CLASSROOMS IN 2009

Having regularly used the Virtual Classroom in my writing courses for nearly 10 years, I've noticed the gradual change in the way students interact in that environment. Initially, in 2003, I too experienced the difficulties of maintaining a purposeful discussion, while students were more interested in the novelty of the virtual space. However, within the past 10 years, students have become increasingly capable of sustaining and leading class discussion online, which gradually changes the classroom dynamic. Using Kirkpatrick's (2005) four categories of time spent in the virtual classroom, I categorized the ways in which my Technical & Scientific Writing students utilized time in the virtual classroom on their initial visit.

For my own analysis, I retrieved three previously recorded sessions of the virtual classroom, each with a different class of predominately freshmen using the media for the first time, and many of whom regularly discussed their online gaming habits. These Technical and Scientific Writing courses cater specifically to students majoring in the sciences and engineering. They were also hybrid online courses, so in addition to regular classroom meetings, we met once per week for 6 weeks in Blackboard's virtual classroom. Additionally, students submitted weekly reading responses to the discussion board for 13 weeks.

There were a total of 55 students (24 males and 34 females) across the three courses. All were predominately freshmen majoring in various engineering and scientific fields. In a class discussion centering on the iGeneration's (Jayson, 2009) use of the Internet, students openly discussed their experience with gaming online in multiple user settings in games like World of Warcraft and Sims Online, playing Facebook games asynchronously with friends, or engaging in military combat simulations with clan members in games like Call of Duty. In classes 1 and 2, only one student from each said she never participated in online gaming. In class 3, two female students said they did not game online. Across three classes, I learned that 93% of the students were online gamers. (The definition of gamer varies from gamer to gamer, but it is important to distinguish between casual gamers who play for fun and hardcore gamers who express dedication to the habit. Urbandictionary has 50 definitions for gamer, ranging from "someone who plays games when bored" to "a person who plays video games excessively." Here, I will use the term gamer to refer to casual players.)

To replicate Kirkpatrick's (2005) study, I analyzed each line of recorded text in order to classify it within one of his four categories: Greeting, Work, Self-Conscious, and Irrelevant. Greetings include any "hello" or "goodbye" as well as "how are you?" Work conversation is any comment or question related to the discussion topic of the day or previous lessons. Self-conscious discourse, as Kirkpatrick identified it, consists of questions and statements regarding problems using the technology or virtual classroom specifically. Irrelevant conversation pertains to anything not related to the course or discussion topics, the technology being used, or greeting classmates. Prior to analyzing the conversations, I expected to see a substantial drop in self-conscious discourse, which would be characteristic of students' predilection toward technology. I also presumed I'd see fewer greetings if my theory on the link to gaming discourse proved true, primarily because gamers commonly move from server to server, or room to room, many times during a game and disregard greetings to expedite game play. After categorizing each line of conversation, I counted the totals to calculate percentages for comparison.

Across the three classes, I saw a considerable improvement from Kirkpatrick's (2005) numbers: Class 1 focused on work-related discourse 71% of the time compared to Kirkpatrick's 45%. While Class 1 increased in irrelevant discourse (at 6%), there were marked decreases in time spent greeting (12%) and discussing problems and questions related to the technology and the assignment (11%). I believe the decrease in greeting time could be attributed to students following my lead, where I gave a quick hello and went right into the discussion. Similarly, Class 2 remained slightly more focused, engaging in academic discourse 81% of the time, self-conscious discourse only 12% of the time, and greetings and irrelevant topics only 4% and 3%, respectively. Class 3 also saw improved numbers over Kirkpatrick's 2001 class, but there was a noticeable increase in time spent on irrelevant discourse (18%) due to a comical interruption in the campus library where many students had decided to sit while logged into the chat session. Despite this, academic discourse remained high at 62%, self-conscious discourse increased only slightly at 17%, and greetings remained steady at 5%. Figure 1 summarizes these findings and compares them to Kirkpatrick's 2001 results.

Examining the Conversations

While Kirkpatrick (2005) didn't have much conversation worth sharing by the end of his study, my technical writing students gave me hundreds of lines of text to examine that exposed their interest in the topic, enthusiasm for the venue, and even their desire for proper grammar. For each class, the topic of discussion was the use of technology in writing and in the workplace. I would begin by showing them some virtual poetry and hypermedia, then move on to discuss the changing technology in the workplace while reviewing an article on the topic. All sessions lasted approximately 50 minutes—the typical duration of class time. Each class followed a slightly different path with their discussion: Class 1

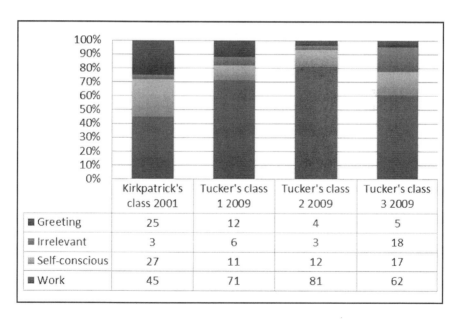

	Kirkpatrick's class 2001	Tucker's class 1 2009	Tucker's class 2 2009	Tucker's class 3 2009
■ Greeting	25	12	4	5
■ Irrelevant	3	6	3	18
■ Self-conscious	27	11	12	17
■ Work	45	71	81	62

Figure 1: Comparison of Kirkpatrick's virtual classroom conversation with my own.

favored a sympathetic discussion on how technology is detrimental to older workers who struggle to stay up-to-date; Class 2 chose to see technology as a benefit in the workplace and in day-to-day communication and writing; Class 3 focused on specific advances in technology, such as Kindle and online journals. As noted earlier, the discussion rarely turned to irrelevant topics, compared to Kirkpatrick's students who preferred not to discuss the assigned readings or remained silent. To contrast my virtual classroom experience with that of G. Kirkpatrick's (2005), I want to share a fragment of Class 2's conversation when the topic turned to how time is spent online:

> Student A: there is nothing wrong with spending a large amount of time on the internet—what matters is whether the time spent was productive

> VT: Good point, [Student A]

> A: and I do not mean only in the business sense of productivity, but was it quality time to add to your mood.

> B: Very true

> A: I don't believe a person can waste time if it is what they desire—the consequences are the only reason desires should change really

> VT: But some social scientists have suggested that we immerse ourselves to the point that we struggle with F2F interaction, is that true? And sometimes the consequences cause people to lose their jobs or loved ones

> A: it is, but imagine a child growing up in a rough area

> C: i agree with you mrs. tucker

> VT: Yet, this kind of tech-savvy person might also be more likely to find certain kinds of work and meets various people from all over the world

> B: Not if someone knows how to balance or manage their time using technology and involving themselves in a social environment

> VT: True, [Student B]. And you make a good point, [Student A], but then that makes me think about the Digital Divide again

> C: i think it can also help us become more open, and with all the different forums, and help sites, people are able to connect over a common hobby

> D: I agree but disagree, because sometimes it can help people be more comfortable when meeting their acquaintance F2F after talking with them for a long period of time over the internet

> B: The majority of college students spend their time using technology yet we are still able to live a fairly healthy social life. So I think it depends solely on the person and whether or not they're willing to break themselves out of the comfort that technology provides.

This discussion confirmed to me that students express their opinions in the virtual classroom with greater enthusiasm than they do in my traditional classroom, where student participation generally hovers around 25% despite my goading. We began the topic of the Digital Divide during the previous classroom meeting, but students showed little interest in sharing ideas at that time. In the virtual classroom, topics were constantly shifting back and forth, and all students present participated. It is evident, too, that the conversation here isn't just about Instant Messaging or some other popular form of writing with technology. The students' argument appears to be about the multiple ways in which we spend time online, from gaming to chatting, wherein the time spent is both social and purposeful. Here these students have engaged in thoughtful discourse using the virtual classroom where they determine the direction of discussion.

While each of the three classes controlled the direction of conversation by choosing what to respond to and what to ignore, it was Class 3 that initiated a language restriction from the onset of the discussion. I assumed that students viewed the virtual classroom as little more than an extension of the actual classroom wherein I was the one who fielded all questions and moderated contributions, so when a student asked, "Do we have to type properly in here, because I really want to text talk," I falsely presumed he was talking to me. I responded that it was not necessary, and the fast-paced environment makes it difficult to vigilantly review one's writing. Simultaneously, another student wrote, "oh no, I hate text talk!" With no one aligning against her, the decision was socially made: there would be no text-talk despite my allowing it. Class 3 then proceeded to correct the bulk of its grammatical and spelling errors, totaling seven corrections, while Classes 1 and 2 had corrected none of their misspellings or sentence errors. With merely one participant saying she did not want to see "text-talk," or Internet-speak, all participants chose to correct their errors. Since there were little more than those seven errors out of several hundred lines of text, I am certain that most errors never even made it to the screen. Perhaps this was a sign that all community members agreed to this stated rule, or perhaps this was, for the students, symbolic of the space as a learning environment in which rules are set and contributions are judged by peers. Either way, it is evident that even in the virtual classroom, socially constructed rules are applied in much the same way that they are in larger online communities.

MEDIATING EXPERIENCES/MEDIATING LEARNING

The ability to use the technology is no longer an issue for students as it once was, and this shift may explain the differences between my students' and Kirkpatrick's virtual class discussions. The problem faced in the past when using virtual environments for classroom instruction was largely one of apathy on the part of students. Even if they were familiar with synchronous and asynchronous virtual spaces, many had yet to experience these as environments in which knowledge could be socially constructed. But as society, particularly the iGeneration, comes to prefer mediated experiences in news, entertainment, and information sharing (Pew Research Center, 2008b), it is quickly becoming an *interface culture* (Stephenson, 1999, p. 47).

It is online gaming wherein we most often witness the social construction of knowledge in a virtual setting. Why gaming and not social media, which has experienced a surge of interest on par with gaming? I believe this is due to gamers having shared goals that are best achieved when all members perform well. In other words, because gamer discourse often meets the standards of "crucial conversations" (Patterson, Grenny, McMillan, & Switzler, 2002) in being high stakes, high emotion, and diversely opinioned, shared goals—in this case the goal of winning the game—create a healthy climate for such discourse. In classrooms and online games, community members progress faster when everyone understands the material/game. Herz (2002) describes this as a kind of interdependence: "Regardless of who wins or loses, they are mutually dependent on the shared spaces where gaming occurs" (p. 184). Social networking sites encourage you to share goals by playing their affiliated games (such as finding a home for someone's newborn cow in Facebook's Farmville), but the main purpose of contributions rarely go beyond socialization. Event announcements, photo sharing, even brief discussions of today's biggest news story do not instigate the kind of learning we look for in a classroom because contributors are not typically invested in their peers' understanding of the content. Social networks can offer more engaging and immersive communication than can a traditional classroom, but they are not immersive learning environments (Rosen, 2010). In fact, social networking sites fail to resemble a true community in which socially interdependent people "participate together in discussion and decision making, and who share certain practices that both define the community and are nurtured by it" (Havelock, 2004, p. 59). To Havelock, learning communities specifically must share a sense of purpose and commitment to the community's values; further, members should share information, support one another, be treated equally, and be able to participate voluntarily. He also notes that participation in these activities fosters respect among members and helps novice members merge into the community. Online games provide that sense of community and greater access to co-learners (of the game or achievement) than do social networking sites.

Further, according to Rosen (2010), the realism of virtual environments provides greater appeal and familiarity for students, and he ranks video games and multi-user virtual environments at the top of his list of technologies that offer realism of simulated environment. It is significant, then, that online games create a collaborative virtual environment using digital representations of people. The creation of a visual and auditory environment in which to socialize and achieve goals allows the virtual environment to construct a sense of place, causing learners to feel more psychologically present (Bailenson, Yee, Bascovich, Beall,

Lundblad, & Jin, 2008a). Bailenson, Yee, Blascovich, and Guadagno (2008b) describe online games as "the best example of social interaction via graphical digital representation" (p. 80). A graphical sense of presence may seem arbitrary, but I would agree with Reid (1995) that "physical context is a dimension of social context" (p. 169), so the effect on student participation is greater in similar synchronous online classroom discussions in which their contributions are immediate and graphical. Similarly, graphical representations provide clearer social cues, which train participants in ways to recognize social constraints in virtual environments where once, as Moran (2001) lamented, there were none. MMOG's, like the MUDs described by Reid (1995), "furnish the void of cyberspace with socially significant indicators," whereas other forms of computer-mediated communication merely provide an interface for written communication (p. 167). The synchronous nature of online gaming mirrors that of a classroom discussion whether face-to-face or online. Students' experience posting to Facebook or Twitter may have more impact on similar asynchronous forms of discussion in which they are asked to make regular posts that may or may not elicit further discussion. It is the particular kind of social construction that takes place in online gaming that I see occurring in my students' online discussions.

According to the PEW Internet & American Life Project (2008a), 78% of 12- to 17-year-olds play online games, and 21% of teens play massively multiplayer online games (MMOGs) that require them to interact online with people they may or may not know outside of the game. In addition, half of all Internet users over the age of 18 play online games. A study of gamer demographics conducted by the NPD Group found that gamers spend 38% of their gaming time playing online (Riley, 2009). Meanwhile, Facebook's Farmville, which allows users to play online with their Facebook friends, sees an average of 32 million players each day (Sheffield, 2010). The most popular MMOG, World of Warcraft, maintains 12 million monthly subscribers internationally (Blizzard Entertainment Europe, 2010), and its competitors see numbers in the millions as well. This information suggests that many incoming students are already well-versed in gaming discourse and likely continue to be online gamers throughout their academic careers. Whether they are defending against the horde in World of Warcraft or fertilizing a friend's crops in Facebook's Farmville, students are immersed in online gaming communities.

Some MMOGs have been maintained on their servers for nearly a decade, suggesting that players can preserve their pseudo-self in the online gaming community throughout their adolescence and young adulthood. These games necessitate active integration into a community in which players must work together toward a common goal and help one another enter into and adapt to the community. Gaming is a learning experience: one must learn how to play the game in order to succeed at it, and the game is best learned from the veteran members. Ian Bogost (2008), in his analysis of gaming rhetoric, describes gaming as a process of exploring and manipulating symbolic systems in order to make meaning (p. 121). We learn the rules as we explore the game, but in MMOGs, rules can be created, enforced, and communicated by one's peers. Consider online player guides and walkthroughs, which are always composed by and for gamers. MMOGs present a unique social context for writing that demands its participants be at least adept rhetoricians and grammarians as they communicate methods for effective cooperative game play that benefits the community as a whole.

As more students are logging into virtual game worlds, they are participating in knowledge making beyond the capabilities of learning-centered games like Oregon Trail. As knowledge in online games is socially constructed, then it is reasonable to agree with Kurt Squire (2006) that "The most intense social learning is found in massively multiplayer games" (p. 23). Squire has called typical gamer practices *leading activities* that "orient learners to academically valued practices and their underlying purposes, both of which are critical for academic success" (p. 23). Essentially, not only does social gaming engage participants in knowledge making, but it prepares them for the challenges of academic discourse. The outcome is one in which, nearly 10 years after Kirkpatrick's (2005) case study, our students are able—if not eager—to meet the expectations of their professor in the virtual classroom.

THE NATURE OF SOCIAL CONSTRUCTION OF KNOWLEDGE IN ONLINE GAMING

As gaming engages participants in knowledge making and rule construction, it does so through social discourse that avoids simplified Internet-speak. Internet-speak, also known as text-talk, *leet* speak, or *1337* speak, is an Internet-based language that replaces letters with numbers, switches the order of letters in commonly misspelled words (*teh* rather than *the*), or spells words phonetically. Sven Birkerts (1994) described Internet-speak as electronic communication's erosion of language by the gradual *dumbing-down* of discourse (p. 129). Birkerts wrote, "There is no question but that the transition from the culture of the book to the culture of electronic communication will radically alter the ways in which we use language on every societal level" (p. 128). Indeed, gaming discourse is altering language, and it is becoming clearer that many gamers, like my class 3, do not condone the dumbing-down of language. The interdependent nature of online gaming invites conversation among community members about how to communicate effectively, indicating that issues of verbal intelligence are important to online communities as they construct the rules or norms that influence immersion into the community.

Both synchronous and asynchronous gaming discourse take on many different topics, including advice-giving and strategy, "LFG" (looking for individuals with whom to accomplish tasks), sales and trade, and, most commonly, bragging and conflict. Figure 2 is an in-game screenshot of the MMORPG Final Fantasy XI, which requires players to team up in order to complete shared goals in this

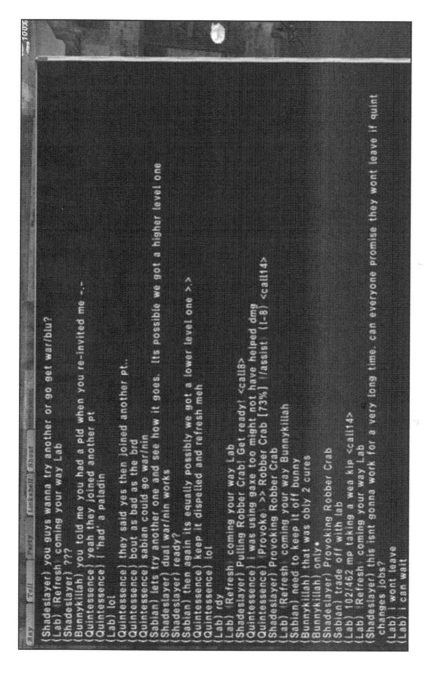

Figure 2. In-game strategy discussion resembles collaborative learning [Bkasura].

rather epic game. The figure illustrates how in-game conversations on topics such as gaming strategy are composed of back-and-forth decision making (as in Shadeslayer's solicitation of opinions from party members), correction of confusing spelling errors (as in Bunnykillah's correction of "only" when trying to provide instruction to his teammate), and language use in a conversational style rather than Internet-speak (although "'bout" and "rdy" are used, there is little Internet-speak beyond shorthand).

While the source of conflict is often game-related, as in this example, the argument often descends (or ascends) into a literal war of words wherein the individual with the most misspellings or misused grammar is consequently considered "in the wrong." This is where the dispute may turn to the boards, where participants can provide a grammar- and spell-checked argument fully supported with screenshots from the in-game conversation. These conversation screenshots are frequently broken down sentence by sentence, annotated, and analyzed by the poster to support his claim. The message boards dedicated to gaming discourse, sites like Allakhazam.com or sites maintained by individuals in the community, are often abuzz with discourse in which participants are posting responses within seconds of the previous post. Users can typically see who is presently viewing the thread, and it is not uncommon for users to remain logged into a forum for several hours outside of or during game play. Because the asynchronous conversation on gaming forums is often as dynamic as the synchronous in-game conversation with hundreds logged in and posting at once, I will be using the examples interchangeably.

The most notable topic of writing discourse that takes place in the gaming community is arguably the misuse of grammar and spelling. In any dispute, an opponent finds that she can immediately debunk the argument of the other by pointing out his flaws in spelling, grammar, or usage. In Figure 3, a game strategy argument has been redirected to a grammar lesson.

Assuming the game itself is the main topic of much gamer discourse, why then is a discussion on grammar of any importance in a virtual world? There was also a very clear indication that proper English was more desirable in my virtual class discussions when students corrected their errors and condemned "text-talk." Essentially, when writing is all one has, then credibility depends upon eloquence and precision of language. Or rather, the ability to be perceived as an eloquent writer is equal to one's success in an argument. Thus, in online discourse, ethos is dependent upon one's writing ability. Enos and Borrowman (2001) described this as the construction of credibility: "Credibility that has not been earned in the traditional senses of education, publication, or experience can be created from nothing—constructed through a few keystrokes in a setting wherein the checking of credentials is difficult at best" (p. 95).

The exploitation of incorrect grammar and spelling to damage credibility can be observed in any message board or chat room where heated debate takes place (however, this may not be considered a "crucial conversation" as it may be high

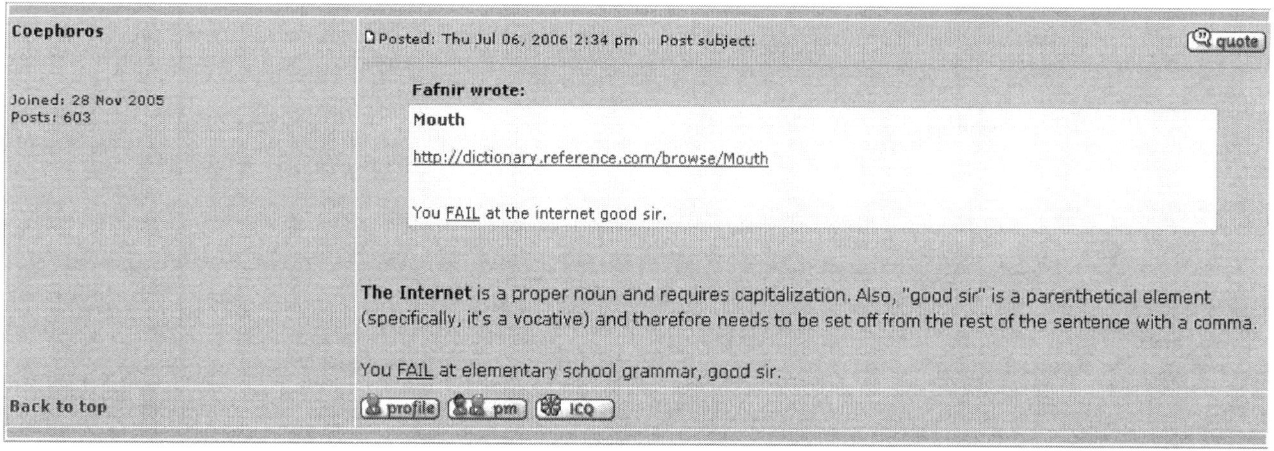

Coephoros

Joined: 28 Nov 2005
Posts: 603

Posted: Thu Jul 06, 2006 2:34 pm   Post subject:

Fafnir wrote:

Mouth

http://dictionary.reference.com/browse/Mouth

You FAIL at the internet good sir.

The Internet is a proper noun and requires capitalization. Also, "good sir" is a parenthetical element (specifically, it's a vocative) and therefore needs to be set off from the rest of the sentence with a comma.

You FAIL at elementary school grammar, good sir.

profile   pm   ICQ

Back to top

Figure 3. A grammar lesson in a gaming forum reroutes a heated debate, discrediting the opponent and ending the discussion [Coephoros].

emotion and diversely opinioned, but is not high stakes, and there are no shared goals). To better exemplify the social construction of knowledge in a virtual community, I want to share a conversation that took place on August 29, 2009, on the computerandvideogames.com forums. This thread begins with a question made by new member Traversman using Internet-speak: "wat game did u look forward 2 and u were den dissapointed wit mine was resi 5 coz i thought it wod b a lot better." With only one true response to his question, the following posters focused their attention on his incomprehensible language, inciting an in-depth conversation on grammar and spelling in forum environments (All spelling and punctuation are the original authors' with the omission of repetitive content):

Poster A: Does an argument against bad grammar demean the recipients ability to spell or the ability of the interrogator's brain.

B: You cant get opinions, or ideas correctly across unless you use english properly. Its also unnecessarily hard to read, regardless of the actual difficulty. Think of it as a courtesy, for our benefit.

A: Yes, all true but text speak is becoming a part of language as it evolves . . . I know what you mean about legible typing being a common courtesy but you can't know everyone's background, for every ten lazy typers you insult you could insult someone who had a hard upbringing and missed out on decent education.

C: Hardly any of us here know anyone else's background, education or even age or nationality. All we've got to go on is what people write and how they write it . . . Aside from the spelling, let's look at the actual content . . . If you want to have any sort of significant discussion, how about expanding on that a little? What wasn't as good as you were expecting? The story? The graphics? The gameplay?

D: Proper English equals common curtosy on a forum.

A: Should I tell any of you off for using acronyms? Where is the line drawn?

E: When letters get turned into numbers. Imagine if the developers of the recent batman game had subtitles like.."2 da b8cave b8man!" (2009)

This conversation shows us how members of the online community control the language used by its participants, similar to the way in which my own student restricted the use of text-talk in our online class discussion. While foul language is typically acceptable to gamers, letters turned into numbers are not. These language rules are not explicitly set forth by forum administrators; the responsibility of language rule making belongs solely to the participants. This explains why my student's protest regarding text-talk superseded my tolerance of it. Those who abide by the socially constructed rules can consider themselves part of that community, and they will acquire knowledge through interaction within the group (Howard, 2001). Those who enter the community anew are required to learn that the nature of gaming discourse goes beyond advice and strategy, and that valuable contributions will necessarily be constructed using proper English grammar and punctuation. Even in the aforementioned forum conversation, poster E was eventually corrected that "B@man" was more appropriate in his example.

When gamers control and restrict language, they set a social standard for the gaming community that will be respected by its peers. What was once feared as the dumbing-down of language, to use Birkets's (1994, p. 129) phrase again, has now returned to adherence of the rules of proper English in an effort to demonstrate respect and trust, but also to gain them as a participant. Individuals who use this form of language, like Traversman in my earlier example, are often symbolically cast out of any serious gaming communities by being ignored entirely (hence only one answer to his question). The post shown in Figure 4 is another example of community-developed rules for writing as a forum member explains when such shorthand is acceptable for this particular group and what role respect plays in the choice to use it. He even recommends posts be spell checked.

In addition to the importance placed on grammar, spelling, and punctuation, speakers in virtual worlds also value the use of supporting material and evidence in argument. This is where the conversation crosses synchronous and asynchronous venues. A discussion that would begin in-game would promptly turn to the forums where evidence can be shared with members. The demand for proof is a common one. For example, a conversation may ensue in-game concerning methods for accomplishing a task that results in a minor disagreement. Using links to resources and screenshots taken of the in-game conversation, a gamer can provide enough proof to "win" the argument. And for gamers, isn't it usually about winning?

APPLYING "GAMESPEAK" TO THE
ONLINE CLASSROOM

But what does all this have to do with college students in a technical writing class? Essentially, student writers in the virtual classroom no longer feel that the chat medium is trivial as Kirkpatrick's (2005) class did. Proximity is not an issue, as students now regularly play online with people they know in real life. Gamers easily maintain the pace of typed conversation, which was at one time students' principal criticism of the virtual classroom. Students sharing discourse digitally may be more willing to proofread their writing to enhance credibility, feeling that they have a real audience in their peers. This would explain why my class discussion board threads are represented by more interesting and thoughtful titles than submitted formal essays; they understand that an audience of their peers must be intrigued into reading the content. But most importantly,

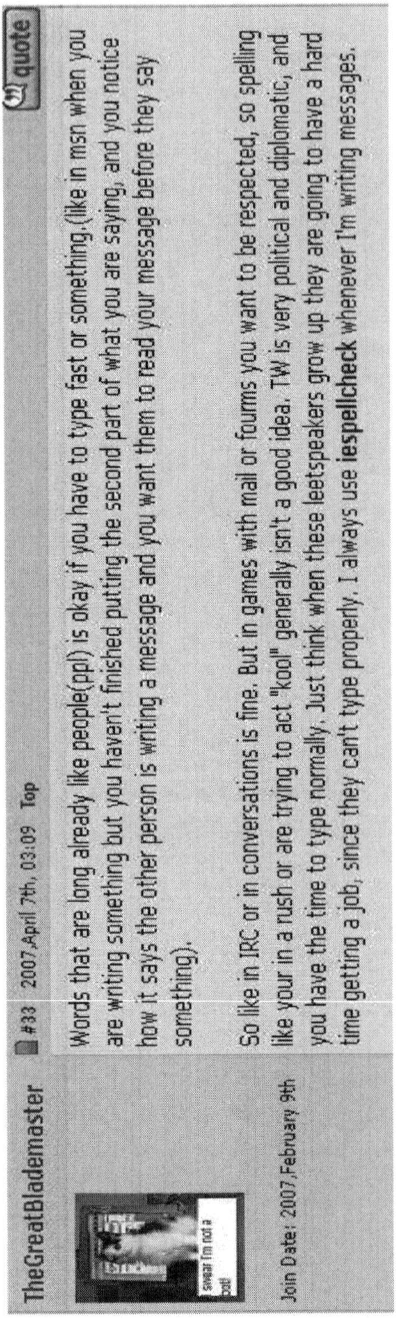

TheGreatBlademaster

Join Date: 2007,February 9th

I swear I'm not a bot

#33 2007,April 7th, 03:09 Top

quote

Words that are long already like people(ppl) is okay if you have to type fast or something,(like in msn when you are writing something but you haven't finished putting the second part of what you are saying, and you notice how it says the other person is writing a message and you want them to read your message before they say something).

So like in IRC or in conversations is fine. But in games with mail or foums you want to be respected, so spelling like your in a rush or are trying to act "kool" generally isn't a good idea. TW is very political and diplomatic, and you have the time to type normally. Just think when these leetspeakers grow up they are going to have a hard time getting a job, since they can't type properly. I always use **iespellcheck** whenever I'm writing messages.

Figure 4. Acceptable use of shorthand is explained by a forum member, not an administrator [TheGreatBlademaster].

they are more confident in their abilities to write, argue, and respond critically to their peers in online conversations than they are in face-to-face discussions because they have already established themselves as members of the online community—a community that clearly values strong writing and rhetorical skills. By bringing our face-to-face students into a handful of virtual classroom sessions, we essentially merge this sense of community with the writing class and show our students that academic discourse communities are not as difficult to enter into as they may have perceived.

Virtual communities that exist in online games, and even Facebook or MySpace, ease students' transition into academic communities in virtual spaces. In the classroom, they are apprehensive about participating in the discourse, but in the virtual classroom they are now accustomed to engaging in heated discussions with a vigilant eye on their use of rhetoric and language. As gamers, they are already members of a discourse community, described by Kenneth Bruffee (1997) as a group wherein members "establish knowledge or justify belief collaboratively by challenging each other's biases and presuppositions, [and] by negotiating collectively toward new paradigms of perception, thought, feeling, and expression" (p. 405). In other words, they are more aware that learning is a social process and are becoming increasingly capable of "joining larger, more experienced communities of knowledgeable peers" (p. 405), such as those existing knowledge communities of the classroom. On the first day of a new class, students certainly do not feel that sense of community with their peers, but they know a knowledge community exists, because I represent it. Several in-class discussions later, they still don't feel part of the community because they interpret all rules and knowledge to be directed by me, as the teacher and leader of the conversations. In my experience, once students are "reintroduced" in the online classroom, their sense of community is heightened and the level and depth of in-class discussions increase thereafter. This could be a result of either their communal bond as a group or their newly realized sense of being part of the academic community as a whole. The nature of a virtual chat allows us all to speak at once: I do not choose who speaks and in what order based on the order of hands raised. Similarly, students cannot observe my facial expressions in order to gauge what their reaction should be to another's contribution. They accept that, in the virtual classroom, they are the ones responsible for determining the direction of the conversation and the rules by which they will all abide. Once they immerse themselves in this academic community the way they would in a gaming or online social community, they realize that the community still exists in the face-to-face venue, and in-class participation increases as a result. In my general education English courses, I have found that voluntary participation in a class of 19 jumps from an average of 5 to roughly 16 (more closely resembling the number of online participants) after just two sessions in the virtual classroom. This is consistent even when students are introduced to the virtual classroom late in the semester. Their sense of community within the classroom is strengthened only after participating in a shared virtual community in much the same way they do every time they play online games.

SILVER LINING OF THE GAMING COMMUNITY'S IMPACT ON THE CLASSROOM

Though many of us may be somewhat fearful of the ways in which Internet-speak has affected our classrooms and have subsequently steered away from employing much technology in our lessons, we are beginning to see a shift in the way students use the virtual classroom that may suggest gaming is not having the negative effect on language we once believed. It is apparent that our students, as avid gamers and users of social networking sites, are participating in complex virtual societies in which language affects not just their message but their credibility in this digital world. The more seriously a gamer takes his gaming, the more seriously he takes his discourse on gaming. If one is to see him as a good, knowledgeable player in the game, then he must exhibit himself as a knowledgeable human being when engaging in discourse. This is similarly true for our students and their projection of a knowledgeable self in the virtual classroom. Further, such discourse should reflect respect for his fellow players by utilizing correct grammar and punctuation (to his best effort). Gamers, like our students, no longer place value on the type of Internet-speak that was once taking over online discourse.

The growing popularity of multiplayer online gaming suggests that future generations of students will be increasingly capable of participating in a community of thinkers that utilizes the virtual spaces for knowledge-making activities. This is essential to our Technical Writing classes as social construc- tionism pedagogy "offers students practice in common forms of work-place writing" (Howard, 2001, p. 57) in which collaborative research and project development is common (and on the Web). In our future use of the virtual classroom, it remains important to open a dialogue with students about how they use the virtual classroom, perhaps in the form of a discussion thread posted after a class session. The topic of discussion for a virtual classroom session should be chosen carefully, favoring issues in which students can freely express opinions rather than having to analyze a reading. This allows students to focus more on the chat log and shared ideas than on outside sources in other windows. It is also useful to bring students into the virtual classroom early in the course and on more than one occasion in order to use it as a learning and discussion tool rather than a novelty. Lastly, if students set their own rules for online discourse (regarding grammar, spelling, and use of proper English), then we may be surprised to find that they will tend to set the bar very high. In allowing them to do so, we enable them to socially construct the rules of their own discourse as they would in a gaming environment and strengthen their bond as a knowledge-making community.

REFERENCES

Bailenson, J. N., Yee, N., Blascovich, J., Beall, A. C., Lundblad, N., & Jin, M. (2008a). The use of immersive virtual reality in the learning sciences: Digital transformations of teachers, students, and social context. *The Journal of the Learning Sciences, 17,* 102–141.

Bailenson, J. N., Yee, N., Blascovich, J., & Guadagno, R. E. (2008b). Transformed social interaction in mediated interpersonal communication. In E. Konijn, S. Utz, M. Tanis, & S. Barnes (Eds.), *Mediated interpersonal communication* (pp. 77–99). New York: Routledge/Taylor & Francis.

Birkerts, S. (1994). *The Gutenberg elegies.* New York: Fawcett Columbine.

Bkasura. (2007, June 13). *Player warning: Noobs.* Message posted to http://killingifrit.com/forums/forum/31-asura/

Blizzard Entertainment Europe. (2010, October 7). *World of Warcraft subscriber base reaches 12 million worldwide.* Retrieved from http://eu.blizzard.com/en-gb/company/%20press/pressreleases.html?id=2443926

Bogost, I. (2008). The rhetoric of video games. In K. Salen (Ed.), *The ecology of games: Connecting youth, games, and learning* (pp. 117–140). Cambridge, MA: MIT Press.

Bruffee, K. A. (1997). Collaborative learning and the "conversation of mankind." In V. Villanueva, Jr. (Ed.), *Cross-talk in comp theory* (pp. 393–414). Urbana, IL: NCTE.

Coephoros. (2006, July 6). *Mouth* [LS members only]. Message posted to http://nantekottals.net

Enos, T., & Borrowman, S. (2001). Authority and credibility: Classical rhetoric, the Internet, and the teaching of techno-ethos. In L. Gray-Rosendale & S. Gruber (Eds.), *Alternative rhetorics: Challenges to the rhetorical tradition* (pp. 93–110). New York: SUNY Press.

Havelock, B. (2004). Online community and professional learning in education: Research-based keys to sustainability. *Association for the Advancement of Computing in Education, 12*(1), 56–84.

Herz, J. C. (2002). Gaming the system: What higher education can learn from multiplayer online worlds. The Internet and the University: 2001 Forum. *EDUCAUSE,* 169–191.

Howard, R. M. (2001). Collaborative pedagogy. In G. Tate, A. Rupiper, & K. Schick (Eds.), *A guide to composition pedagogies* (pp. 54–70). New York: Oxford University Press.

Jayson, S. (2009, January 29). From business to fun: What different generations do online. *USA Today.* Retrieved from http://www.usatoday.com/tech/webguide/internetlife/2009-01-28-online-generations_N.htm

Kirkpatrick, G. (2005). Online "chat" facilities as pedagogic tools. *Active Learning in Higher Education, 6*(2), 145–159.

Moran, C. (2001). Technology and the teaching of writing. In G. Tate, A. Rupiper, & K. Schick (Eds.), *A guide to composition pedagogies* (pp. 203–223). New York: Oxford University Press.

Patterson, K., Grenny, J., McMillan, R., & Switzler, A. (2002). *Crucial conversations: Tools for talking when stakes are high.* New York: McGraw-Hill.

Pew Research Center. (2008a, September 16). Pew Internet project data memo. *Pew Internet & American Life Project.* Retrieved from http://www.pewinternet.org/

Pew Research Center. (2008b, December 23). Internet overtakes newspapers as news outlet. *The Pew Research Center for the People and the Press.* Retrieved from http://www.pewinternet.org/

Reid, E. (1995). Virtual worlds: Culture and imagination. In S. G. Jones (Ed.), *Cybersociety: Computer-mediated communication and community* (pp. 164–183). Thousand Oaks, CA: Sage.

Riley, D. M. (2009, June 29). Video gaming attracts larger female audience in 2009. *The NPD Group.* Retrieved from http://www.npd.com/press/releases/ press_090629b.html

Rosen, L. (2010). *Rewired.* New York: Palgrave Macmillan.

Sacks, H., Schegloff, E. A., & Jefferson, G. (1978). A simplest systematics for the organization of turn taking for conversation. In J. Schenkein (Ed.), *Studies in the organization of conversational interaction* (pp. 7–55). New York: Academic.

Sheffield, B. (2010, March 9). GDC: Farmville reaches 32 million daily users. *Gamasutra.* Retrieved from http://www.gamasutra.com/php-bin/news_index.php?story=27593

Squire, K. (2006). From content to context: Videogames as designed experience. *Educational Researcher, 35*(8), 19–29.

Stephenson, N. (1999). *In the beginning . . . was the command line.* New York: Avon.

TheGreatBlademaster. (2007, April 7). *Grammar, spelling, etc.* [World 5]. Retrieved from http://forum.tribalwars.net/

Traversman. (2009, Aug. 23). *wat game did u look forward 2 and u were den disappointed* [General gaming]. Retrieved from http://forums.computerandvideogames.com/viewtopic.php?t=97377&highlight=wat+game++forward

http://dx.doi.org/10.2190/OE2C9

CHAPTER 9

Cybergogy, Second Life, and Online Technical Communication Instruction

Lesley Scopes and Bryan Carter

Over the past few years, virtual environments have captured the pedagogical and creative imagination of educators around the world as their access and availability have increased. These environments present an opportunity to engage students differently, but they also provide a platform on which new theories of teaching and learning may be explored. Cybergogy is the study of how environments like these are being used for teaching and learning. The following case study illustrates how to engage learners through cognitive, social, and emotional factors within virtual environments, such as Second Life®, while focusing on technical communication.

VIDEO GAMES, SERIOUS GAMES, VIRTUAL WORLDS

Video games are often regarded as violent in nature and are perceived to encourage aggressive, antisocial, and addictive behavior or desensitized responses to scenes of violence, as reported in *New Scientist* (Motluk, 2005). Consequently, many teachers and parents frown on the use of video games in the classroom because they believe that games are fundamentally opposed to serious endeavors—that they are superfluous, frivolous, and lacking morality. Notions such as these are not without substance, and there is a shortage of research to counter them. However, video games that possess an educational quality, also termed "serious games," are becoming part of the future landscape for education.

Wexler, Aldrich, Johannigman, Oehlert, Quinn, and van Barnveld (2007) define serious games as "an optimized blend of simulation, game element and pedagogy that leads to the student being motivated by and immersed into the purpose and goals of a learning interaction." Hackerthorn (2007) describes a serious game as "a game which has enduring value beyond that of entertainment," going on to explain that, for a game to possess enduring value, it should demonstrate a direct relevance to the real world as opposed to being based in pure fantasy, preferably with an explicit connection to a real world system. Although there are a number of effective interactive educational titles, they are rarely used for an extended period of time, and often they are "static" titles that, when played once, tend to lose their luster.

Virtual worlds provide an alternative to games. Unlike most games, virtual worlds cannot be paused or restarted; they persist, which means they continue to exist and function dynamically whether the user is there or not (Bell, 2008). Although the various categories of virtual world and online games are not clearly distinguished, we want to differentiate game-centric virtual worlds, which include Massive Multi-player Online Role Playing Games (MMORPGs) such as *World of Warcraft*, from social-centric, 3D immersive (3Di) virtual worlds such as Second Life. Game-centric virtual worlds are narrative driven, orchestrated by the game designers. Similar to video games, they are constrained by rules and game mechanics, they are competitive, and they are driven by the goal of winning. MMORPGs are becoming ever more popular among adolescents and adults due to their social context, while at the same time they offer an array of complex activities and objectives that players must accomplish in order to "succeed" in the game. Several recent studies have examined the teaching and learning potential of this particular genre of video game most specifically to teach science and physics (Recent University of Central Florida NSF grant award number 0537078). These efforts are important in that they suggest that sound pedagogical methodology can be incorporated into these games and that more researchers are exploring their potential.

With an increase in high-quality graphic computing and faster networking capability now becoming more commonplace in homes, the "pre-scripted," often rendered versions of the most popular games (note the advanced graphics in games such as *Medal of Honor*, *Grand Theft Auto*, and *Madden Football*) have given rise to an even more interactive, completely unpredictable environment called a micro-world. The term "micro-world" was coined by Lloyd P. Rieber and is defined as "a small but complete subset of reality in which one can go to learn about a specific domain through personal discovery and exploration" (Rieber, 1992). Micro-worlds allow users to interact with others and build objects within the environment, thus adding to the interactive nature of the world. Through the creation of a number of environments where Rieber's son could determine his own direction and make decisions regarding his learning that changed based on the decisions he made, Rieber suggests that visually based virtual environments are an extension of constructivist learning theories (Rieber, 1992). Ludlow and Wallace (2007) observe that

> People come to virtual worlds because in them they find more than games; among other things, they find other interesting people. They come to compete with each other, to collaborate with each other, to learn from each other, to profit from each other, and to talk to each other at the coffee machine at work or in chat rooms on the Internet. Players come to interact with other players, and in that way, these games are a very special form of interactive entertainment, in that they derive their value *mainly* from the fact that there are other players there. Without other players, MMOs would be—well, they would be empty.

Between social networking sites like Facebook and collaborative video games like Halo, Second Life is an ideal platform combining elements of both. The attraction to the social, non-competitive aspects of MMORPGs suggests why a social-centric, 3Di virtual world like Second Life appeals to users, and Second Life's similarities to serious games suggest that it might offer an almost unlimited number of teaching moments and learning possibilities for technical writing classes. Second Life is a Collaborative 3D virtual environment designed by and supplied from streaming servers owned by Linden Lab™. It is an immersive environment consisting of over 5 million residents from almost every walk of life, from around the world, including a small but growing cadre of educators who recognize how a 3Di environment can affect the educational experience in a positive way. Most educators have never experienced an interactive 3D environment where real learning can take place and where striving for authenticity is an ongoing battle in which credibility and validity are the major stakes.

In contrast to MMORPGs and "micro-world" video games, Second Life is not constrained by a game designer's master narrative or by goal-oriented game rules; rather and it is open-ended, without the conclusions typically found in competitive games. It actively supports human-human communication in addition to human-machine communication and uses a virtual or "synthetic" world as the user interface. As a milieu for social construction of knowledge, Second Life is ideally suited to facilitate Wenger's (2006) notion of "Communities of Practice," which describes groups of people with a common interest, a shared history, a shared sense of identity, and a similar knowledge set that has been derived over time. Lombardi and McCahill (2004) explain that, "In pursuing their interest in their domain, group members engage in joint activities and discussions, help each other, and share information. They build relationships that enable them to learn from each other." Our experiences in Second Life suggest that social interaction between participants is almost inevitable. Faculty at Drury University, MO report that learners seem to break out of their normal roles and dismiss the social norms and protocols that we are used to in a traditional classroom.

Students who would not normally communicate in class are now dominating the virtual classroom (Scopes, 2011a, p. 21). The environment supports multiple communication channels across a broad spectrum, including asynchronous text messaging, synchronous, and asynchronous Instant Messaging, synchronous public-typed chat, distributable text-based note cards, and real-time voice conversation using Voice over Internet Protocol (VoIP), in which it is possible to address an individual user in a private call or a group of almost unlimited size within the local vicinity. Users can communicate with virtual 3D objects that have been scripted in Linden Scripting Language (LSL) to perform certain functions on touch, such as, most simplistically, to dispense a note card or open a door, or, more sophisticatedly, to react to and acknowledge the presence of the user's avatar. Similarly, Second Life objects can communicate by linking to web sources such as YouTube® to enable external data to enter the virtual world. At one point, Linden Lab implemented a trial of SLim (Second Life Instant Message), which extended the range of communication opportunities by allowing users logged into Second Life (in-world) to receive and respond to instant messages from users not simultaneously logged on in-world. In effect, during the beta testing of SLim, communication channels that were once contained entirely in-world could extend between both worlds synchronously. In short, Second Life combines the educational value and the real world relevance of serious games with the persistent, unconstrained environment of a social-centric virtual world.

Virtual Worlds and the Online Classroom

Online educators face a common and often perplexing question: how to engage their students. Jones (1998) has suggested that learners are not intrinsically motivated unless the learning environment offers motivational features. He further stipulates that learners need to have a reason for entering the computer-based environment but then also need to find it stimulating enough to engage in the environment. In order for knowledge and skills to come together in interactive learning, students need practice and experience (Jones, 1998). Students also need opportunities to feel safe to learn in an environment that provides them with experiences that allow them to apply existing knowledge and succeed in successive steps. Games and simulations can provide such a "world" for students (Gredler, 2001). Simulations have been used to enhance adult learning in corporate and military settings for over a half-century, but the use of games in traditional educational settings has only recently received attention (Thompson & Rodriguez, 2004). Recognizing the motivational and instructional power of games and simulations moves educators into a new realm for delivery of learning outcomes (Jenkins, 2005). Jenkins recently proposed several aspects of games that make them a viable approach to promote student academic learning. He suggests that serious games offer the following advantages to their players:

- Lower the threat of failure
- Foster engagement through immersion
- Manage levels of attainment to prevent users from feeling overwhelmed
- Link learning to goals and roles
- Create a social context with shared interests
- Present multi-modal learning environments
- Support a framework of inquiry (pp. 49–50)

The use of games and simulations capitalizes on the motivational factors necessary to engage the learner. Embedding learning activities into games and simulations in an online environment will offer students socially acceptable and personally gratifying opportunities to learn (Thompson & Rodriguez, 2004).

Well-designed social learning environments also foster increased opportunities for collaborative activities. Socialization between humans uses many cues to provide the intended message. With the latest developments in 3Di virtual worlds, which are now available to anyone with a relatively recent computer and high-speed connection to the Internet, technology is now able to provide much more immersive experiences, incorporating rich visual elements and multimedia artifacts that present a full-featured social learning environment. When enhancements to virtual worlds are made that mimic real life, users become more enmeshed or immersed with the content and less focused on user interface issues that sometimes plague advanced virtual environments. In traditional classroom settings, there tend to be fewer opportunities to collaborate with students from other classes, other schools, or other countries. Aggravating circumstances include lack of Internet connectivity, fewer computers in the classroom, or a curriculum that does not include such interaction. However, when these factors are in place, the chances of students meeting and collaborating from within these virtual spaces increases dramatically, encouraging students not only to learn and communicate with those from other physical locations but also to define their own path regarding how they wish to engage one another in the process.

CYBERGOGY OF LEARNING ARCHETYPES AND LEARNING DOMAINS

Underpinning the use of virtual worlds as pedagogical platforms is a theory, the Cybergogy of Learning Archetypes and Learning Domains (Kapp & O'Driscoll, 2010; Scopes, 2009, 2011a). Based on social constructivist learning theory, this theory posits that knowledge is constructed when individuals in a group engage socially in solving shared problems and where there is an opportunity for more skilled members to contribute their knowledge to the group. The model of cybergogy is composed of two interacting components, Learning Archetypes and Learning Domains. Learning Domains are strands drawn from established real-world paradigms, adapted to become felicitous to the nature of a virtual world and blended into a Taxonomy of Learning Domains that forms the essence of the scientific validity of this model (see Figure 1). The model addresses Cognitive, Emotional, Dextrous, and Social Learning Domains, with the intention of drawing forth all of a person's sensibilities through their avatar into the virtual environment, all which should be engaged using combinations of Learning Archetypes as a vehicle toward attaining a condition of immersion.

Learning domains pivot upon desired learning outcomes, and learning archetypes can be crafted to elicit responses from the learning domains at the required level of implementation as indicated by the blended taxonomy in Figure 1 and explained in more detail in Scopes (2011a, p. 11). As a pedagogic rationale, learning archetypes are building blocks described as "instructional strategies, methods or archetypes for facilitating learning" (Kapp & O'Driscoll, 2007). Learning Archetypes can be categorized into five different activity types (Kapp & O'Driscoll, 2010; Scopes, 2009):

1. **Roleplay**: *To assume a role in an alternative form (living or inanimate) with the objective of undertaking aspects of action, interaction or portrayal*

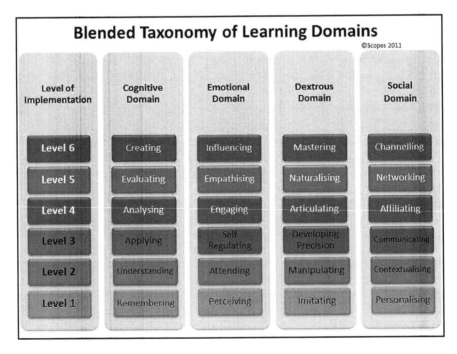

Figure 1. The Blended Taxonomy of Learning Domains (Scopes, 2011b).

of emotions. Roleplay can be freeform, structured, semistructured, drama-tized, or conducted by an individual or collaboratively with multiple role players.

2. **Peregrination**: *Traveling to locations or the very action of journeying to a destination provides the circumstances under which learning can take place.* Activities can include a Treasure Hunt or a Guided or Independent Tour, and the context can vary from factual and historical to futuristic and phantasmagorical.

3. **Simulation**: *The implementation of an environment designed to represent real or virtual conditions for the purposes of imitation, enactment, explor-ation, rehearsal, and evaluation.* A virtual simulation activity can support the rehearsal of a physical world task and is useful for familiarization, prototyping, and testing.

4. **Meshed**: *The creation of opportunities not simply to network but to com-bine and interconnect individuals and groups in various ways for desired purposes and outcomes.* Activities such as co-creation, group forums, small group work, and social networking can be conducted synchronously, asyn-chronously, and in mixed reality event blending real life and Second Life activities as part of the learning experience. For example, a real-time, live presentation can be video streamed in-world to an audience of Second Life avatars. The audience is often able to relay questions and comments to the speaker regardless of the geographical locations of all involved.

5. **Assessment**: *Execution of appropriate methods of assessment, evaluation, and feedback as part of the learning process.* Formative and summative assessment of learning can be conducted in Second Life with the use of available assessment and survey tools or by engineering any of the arche-types to serve as an evaluation mechanism.

Learning Archetypes can be crafted in terms of type of content, degree of sophistication, or level of complexity to generate the desired learning experiences at the required level of implementation dependent upon intended outcomes. Several different Learning Archetypes can be orchestrated into a series of activ-ities, producing a rich cybergogy composed of varied learning experiences that form the content of a single lesson or the structure of an entire course curriculum. Some Learning Archetypes can be designed to be conducted synchronously with a group of learners or in other cases asynchronously to allow individual learners to revisit the learning opportunity for self-paced acquisition of information within the 3Di environment. It is possible to identify a broad set of options in which Learning Archetypes can be administered. These include, at the most elementary, a classroom scenario. A virtual classroom can be used to deliver content in a traditional pedagogic style, but it has no essential advantage over any other more stimulating setting that can be created for the same purpose along a spectrum from the mundane to the sublime, other than that a replication of a classroom may serve to maintain a "reassuring" element of the familiar in a somewhat unfamiliar new world. Our chapter focuses on more innovative environments than the virtual equivalent of the traditional classroom.

As pedagogical strategies, Learning Archetypes form an ideal tool for eliciting desired student learning experiences and outcomes. For example, the Roleplay Archetype can be free-form, allowing the actors to spontaneously co-create a scenario; designed according to a scripted narrative leading to a predetermined outcome; or engineered to involve students in an immersive re-enactment of a real event. The Peregrination Archetype (travel to locations) can serve as an aid to orienting users to a localized environment and encourage them to dig below the surface of the initial visual impact presented. Within the Peregrination Archetype, a Treasure Hunt activity can enable learners to explore an area in detail with the quest of searching for specific objects, perhaps with an objective of taking a snapshot of the object as evidence of a successful find. Treasure Hunts can be timed or rewarded to add a competitive edge or to enhance the sense of play-fulness or employed as a collaborative team-building exercise. Also within the Peregrination Archetype are Guided Tours and Independent Discovery activities for exploration of areas of pertinent or general interest. These activities serve to broaden awareness of the work and interests (and sometimes passions) of other Second Life contributors who are often available to speak with authority on the subject matter in hand. Learners can visit places not possible in the real world, travel forward or backward in time to get a "feel" for some event, item, or environment it would not be possible to experience otherwise.

In practice, within the Meshed Archetype, a Co-Creation activity requires two or more learners to actively work together to produce an artifact of worth or meaning. In this context, learners might produce in collaboration with one another a dramatic stage set to sustain the role-play activity or to compose a scripted, informed narrative for the role-play re-enactment. A social networking activity (also falling within the Meshed Archetype and engaging the Social Learning Domain) is an important activity to incorporate into any learning event, especially within a Social Constructivist paradigm. Within this networking activity, students can access appropriate Web-based mediation tools (such as wikis and social net-working sites) within Second Life to interact with one another. Using voice-over Internet protocol (VoIP), instant messaging (IM), and other communication appli-cations, it is possible to trigger an exchange of information and ideas by asking expansive, general questions. Instructors can use the Assessment Archetype by means of assignments perhaps in conjunction with an institutional learning man-agement system. Assessment methods employed should be capable of reflecting the impact made within the Learning Domains inasmuch as evaluating what a learner learned (cognitive), experienced and felt (emotional), manipulated and interfaced with (dexterous), and fostered (social). The Assessment Archetype will contain Assessment methods, which, despite being dreaded by most, are useful for progress-checking by the instructor. They allow constructive, learner-focused guidance and stimulate the opportunity for the learner to monitor, manage, and self-direct their own learning in line with the "Re-Engineering Assessment Practices" (REAP). The REAP model emphasizes students' responsibility for their own learning by helping to raise awareness of gaps in their knowledge. The key to successful implementation of any of these archetypes is to enmesh them directly into a curriculum designed specifically for a virtual environment. Virtual Harlem is a good example of such a design.

The Virtual Harlem Project was created in 1998 at the University of Missouri-Columbia, first using very high-end computers and later ported to the virtual world of Second Life. The project is comprised of two simulated virtual spaces (commonly referred to as "sims"). They represent Harlem, NY as it existed during the Jazz Age and Harlem Renaissance, circa 1920s and part of the 18th Arrondisement, Montmartre, in Paris, where jazz was introduced during the same period after World War I (see Figure 2). The project is rather different from other educational settings in Second Life. For one thing, it is used to teach/experience the literature and history of the period, and for another it is connected very strongly to the Second Life community but not necessarily to any educational entity. Role-play occurs quite frequently when "period-oriented" events occur, such as Jazz Night at Bricktop's (see Figure 3) in Virtual Montmartre or Josephine Baker offering a tour of her mansion in the same area. A role-play experience is also being designed by students over a period of several semesters that encourages participants to become a part of the community through their role

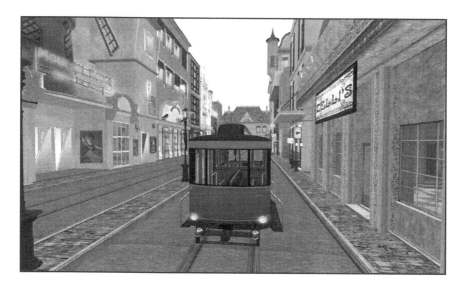

Figure 2. Virtual Montmartre, in front of Zelli's Cabaret and the Moulin Rouge (Carter, 2011a).

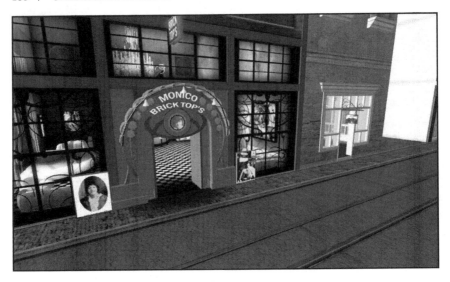

Figure 3. Virtual Montmartre, Bricktop's Cabaret (Carter, 2011b).

in order to solve an ever-changing mystery. The role-play mystery is also designed to encourage travel within the Peregrination Archetype to a variety of destinations in addition to New York (Virtual Harlem) and Paris (Virtual Montmartre). While visiting these and other locations, students learn about those places through text, audio, and visual artifacts while participating in the experience or even while interacting with students, researchers, or residents of Second Life who are from those real-life locations. An example of this sort of interactivity is seen in the construction and enhancement of a number of locations on Virtual Harlem and Virtual Montmartre to include students from the University of Paris-Sorbonne and those at the University of Central Missouri. Students at these two schools worked together on the Hellfighter Museum, a museum dedicated to the African American troops who were allowed to fight in World War I but only under the French flag (see Figure 4). Students at both locations met within the environment and through the use of video, audio, images, and text. Using the Meshed Archetype, addressing the Social Domain, they co-constructed an interactive experience that related the experience of the soldiers from the 369th and 370th regiments. The Assessment Archetype was implemented, addressing the Emotional and Dextrous domains to ascertain learning. They were assessed by looking at the accuracy of the content and at the interaction of museum visitors with the content.

Designing activities using combinations of these five Learning Archetypes allows instructors to engage and immerse students in ways that are impossible in physical classrooms. While these activities move students beyond the limits

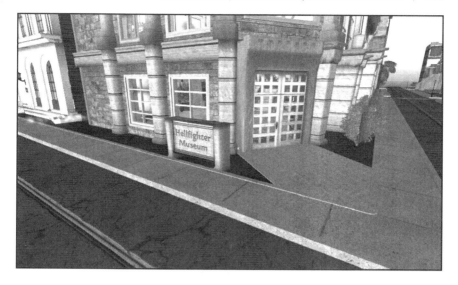

Figure 4. Virtual Harlem, Hellfighter Museum (Carter, 2011c).

of physical, real-life activities, they also build and strengthen the connections between students through social activities and dialogues. Palloff and Pratt (2007, p. 171) suggest that the instructor should facilitate these dialogues without dominating to allow for a "volley of views" in response; and Etienne Wenger (1991, p. 5) encapsulates the value of social networking in the learning process: "Be aware that the social world is where work gets done, where meaning is constructed, where learning takes place every day, where innovation originates and where identities are formed."

TECHNICAL WRITING IN VIRTUAL ENVIRONMENTS

Employing the Learning Archetypes to promote student learning in our courses, we have found that virtual worlds have the potential to inspire levels of creativity among our students that we are sometimes hard-pressed to bring out in a traditional classroom environment. Taking full advantage of this potential is no easy challenge. For the last 5 years, Dr. Carter has been teaching literature and writing classes that meet fully within the virtual environment of Second Life. Through this platform he has read some of the most interesting and well-written essays by students in a number of years. The writing course introduces two additional objectives to the traditional set of those normally found in many courses: students learn through "experiential writing" and by writing for "machinima." Machinima is a video art form in which the actors/characters are represented by avatars within a given virtual environment. Scenes are shot on sets also found in the virtual worlds, including game-centric virtual worlds such as EVE Online. For example, Ian Chisholm, an EVE Online user, produced a machinima that started as a pilot episode of a story in the EVE virtual world but proved so popular with other users and YouTube viewers that he went on to produce two more episodes. The three-part series is called Clear Skies (http://www.clearskiesthemovie.com/about.htm).

Experiential writing is not a new concept. Writing about that which we experience often encourages a different level of detail, interest, and even excitement about a topic. The idea is simple. At the beginning of the term, students are asked if any of them have visited a nuclear power plant or know anything personally about the meat packing industry. Usually no hands go up. However, when asked who has visited Florida or California, quite a few of them voluntarily describe their adventures, how the air smelled, the traffic, or even the beach. Students quickly realize that it is easier to write about something done or "experienced" rather than writing about something from a third-person perspective. Writing in this way, students are tasked to select a topic from those predefined at the beginning of the term, visit locations in Second Life related to their topic, and research outside sources to support their chosen topic. For those who chose machinima as their topic, the assignment also requires a précis, a preliminary script, shooting location scouting report, and camera angle brief.

In this final section of the chapter, we demonstrate how these activities can be designed to engage students and promote their achievement of learning outcomes. The first assignment described in this section illustrates how both experiential learning and writing for machinima can be combined in a technical writing assignment; the second describes how to promote technical writing through simulation development.

WRITING FOR MACHINIMA

Machinima within virtual environments is quickly becoming one of the most interesting and cost-effective ways for both students and aspiring new media professionals to produce high-quality film projects instead of, or prior to delving into, higher-budget productions. Machinima is a film genre in which the actors are characters from any virtual environment, including video games or 3D virtual worlds like Second Life, and the sets are the multiple locations found within these platforms. When students select this topic as their writing assignment, there are several writing "milestones" that must be completed as part of their overall assignment.

As with almost any writing class, students must of course write either a thesis statement or research question as part of the beginning of their assignment. This, along with a preliminary outline, forms the basis of what direction their final report will take. As with all other topics from which students have to choose, those writing about machinima must visit locations in Second Life related to the topic. There are many locations in Second Life where machinima is not only practiced but is a part of the business model of some residents and/or groups. For example, the Metaverse Broadcasting Company in Second Life regularly hosts in-world shows very similar to talk shows with which we are all familiar, interviewing "A-list" personalities in Second Life. The Second Life Theater Company performs plays in-world that are often filmed and placed online for those not in Second Life to enjoy on the Web.

When visiting, students are tasked not only to describe the location and what they experience in the Emotional Domain but they are also asked to engage in the Social Learning Domain by conducting interviews with those who work there, and they may even participate in some of the creative endeavors happening at the locations they visit within the Peregrination Archetype. Furthermore, selecting this topic necessitates learning how to prepare for and create a very short machinima. Students learn how to use free screen capture applications, either Web based like Screenr, or stand-alone applications like Fraps or Screen Flow. They also learn how to configure their audio settings to capture both their voice and that of other avatars in the shoot. Finally, they are taught how to output that screen-captured video to a format that can be imported into a non-linear video editing program for processing and further editing. Their completed video is placed online using one of the many video-streaming services like YouTube or Blip.tv. Doing this work requires quite a bit of planning, demonstrated not only through their milestone writing assignments but also in their own machinima.

Milestone writing assignments are, we believe, crucial in keeping students on track but also impress upon them that, because there are many steps in completing a machinima, organization is key. The first milestone assignment that students must complete is a précis describing what their machinima will be about—their overall theme or objective to be realized through their creation. This detail serves as a textual description of what they hope to accomplish in a machinima lasting approximately 3–5 minutes. In addition to their précis, they must also complete a preliminary script, detailing how many actors will be involved and some idea of any dialogue that will take place. These two assignments are usually spaced one week apart so that students will have an opportunity to consider carefully that which they really wish to say through their machinima as well as how many others they will need to complete their project.

Within the Meshed Learning Archetype, attending particularly to the Social Learning Domain, students are encouraged to work together on these projects. Although every project must be different from that which is submitted by their peers, it is unrealistic to expect students to complete an individual assignment like this in such a short period of time. This model also mirrors how much of the world outside academia works with regard to collaborative teams or groups. After a précis and preliminary script are submitted and approved (students post these assignments on their personal blogs for comment), within the Peregrination

Archetype they move to scout locations in Second Life where their machinima can be completed. This shooting location scout report must also be posted on their personal blog site. Their scout report must include 2–3 locations in Second Life where they would like to shoot their machinima, a justification as to why those locations were chosen, proof that they have contacted the "sim" owner to ask permission to film there and any response received. Finally, students must post on their personal blog a camera angle brief that offers a preliminary idea of not only what will be shot but also from where filming will take place. This textual camera angle brief must be accompanied with pictures from the angle they will be shooting, along with a very brief description of what that scene will entail.

These assignments, spaced approximately one week apart, offer students ample time to do what is necessary to complete each milestone assignment but also encourage them to use their time in class and in Second Life efficiently. The class meets twice weekly, and within the Meshed Archetype meetings are composed of announcements, micro-lectures on some aspect of the writing process, oral reports from collaborative groups, and questions; the remaining hour or so is used for students to work on their projects. In the micro-lectures, students are taught the basics of machinima filming, including camera movements in Second Life, screen capture, and incorporation of audio. Students also learn how to use a basic video-editing program.

Students who complete this assignment are typically already very comfortable with virtual environments, gaming, and computers. They are also very interested in new media and in creating machinima, and they are somewhat familiar with the film genre. The authors believe this familiarity with computers and the genre, along with interest in the medium, encourages students to produce very high-quality projects, suitable for inclusion on their electronic portfolio.

Simulation Writing

The second topic choice that includes a high degree of technical writing is the simulation writing assignment. This assignment is quite different from the machinima topic in that what they complete for this project may be included in the long-term development of a simulation. Dr. Carter's use of this assignment centers on the Virtual Harlem Project described earlier, with its two simulations—Virtual Harlem and Virtual Montmartre. This assignment requires students first to wander the streets of Virtual Harlem and Virtual Montmartre and observe what is already present on both simulations—museums, art galleries, cabarets, period businesses, open spaces and locations where live or creative events can take place. They then are required to write a proposal for an addition to one of the simulations that fits with the period or some theme that is relevant to the overall Virtual Harlem Project. Past proposals have included a museum dedicated to a particular performer of the period like Josephine Baker or a film maker of the period like Oscar Micheaux, an art gallery dedicated to one or more artists of the period, or even an event on one of the simulations that they would organize and publicize, and in which they would perhaps even participate. This proposal must include their idea, how it would enhance the Virtual Harlem project, and what resources they would need to complete their project. In addition to their proposal, students must also complete a location scout report, showing where their project would be housed on either Virtual Harlem or Virtual Montmartre. Finally, students undertake some preliminary research on their subject/personality and document how and where their project will fit on Virtual Harlem or Virtual Montmartre. The final report that students submit includes all these parts along with a description of what they did, how they did it, and some assessment of how well it fits into the Virtual Harlem Project. For instance, it is important for students to document how they added images to a rotating picture frame in Second Life and all the steps involved in finding suitable images online, importing them into Second Life, and then adding them to the frame. Students who select this particular assignment are usually already interested in some aspect of the Jazz Age or Harlem Renaissance. They have been English or History majors and have used what they have contributed to the Virtual Harlem Project to add to their personal portfolios as examples of creative ways to demonstrate their understanding/research of the period and/or their subject.

While Dr. Carter's assignment focuses on a project that he uses for many courses he teaches in Second Life, instructors interested in using a comparable assignment for their students can introduce Second Life at little or no upfront cost and focus their efforts on the processes described above for machinima-making. Most simulation owners welcome the additional traffic and, if approached by an instructor explaining the objectives of a unit or course, would have little objection to students filming on their simulation. Also, many universities have established a presence in Second Life yet make little use of their simulations on a regular basis. Again, many would welcome constructive activities on their virtual premises. Finally, students may also join a theater group or a subculture or role-playing group in Second Life and experience the world through a role, thus making their own presence in Second Life even more complex—that is, playing a role within a role. By having students co-create an event or period with other students, instructors can incorporate interesting methods of assessment to gauge student understanding of a concept, based on accuracy or how well they play the role or re-create an event. This will necessitate instructors not just to be familiar with what they want students to master (the content) but also to be aware of how that mastery is expressed through a mediated environment like Second Life to include various levels of communication and interactivity.

CONCLUSION

A result of teaching within a virtual world is an expansion of how students are encouraged to view the interconnectedness of the various systems that serve to make these worlds work. Discussing assets, inventories, communication, and access to information from within Second Life is only one way students can begin to understand how computing has evolved past the once-passive aspects of Web 1.0, referred to as "Flatlands" (Kapp & O'Driscoll, 2007). Further analysis of personas existing within Second Life often yields insight into how one is represented and how identities are formed, modified, and evolve. When students begin to consider the true meaning of "presence" within a virtual environment, it can often lead to interesting discussions. Another one of the very interesting by-products of virtual worlds in education is the evolution of a new type of faculty member using them as well as other rather experimental technologies for teaching and learning. We like to refer to these faculty as "New Digitals"— faculty members who may or may not have tenure, but who are seeking to legitimize the use of advanced technologies in their fields, as discussed in detail by Scopes (2011a). This type of teacher is willing to take chances with platforms that may not be widely used or even considered in the discipline in which he or she is a specialist, but because of the interest in advanced technologies, a new level of creativity is enabled. *Enabling* is the key word here because of the many activities we wish we could do in a traditional classroom space but because of a number of reasons, these activities are utterly impossible. Collaborating with students or colleagues at other universities from around the world; interacting with those outside academia, and traveling to distant locations that enhance learning, multi-modal communication, and an alternate sense of presence when physicality is not always possible are just a few of the possibilities made available to those using virtual environments.

REFERENCES

Bell, M. (2008). Toward a definition of virtual worlds. *Journal of Virtual Worlds Research, 1*(1), 1–5. Retrieved February 12, 2009 from http://journals.tdl.org/jvwr/article/view/283/237

Carter, B. (2011a). *Virtual Montmartre, in front of Zelli's Cabaret and the Moulin Rouge.* Retrieved December 15, 2011 from http://slurl.com/secondlife/Virtual%20Montmartre/194/194/30

Carter, B. (2011b). *Virtual Montmartre, Bricktop's Cabaret.* Retrieved December 15, 2011 from http://slurl.com/secondlife/Virtual%20Montmartre/133/201/30

Carter, B. (2011c). *Virtual Harlem, Hellfighter Museum.* Retrieved December 15, 2011 from http://slurl.com/secondlife/Virtual%20Harlem/128/128/30

Gredler, M. E. (2001). Games and simulations and their relationships to learning. In D. H. Jonassen (Ed.), *Handbook of research for educational communications and technology* (2nd ed., Vol. 2, pp. 571–581). Hillsdale, NJ: Erlbaum.

Hackerthorn, R. (2007). Serious games in virtual worlds: The future of enterprise business intelligence. Beye Network. Retrieved February 16, 2009 from http://www.b-eye-network.com/view/4163

Jenkins, H. (2005). Getting into the game. *Educational Leadership, 62*(7), 48–51.

Jones, M. G. (1998). *Creating engagement in computer-based learning environments.* University of Memphis. Retrieved January 10, 2011 from http://it.coe.uga.edu/ itforum/paper30/paper30.html

Kapp, K., & O'Driscoll, T. (2007). *Escaping flatland: The emergence of 3D synchronous learning.* e-Learning Guild Immersive Learning Simulations Report.

Kapp, K., & O'Driscoll, T. (2010). *Learning in 3D: Adding a new dimension to enterprise learning and collaboration.* San Francisco, CA: Pfeiffer.

Lave, J., & Wenger, E. (1991). *Situated learning: Legitimate peripheral participation.* New York: Cambridge University Press.

Lombardi, J., & McCahill, M. (2004). Enabling social dimensions of learning through a persistent, unified, massively multi-user, and self-organising virtual environment. In *Proceedings of the Second Annual Conference on Creating, Connecting, and Collaborating through Computing, January 29–30, 2004, Japan.* Retrieved April 16, 2007 from http://www.opencroquet.org/index.php/About_the_Technology# Education

Ludlow, P., & Wallace, M. (2007). *Second Life Herald: The virtual tabloid that witnessed the dawn of the metaverse.* Cambridge, MA: MIT Press.

Motluk, A. (2005). Do games prime brain for violence? *New Scientist, 186*(2505), 10.

Palloff, R. M., & Pratt, K. (2007). *Building online learning communities* (2nd ed.). Hoboken, NJ: Wiley/Jossey-Bass.

Rieber, L. P. (1992). Computer-based microworlds: A bridge between constructivism and direct instruction. *Educational Technology, Research, and Development, 40*(1), 93–106.

Scopes, L. (2009). *Learning archetypes as tools of cyberology for a 3D educational landscape.* Master's thesis, University of Southampton. Retrieved January 10, 2011 from http://eprints.soton.ac.uk/66169/1.hasCoversheetVersion/Learning_ Archetypes_as_tools_of_Cybergogy_for_a_3D_Educational_Landscape_-_Lesley_ J.M._Scopes_2009_V2.0.pdf

Scopes, L. (2011a). A cybergogy of learning archetypes and learning domains: Practical pedagogy for 3D immersive virtual worlds. In R. Hinrichs & C. Wankel (Eds.), *Transforming virtual world learning: Cutting edge technologies in higher education* (pp. 3–28). United Kingdom: Emerald.

Scopes, L. (2011b). *The blended taxonomy of Learning Domains.* Retrieved December 15, 2011 from http://maps.secondlife.com/secondlife/ARCHI21/149/35/88

Thompson, A., & Rodriguez, J. C. (2004). Computer gaming for teacher educators. *Journal of Computing in Teacher Education, 20*(3), 94–96.

Wenger, E. (1991). Communities of practice: Where learning takes place. *Benchmark Magazine,* Fall issue. Retrieved December 1, 2011 from http://www.ewenger.com/ pub/index.htm

Wenger, E. (2006). *Communities of practice: A brief introduction.* Retrieved April 15, 2007 from http://www.ewenger.com/theory/index.htm

Wexler, S., Aldrich, C., Johannigman, J., Oehlert, M., Quinn, C., & van Barnveld, A. (2007). Immersive learning simulations: The demand for and demands of simulations, scenarios and serious games. Santa Rosa, CA: e-Learning Guild.

http://dx.doi.org/10.2190/OE2C10

CHAPTER 10

From Divide to Continuum: Rethinking Access in Online Education

Keith Gibson and Diane Martinez

Technology and education, especially online education, are topics of great interest in higher education due to changing student demographics, university budgets, and competition. The academic community is clearly open to online learning: enrollments have seen steady increases over the past decade, including a 12% increase in 2007 in the number of students taking an online course (Allen & Seaman, 2008). Many instructors are fully embracing this new medium, delivering their courses using a variety of technologies from the simple to fringe and experimental. In our enthusiasm, however, we cannot ignore that even though 57% of American households today have access to the Internet (Kruger & Gilroy, 2009), the digital divide is still a significant factor in the effectiveness of innovative technology in the online classroom. The impetus behind online education has always been increasing the availability of education to those who would otherwise not have access, and in a physical sense, it has been very successful: thousands of students who would not be able to physically attend a face-to-face class have earned college degrees online. If, however, our online classes employ technologies that many online students cannot fully participate in, we may be causing an electronic version of the physical problem we have worked so hard to solve. And it is the innovative use of technology as well as the incorporation of new and advanced technologies in education that complicate the concept of the digital divide today beyond its original meaning of access. In this chapter, we will examine ways the digital divide has changed over the past decade, analyze some of the more prominent new technologies being employed in online education, and discuss how the more complicated issues of the digital divide today give educators more to consider when introducing or requiring these new technologies in their courses.

Though total Internet access has increased significantly over the past decade (up 138% since 2000), there is still disparity in the "presence of computers in the home" (Kruger & Gilroy, 2009, p. 1), training, and affordable Internet access. And despite government initiatives to reduce the digital divide, broadband access is far from universal. While 74% of Americans have Internet access through home computers, school computer labs, or mobile devices, a Pew survey reports that broadband service is available to 60% of suburban households, 57% of urban households, and only 38% of rural users (Horrigan, 2009, p. 3). The trend of increased Internet access is certain to continue, but the relative paucity of broadband access suggests there will always be stark differences in the way significant portions of the population access and use the Internet: those with more youth, money, and education will tend to be leaders in acquiring and using new technology, and they will always be ahead of a sizable percentage of our potential students precisely because online college students tend to be those who are a bit older and striving to attain money and education. As we will show below, this is particularly true in online education, and if we do not take these differences in access seriously, we risk making their quest for education more difficult than it needs to be.

The persistence of the digital divide is an important issue for online education. Pedagogical innovation is clearly a positive for the continued growth and vitality of our field, but innovation in online education generally requires access to and knowledge of cutting-edge technologies. For instance, classes that use Second Life require a robust computer system with more than average memory and a high-speed Internet connection; and to feasibly access and participate in classroom activities via mobile devices most would have to have a smart phone instead of a regular cell phone with simple texting capability, that is, using a number pad instead of a keyboard like on an iPhone. When considering accessibility and fairness against innovation, some people will always be left behind; thus, we have to ask if innovation is still positive and advantageous if only those students and instructors who have the ability to delve into such endeavors are the only ones benefiting from it when others are merely overlooked or omitted, whether intentionally or not. One of the key benefits of online education is the way it spreads access to those who are not ordinarily able to attend accredited universities, but if our new pedagogical strategies require broadband access or other technologies that poor and rural students do not have, we may be leaving out the students who need online education most.

Some educators, however, may not experience as much disparity among their students when it comes to access to, familiarity, or comfort with using new technologies as presented in some of the statistics in this chapter. And so the question arises that when these factors are not an issue for the majority or all of the students in a class, should we as educators take advantage of this homogeneity and push ahead using advanced technologies for educational purposes even if those in less advantaged areas or schools that have a wider technologically heterogeneous student body may not ever have the same opportunities? In other words, is it ethical to take advantage of those instances in which our students can overcome any minor disadvantages they may have between one another and create a relatively equitable environment if doing so perpetuates or even widens the gap on the digital divide? Should advantaged students be denied the use of advanced technologies, especially if such technologies are shown to improve learning, simply because less advantaged students may not have access to the same technology? Responses to these questions have serious implications because they raise the issue of what it means to have an equitable and fair education. Should all online education practices be dictated by the most disadvantaged students? This certainly is not the case in traditional educational settings; chemistry lab facilities at Harvard are not dictated by the budgets at a small community college. Similarly, we want to look at the advantages and disadvantages of a flexible approach to technology use in online education, particularly with advanced technologies, especially when the majority of students in online classes are not traditional students.

These are difficult questions, and we do not claim to be providing easy answers. Our goal for this chapter is to provide a more complete picture of the evolving digital divide and complicate the use of cutting-edge technologies in online education in light of that picture. To these ends, we will explore some of the latest educational surveys and government reports on the use of technology in the home and for educational purposes. The intent is not to dissuade readers from using technology in experimental or creative ways in the classroom, but instead to consider the audiences who are being served and those who are not able to take advantage of such efforts.

FROM DIGITAL DIVIDE TO DIGITAL CONTINUUM

A mere 10 years ago, the digital divide was a straightforward phenomenon defined by access: some people could get online and some people couldn't. President Clinton called for steps to narrow the divide by expanding networks of Community Technology Centers in low-income areas to provide workers with skills needed for employment in information technology fields (Brooks, 1999). In a Memorandum for the Heads of Executive Departments and Agencies, Clinton cited the findings from a study by the National Telecommunications and Information Administration that found minority (African American and Hispanic) and low-income populations less likely to have Internet access than White households and those who were making $75,000 or above at the time (Clinton, 1999). In one sense, this has worked very well: the percentage of

Americans who can get online is much higher than it was a decade ago, as noted above. This does not mean, however, that there is anything approaching homogeneity in the kind of access Americans have. Internet access is much more complicated than it was 10 years ago, and the metaphor of a digital divide paints too simple a picture for our current situation. Instead, we propose a digital continuum that will allow us to describe two important variables that define the quality of access and the three factors that affect each of those variables. Specifically, we will describe the digital continuum in terms of speed and mobility, and we will examine the way these variables can be understood in terms of cost, availability, and age.

One defining characteristic of the digital divide today is speed. Broadband, high-speed Internet access allows users to send and receive data at high rates of speed, much faster than dial-up provided and still provides today. So while access has increased steadily over the last 10 years, speed is now one of the dividing lines as low-income and rural areas are most affected because they often lack the ability to connect to broadband technologies such as satellite, cable, and wireless (Kruger & Gilroy, 2009). Speed varies from state to state and even one region to the next. For instance, the Northeast and Mid-Atlantic regions are generally faster than the South or rural areas of the United States, and Delaware has an average download speed of 9.9 mps, while Idaho averages 2.6 mps (Cauley, 2009). Taking advantage of speed, whether or not it is available in one's area, is another thing. "Non-broadband users tend to be older, have lower incomes, have trouble using technology, and may not see the relevance of using the Internet to their lives" (Kruger & Gilroy, 2009, p. 2).

Mobility is currently another variable of the digital divide. While access for minority and low-income populations has increased over the last decade, the type of devices with which they access the Internet has changed as well, and these devices are shaping the way these groups can utilize the Internet. A 2009 Pew survey showed that mobile devices are now more commonly used for access to the Internet than traditional connections in the home, but these devices are not spread evenly among the population: half of African-Americans and Hispanics used handheld devices to access the Internet, whereas only 28% of White Americans used them (Wortham, 2009). These devices are useful for many things, but when a handheld device is the only or primary tool to access the Internet, the potential uses of the Web fall dramatically due to the smaller screen and limited interface. A college student who can access the Internet only via their cell phone, for example, would experience an online class in a much more limited way than a student with a traditional home broadband connection and a computer.

The first two factors affecting the breadth of the digital divide are price and availability. In 2009, broadband Internet access cost nearly twice as much as dial-up access, with national averages of $38 and $20, respectively. This significant difference in price is the main barrier to broadband adoption: a Pew survey found that 35% of dial-up users would switch to broadband only if the price fell (Horrigan, 2009). Not even a price drop will help where no broadband access is available, and that remains the case for large portions of the rural United States. In fact, 17% of dial-up users cite availability as the only reason they have not adopted broadband service (Horrigan, 2009). The combination of price and availability, then, compose more than half of the barrier to broadband access in America.

A third factor is especially important for thinking about online education: age. The 2009 Pew survey found that the factor second-most negatively correlated with home broadband access is age; older Americans are less likely to have broadband access at home. This is noteworthy for online educators because students in online college courses tend to be significantly older than students in face-to-face classes. U.S. Census figures for 2008 indicate that of the 7.1 million college students in the country, only 1.8 million are age 25 or older. This rate is half what online colleges typically report; 52% of the students in online courses at the San Diego Community College are 25 or older (San Diego Community College District, 2010). The average age of students at the University of Phoenix is 35–37 (Edvisors, 2009). And Barbara Belzer, the Assistant Dean of Distance Education at the University of Memphis, while noting that exact figures are hard to come by, points out that their "typical online student" is "a middle-aged female with children" (Otwell, 2008). Since the likelihood of broadband access decreases with age, the older students in online classes are less likely than their face-to-face counterparts to have high-speed Internet access at home.

Online education, from its inception, has been designed to attract students unwilling or unable to attend face-to-face courses for any number of reasons. Some of the most common factors for choosing online courses have always been the age of the student, the cost of the courses, and the ease of access. These three factors combine to create a student demographic much more likely than those in face-to-face universities to be on the far end of the digital continuum that has limited access. This would not necessarily be a problem; there are plenty of educational technologies that work well with low-speed Internet. The current push in online pedagogy, however, is toward technology that requires more expensive hardware and faster download speeds, and this trend could leave some of the very students online education intends to serve excluded from class. In the remainder of this chapter, we examine four technologies currently in use in educational settings: mobile applications, social networking, interactive videoconferencing, and massively multiplayer online games (MMOGs). These technologies have appeared prominently in online education scholarship, as described below. These appearances have been largely positive, and they have effectively persuaded many online instructors to employ more and more cutting-edge tools in their pedagogies. With this chapter, we are trying to not necessarily discourage their use but rather to complicate our thinking about these technologies specifically and new technology generally in online education. What we discuss in the sections below are the current uses of these technologies, the advantages of these technologies for educational purposes, and then the considerations or possible disadvantages of using these technologies, including an evaluation of whether or not such use is available to all online students or if they cater to those on one end of the digital continuum.

TECHNOLOGY IN THE CLASSROOM

Various technologies offer a wide range of mediums to deliver information to students who have different learning styles. Even the generic concept of online education allows independent learners more flexibility in their pace and schedule and level of engagement than some face-to-face courses. Innovative experimentation and research in technology and education can be exciting for both instructors and students, and there are some truly worthwhile uses of technology in both online and face-to-face courses. Some work quite well and require minimal cost and effort for students, such as mobile applications and social networking, while other courses are so technologically advanced (when using Second Life, for instance) that some students are unable to participate merely because their access is restricted (or even unavailable) or their connection and download speeds are not fast enough for the programs. In this section, we discuss the use, justification, and technical requirements of mobile applications, social networking, interactive videoconferencing (IVC), and massively multiplayer online games (MMOGs).

Mobile Applications

Mobile applications are an area of educational innovation that is being explored in both face-to-face and online classrooms. Mobile learning, or learning that takes place using handheld devices, such as cell phones, PDAs, and iPods, opens up a new arena for learning and a whole new market of adult learners. "Wireless devices have the potential to give instant gratification to students by allowing them to interact with the Internet, access course materials, and retrieve information from anywhere" (Liaw, Hatala, & Huang, 2010, p. 446). Clearly, one of the biggest attractions for mobile learning is the continuation of technology that provides learning opportunities anytime and anywhere.

There are many advantages to mobile learning in online education. From a pedagogical standpoint, the convenience of being able to download or listen to course material at any time supports the idea of self-paced education, which is popular among busy adult learners. Furthermore, the technological aspect of mobile learning makes students active learners, and they "acquire new knowledge within meaningful learning activities" as they "begin to adapt their communication and learning activities accordingly" (Liaw et al., 2010, p. 447). Other educational researchers have found mobile applications used for educational purposes can provide students with engaging problem-based learning activities (Massey, Ramish, & Khatri, 2009). For instance, Massey et al. (2009) reported on a graduate course in which students worked directly with mobile applications industry partners in evaluating and assessing the design, development, and "value of mobile technologies for the associated stakeholders, e.g., students, faculty, and the broader university community" (p. 183). In this course, students were using mobile technologies while also learning how to problem-solve and provide real-world industry sponsors with feedback about possible uses for these technologies in educational settings.

The disadvantages of relying on mobile applications for online courses are probably obvious to anyone who has tried to send a long text message. Although most mobile devices include texting features, not all are keyboards, and the time and tediousness of writing a complete and thoughtful response that refers to reading assignments may be so difficult as to discourage students from actively participating in the discussions. If students can persevere through the thumb cramps, the time required to be active in class could easily push the student into a higher, more costly service plan, increasing the price of the course and further discriminating against the poorer students. If students want to download course materials, then they will need Internet access; however, if they are able to download the material onto the handheld device via a home or work computer, then all they need is the ability to access the files on the device, whether it is a written file, video, or maybe even a podcast, in which case all they need is audio capability, which most handheld devices have anyway. Depending on the speed of the device, downloading from the Internet may be slow and time-consuming, so file size and mobile device download speed are certainly considerations. Another aspect about using mobile technologies for coursework is the ability to multitask, such as referring to an electronic reading file while composing a post to a discussion board. Multitasking on a mobile device is difficult because not all of these devices allow a user to have two or more applications open at the same time. Imagine trying to refer to a reading assignment while composing a discussion board response on a cell phone, even something as advanced as the iPhone or iPad. The lack of visual space alone can be cumbersome. Add in the tediousness of composing a long response as mentioned above, and one result could be discussion questions that are composed similarly to text messages, which is not academic writing or what is expected in a discussion question response. In fact, using mobile devices for academic purposes could result in abbreviated writing in all areas of school, which then opens up further discussions about comprehension, learning, and demonstration of knowledge.

Social Networking

Social networking is also of interest in education because it is currently one of the main forms of communication for traditionally aged college students (18–24 years old; Bradley, 2009); however, older students find just as many uses for social software as traditionally aged students. Social software is Web 2.0

technologies intended to build community, share interests and information, and invite interactivity among like-minded groups of people. Examples of social networking technologies include Facebook, Twitter, LinkedIn, blogs, wikis, and YouTube.

The main advantage of social networking tools is the familiarity many online students already have with them. Bradley (2009) reports that traditionally aged students use social networking tools several times a day and even rely on them to communicate with other students and instructors about their courses. A study by Jones, Blackley, Fitzgibbon, and Chew (2010) shows that students find social networking platforms enjoyable to use, and that they increase communication and encourage sharing. For instance, course and program feedback can be facilitated to a greater degree when social networking tools are used. In 2009, the feedback on Texas Tech's PhD summer conference "took on a uniquely digital and more permanent form . . . [in which] tweets generated a unique online community for faculty and students" (Hosterman, 2009, p. 13). This sense of community drives many university offices and departments to utilize social networking tools as a way to build a sense of belonging and increase participation and attendance. And because of its social nature, social software is of particular interest to those who subscribe to social constructivist pedagogy and for those interested in creating life-long learning experiences for students (Jones et al., 2010). Social software takes full advantage of the concept of learning from one another as users in a social community are encouraged to post and respond to one another on even the most seemingly trivial aspects of their lives and learning. In social networks, members are fully immersed in social connections, and communication among members is paramount because that is the nature of social networking (Jones et al., 2010). Additionally, social networking supports life-long learning habits because students are encouraged to learn things on their own. This independent learning, students believe, will increase their employability (Jones et al., 2010).

What is required of learners when employing social networking tools in a curriculum? Beyond the use of a computer with Internet access, little more is required; however, there are sensitive issues to consider. For example, when signing up for an account on Facebook, usually personal information is requested, such as name and e-mail. While this information is not necessarily available to others in the class, forcing students to participate in such activities as a class requirement when personal data is collected could be construed as an invasion of personal privacy, especially when most sites cannot guarantee data protection (Jones et al., 2010). Additionally, research by Jones et al. showed that some students, about half of those interviewed, were not happy about the invasion of education into social spheres. Those students who objected to having social networking tools used for educational purposes cited separation of school and personal life as their main objection.

Perhaps the most important disadvantage to consider is the potential for privacy issues. Belonging to a somewhat public community, such as a classroom page on

Facebook, means that students who want to be part of the class's Facebook page will have to use their personal Facebook accounts to join unless they create a separate school account, which can be time-consuming to set up or maintain. If students use their personal Facebook accounts, then anything they post about their personal lives becomes the business of classmates, even when it has no relevance to the course. This could have implications for their professional lives as one can never really be certain who they will work with or for in the future. Consequently, it might be worthwhile to consider the advantages of building community using something like Facebook over building community in some other way in the online classroom, such as having a student lounge or online chat area in the online classroom itself instead of going outside where students may be exposing their personal lives to fellow students.

Interactive Videoconferencing

Scholars have long maintained that the goal of online education is not to replicate the face-to-face class in an online setting; but the possibility of an occasional face-to-face conference is an appealing one nonetheless. Interactive videoconferencing (IVC), thus, has become a popular addition to many online courses. They are used to connect students collaborating on a project, professors discussing work with students, or faculty collaborating on a class, and they can help students and instructors re-create the feeling of community many online classes lack. There are a number of options for IVC, and many of them are completely free of charge: Adobe Connect, Skype, and Google Video Chat among them. The prevalence of cheap, user-friendly software packages to facilitate IVC has brought it to the attention of many online instructors.

Anastasiades (2007) describes the pedagogical advantages IVC can provide. The collaborative learning environment, so easy to create in a face-to-face classroom, can be difficult to replicate with students learning at a distance. IVC allows students to communicate quickly, discussing projects and assignments in a way very similar to the face-to-face classroom. The desire for this technology is clearly there; Baker and Tonkin (2007) conducted a survey in which the "desire to see more audio and videoconferencing in online courses was the single most commonly cited feature" (p. 129) by faculty asked to describe the direction they would like to see online courses taking. These kinds of experiences are becoming increasingly common in education, even for very young students. Greenberg (2006) reports that 25% of U.S. elementary and secondary schools employ "collaborative learning activities in Distance via Videoconferencing almost every day" (p. 141). This familiarity with IVC for so many students makes it especially attractive for teachers looking to supplement their courses with some face-to-face interaction.

Effective IVC is not a technologically simple task, however; it requires, at minimum, a webcam, microphone, and significant Internet speed. Dooley,

Lindner, Dooley, and Magnussen (2005) detail the requirements for high, medium, and low-speed videoconferencing, and they note that only low-speed videoconferencing is feasible with dial-up connections; due to the slow download speed, "the quality of the signal is poor and the signal breaks up and freezes frequently" (p. 169). Skype, for instance, a common, free software tool for interactive videoconferencing, requires up to 16 kilobytes/second. When a school can provide the bandwidth required on both ends of the videoconference, there is no problem. For students logging into a university from home, however, the individuals become responsible for the download speeds on their side of the conversation. As many of us have experienced, there is little more frustrating than a videoconference with poor video quality. One of us attended a conference last summer in which a presenter was delivering his paper via online video, but the signal broke up so badly, the speaker simply stopped speaking after 10 minutes. Online education that heavily utilizes IVC risks driving dial-up Internet users away from the screen and away from the course.

Massively Multiplayer Online Games

Another increasingly common pedagogical tool is the video game. The pedagogical justification for video games is built largely around James Gee's (2004) contention that the "theory of learning in good video games fits better with the modern, high-tech global world today's children and teenagers live in than do the theories and practices they see in school" (p. 7). Proponents of these games argue that the digital natives who are our students will learn better, more effective lessons if we teach them via these tools that replicate the digital world they will be working in. Steinkuehler (2004) claims we should explore the educational potential of video games because "by far, videogames (MMOGs in particular) are the most important entertainment media in the lives of the millennial generation" (p. 527).

One of the most pedagogically flexible video games is Second Life, a virtual world in which players build identities, get jobs, and live in communities. Bransford and Gawel (2006) are enthusiastic about the possibilities of "true collaboration" in Second Life: "If we can eventually combine the talents of content area specialists, creative designers, learning scientists and assessment experts, we can recognize their contributions by expanding academic peer reviewed products to include learning environments" (p. iii). Mason and Moutahir (2006) point to the potential for multidisciplinary collaboration and meaningful cultural awareness, as students with diverse backgrounds come together in this virtual space. Hayes (2006) notes the more technical educational benefits of Second Life:

> 1. Learning technical and design skills . . . [including] learning how to appropriate and reappropriate tools within and beyond the SL world as well as learning the norms and subcultures of particular user-creation affinity

groups. 2. Learning how to participate in the broader *SL* economy . . . and contending with complex ethical concerns related to such issues as "virtual" property rights. (pp. 155–156)

Childress and Braswell (2006) see Second Life (and other MMOGs) becoming increasingly realistic and interactive, "blurring the line between the face-to-face learning environment and the online virtual learning environment" (p. 194). This blurred line could potentially ease the fears many have of online education, paving the way for more broad-based support of this educational option.

There are, of course, some who are skeptical about the current enthusiasm for MMOGs in education. Michael Bujega (2007) points out that games like Second Life are far from utopian environments, and he wonders if we will ultimately be held accountable "for requiring students to enter a virtual world filled with online harassers" (p. C1). The EDUCAUSE Learning Initiative (ELI) (2006) notes that virtual worlds, precisely because they are new and interesting "present a risk of students simply goofing off, not participating at all, or engaging in inappropriate or offensive behavior" (p. 2). The ELI also points out the technical barriers these games pose for many users:

> The smooth operation of virtual worlds requires robust hardware and fast Internet connections. Some virtual worlds reside on corporate servers, and course activities that use those worlds depend on the availability of the application, which can be spotty. With steep technology requirements also comes a greater burden on support staff to ensure the infrastructure can handle user demands. (p. 2)

Indeed, the Second Life Web site makes it clear that ELI is not exaggerating about the "robust hardware and fast Internet connections" required. It lists among its "Minimum Requirements" cable or DSL Internet access, 512 MB of RAM, and a Pentium III processor. These requirements will exclude far too many potential students in rural areas; since these are the students online education is, in part, designed to serve, we should think carefully about the utility of games like Second Life.

CONCLUSION

The drive to include more cutting-edge technology in our pedagogy is inspired in part by our acknowledgement that many of our students are, in Marc Prensky's (2001) terminology, digital natives, while most faculty are digital immigrants. Sensitivity to this difference in our approaches to technology is wise, and we need to understand these approaches as we build our courses. Accommodating digital natives in our classes does not simply mean using more technology, however. Most importantly, we must let our pedagogy lead the technology in our classes (and not the other way around), but we need to also remember that, although many of our students are digital natives, there is still a sizable percentage who are not. Perhaps ironically, online education features higher percentages of digital immigrants than traditional education since online education caters to nontraditional students. Precisely for this reason, we must be deliberate about considering our online courses from the perspective of these digital immigrants, especially those on the other side of the digital divide.

Technology offers a wide menu of services, resources, and avenues for effective teaching and learning; however, it is advantageous for both instructors and students to understand the implications of including technology in the classroom. Pedagogy and actual learning must be weighed carefully against innovation and enthusiasm. Conole and Culver (2010) claim,

> There is little evidence of learning from past innovation, and hence there is a lot of repetition of mistakes and claims of "innovation" that do not bear witness to close scrutiny. . . . there are few examples of true innovation and new pedagogy, little transfer between pockets of good practice or evidence of scaling up more broadly. (p. 679)

Educators should not be shy about exploring and using technology in the classroom, but they also must understand that implementation of any tool or approach has to be researched and scrutinized for effectiveness and actual learning before putting it in use in the classroom.

The desire to continually explore new technologies and discover pedagogical uses for them is an admirable one. We should certainly be striving to improve our teaching however we can; if cutting-edge computer technology can help us do that, we should not be afraid to use it. Many online educators have shown great enthusiasm for new technology and have quickly adopted it for the distance classrooms. In our excitement for new tools, however, we must not lose sight of the students whom online education was designed to serve, many of whom are on the far end of the digital continuum, without access to broadband Internet or the latest-generation computers. We are arguing that the needs of these students must be considered, and if our online teaching requires computer equipment these students do not have, we will be excluding an important segment of our audience. When we understand the technological state of a nation and the conditions under which a great portion of our population still struggle, then we can discuss and explore a means for wider distribution for cutting-edge advances in educational technology. The potential rewards of new technologies cannot be the only consideration in their adoption; we must consider the risks as well. We are not arguing for an abandonment of new technologies in online education; instead, we are urging a thoughtful examination of the risks and rewards of this technology use. We can imagine a variety of outcomes of this forethought: teachers may decide the rewards for the students who have complete access outweigh the risks of an inequitable experience, and they adopt the new technology; teachers may decide the risks outweigh the potential rewards and continue to use simpler technologies they have previously used; or teachers may decide the risks outweigh the rewards for a specific technology, so they continue searching for other simpler, new technology. As long as teachers are specifically considering their technology choices before adopting them, we believe our students will be better served.

Furthermore, we have good reason to believe that the digital continuum is not a temporary situation. The difference in technological access is simply a specific instance of the general difference in wealth that has existed as long as humans have lived in societies; given that there will always be a rich-poor divide, the rich will always be able (and often willing) to buy newer, better, and faster technology. Thus, even though efforts in the last 10 years to increase access have proven positive in most areas throughout the United States, new technologies will always be adopted at different rates. It is not our intention to say that because this situation appears to be a permanent, albeit evolving, issue that we are going to have to deal with from now on, that education should abandon technology completely or use only the lowest level of technology available. Certainly each situation has to be weighed carefully by individual instructors. Our goal with this chapter is to persuade instructors to pause and think through these issues before they use technology in their classes. Even more importantly, we hope this article and others like it motivate us all to continue discussions about the educational use of technology so our ideas for how we use technology in the classroom are as innovative and intriguing as the very technology that is available to us.

REFERENCES

Allen, E. I., & Seaman, J. (2008). *Staying the course: Online education in the United States*. Needham, MA: Sloan Consortium.

Anastasiades, P. S. (2007). Interactive videoconferencing (IVC) as a crucial factor in distance education: Towards a constructivism IVC pedagogy model under a cross-curricular thematic approach. In E. P. Bailey (Ed.), *Focus on distance education developments* (pp. 41–53). New York: Nova Science.

Baker, J., & Tonkin, S. (2007). Online faculty proficiency and peer coaching. In B. H. Khan (Ed.), *Flexible learning in an information society* (pp. 126–134). Hershey, PA: Information Science.

Bradley, P. (2009, November 16). CCSSE finds increasing use of social networking tools. *Community College Week, 5*.

Bransford, J., & Gawel, D. (2006). Foreword. In D. Livingstone & J. Kemp (Eds.), *Proceedings of the Second Life Education Workshop at the Second Life Community Convention* (p. iii). Paisley, England: University of Paisley.

Brooks, C. (1999, December 23–29). Breaching the digital divide. *The New York Amsterdam News*, p. 34.

Bugeja, M. (2007, September 14). Second thoughts about Second Life. *The Chronicle of Higher Education*, p. C1.

Cauley, L. (2009, August 25). Internet speeds vary across USA. *USA Today,* p. 1B.

Childress, M., & Braswell, R. (2006). Using massively multiplayer online role-playing games for online learning. *Distance Education, 27*(2), 187–196.

Clinton, W. (1999, December 19). Memorandum on narrowing the digital divide. *Weekly Compilation of Presidential Documents, 35*(49), 2554.

Conole, G., & Culver, J. (2010). The design of Cloudworks: Applying social networking practice to foster the exchange of learning and teaching ideas and designs. *Computers & Education, 54,* 679–692.

Dooley, K. E., Linder, J. R., Dooley, L. M., & Magnussen, W. (2005). Delivery technology. In K. E. Dooley, J. R. Linder, & L. M. Dooley (Eds.), *Advanced methods in distance education* (pp. 162–181). Hershey, PA: Information Science.

EDUCAUSE Learning Initiative (ELI). (2006, June). *Seven things you should know about virtual worlds.* Retrieved September 2, 2007, from http://connect.EDUCAUSE. edu/library/abstract/7ThingsYouShouldKnow/39392

Edvisors Online Education Blog. (2009, August 28). *Average student age on the rise.* [Posted message] Retrieved from http://blog.edvisors.com/online-education/ the-average-age-of-students-is-on-the-upswing/

Gee, J. P. (2004). *What video games have to teach us about learning and literacy.* New York: Palgrave Macmillan.

Greenberg, A. (2006). Taking the wraps off videoconferencing in the U.S. classroom: A state-by-state analysis. Retrieved from http://www.wrplatinum.com/content.asx? CID=5912

Hayes, E. (2006). Situated learning in virtual worlds: The learning ecology of Second Life. *Proceedings of Adult Education Research Conference 2006.* Retrieved from March 1, 2010, from http://www.adulterc.org/Proceedings/2006/Proceedings/ Hayes.pdf

Horrigan, J. (2009). *Home broadband adoption 2009.* Washington, DC: Pew Research Center.

Hosterman, A. R. (2009). Tools of the trade: Getting technical about using twitter. *Intercom, 56*(10), 12–14.

Jones, N., Blackley, H., Fitzgibbon, K., & Chew, E. (2010). Get out of MySpace! *Computers & Education, 54,* 776–782.

Kruger, L. G., & Gilroy, A. A. (2009). *Broadband Internet access and the digital divide: Federal assistance programs.* Washington, DC: Library of Congress, Congressional Research Service.

Liaw, S., Hatala, M., & Huang, H. (2010). Investigating acceptance toward mobile learning to assist individual knowledge management: Based on activity theory approach. *Computers & Education, 54,* 446–454.

Mason, H., & Moutahir, M. (2006). Multidisciplinary experiential education in Second Life: A global approach. In D. Livingstone & J. Kemp (Eds.), *Proceedings of the Second Life Education Workshop at the Second Life Community Convention* (pp. 30–34). Paisley, England: University of Paisley.

Massey, A. P., Ramesh, V., & Khatri, V. (2006). Design, development, and assessment of mobile applications: The case for problem-based learning. *IEEE Transactions on Education, 49*(2), 183–192.

Otwell, J. (2008, July 25). Online student demographics vary, from traditional to working moms. *Memphis Business Journal*. Retrieved February 26, 2010, from http://memphis.bizjournals.com/memphis/stories/2008/07/28/focus4.html

Prensky, M. (2001). Digital natives, digital immigrants. *On the Horizon, 9*(5), 1–6.

San Diego Community College District. (2010). SDCCD online student profile. *Office of Institutional Research and Planning*. Retrieved March 1, 2010, from http://research.sdccd.edu/Include/Student%20Profiles/Online%20Demographics/Profile_Online_Fall09.pdf

Steinkuehler, C. (2004). Learning in massively multi-player online games. *Proceedings of the Sixth International Conference on Learning Sciences* (pp. 521–528). Mahwah, NJ: Lawrence Erlbaum.

U.S. Census Bureau. (2009). *School enrollment–social and economic characteristics of students: October 2008*. Retrieved February 27, 2010, from http://www.census.gov/population/www/socdemo/school/cps2008.html

Wortham, J. (2009, July 27). Digital divide, shrinking. *New York Times,* p. 4.

http://dx.doi.org/10.2190/OE2C11

Section III: Reinventing Course Contents and Materials

CHAPTER 11

Adapting Instructional Documents to an Online Course Environment

Jacqueline Cason and Patricia Jenkins

When faculty teach courses online for the first time, they may do so for any number of reasons, ranging from the course having been slotted that way prior to their putting it in their workload, to their wanting more flexibility in their own schedule, to the administration encouraging them to meet the needs of students. And they may be new to teaching a particular course, new to teaching online, or both. Furthermore, their technological comfort zone may range widely depending on their fluency: They may be guided by a strong orientation toward print-based composing, or they may be as technologically fluent as their students. The process we describe below characterizes the experience of teachers who came of age before the emergence of new media and who were encouraged by administration to offer courses that would meet the needs of students and lighten the demand for on-site classroom space. However, our experience may inform younger faculty who have not yet taken the plunge or program administrators who supervise contingent faculty who prefer the flexibility of teaching online. Once faculty have committed to teaching online, many of them most likely begin to familiarize themselves with the campus delivery system available and soon realize that their courses can be ultra-technologically sexy or pretty dang technologically straight-forward, depending on the system, their knowledge, available support—and their comfort level. They should also be aware that as online enrollments have increased, so have distance course attrition rates, so they will need strategies for engaging with their students (Carr, 2000).

In the process of moving a course first created for the face-to-face environment to an online interface, they realize that their course documents, in standing alone, lack the supplemental live presentation of the on-site classroom. Imagine walking into a classroom, distributing an assignment sheet, and exiting the classroom to await questions from a remote location. In the on-site classroom, instructors more often *present* their assignment sheets because meaning inheres not in the document itself but in the complex interrelationships among activities, context, participants, and the discursive signs that articulate those relationships. If the instructor does not attend to those relationships, meaning making on the part of the student may be limited.

As composition studies continues down the innovative path of online education, it is worthwhile to listen to voices like Farber's (2008), who describes the on-site classroom as "a technology whose time has come," a place marked by the "purposeful convergence of people in time and space." He describes the qualities of the on-site classroom as "present, immediate, alive"; "complex, multidimensional"; "physically and socially situated"; "a lively and productive interplay between cognition and affect"; a place where connections can be "integrated, . . . memorable, . . . transformative" (p. 217). By contrast, he describes screen time pejoratively and encourages us to infer that the online course might be "a neutralized version of the real time, real space" of the classroom. Furthermore, Farber's depiction of an enriched learning space reminds us that print-based documents are just one element in the communicative process, combined with multiple nonverbal, verbal, and visual resources. What are instructors to do if they can no longer draw upon the full repertoire of communication strategies available to classroom teachers in a space where physical presence, images, words, sounds, and dialogue are integrated during live presentation? To compensate for the inherent multimodality and synchronicity of the on-site classroom, they will seek a way to establish their physical and social presence, even in the most presentational of documents, the assignment sheet. Our analysis suggests that as online teachers continue to innovate, they will need to rely on a different repertoire.

The principles of multimodal authorship described by Winters (2010) echo the description of Farber's on-site classroom and align well with the work of writing teachers who author texts that are often nonlinear, integrated, and layered, using multiple modalities. Borrowing Winters' principles of authorship, we can describe composition teachers as "meaning-makers" who "orchestrate a multiplicity of modes," who "shift among social (inter)actions of design, negotiation, production, and dissemination," and who "create storylines and subject positions" (p. 2). And the resources for doing that vary according to the spaces in which they teach. What does it mean to adapt materials so that they are suitable for an online course, and how does the new space of the online environment change the nature of assignment documents? What should inform teachers as they create *new* materials for the online environment? How do those materials adapt over time? In other words, what does teaching *online* mean for the materials we create and post?

Understandably, much of the scholarship on online teaching addresses the challenge of developing pedagogically sound, interactive learning environments; it does not, however, address specifically adapting or creating instructional materials. Nonetheless, the instructor concerned about what this means for writing and rewriting materials can glean some useful advice from these broader discussions of course design. For example, in the context of discussing "the problem of designing interactive, collaborative learning online," Grady and Davis (2005) offer criteria for well-designed documents: They point out that "it is important to provide more content and explanation in an online course in order to replace the natural interactions and explanations that occur in a face-to-face class" (p. 109). They also suggest that the syllabus should contain "clearly marked links and connections to other parts of the online course" (p. 109) and that the schedule, too, should contain hyperlinks so students can access places in the online environment as well as documents (p. 110). In the context of examining physical, virtual, and cognitive gaps in the online environment, Carter and Rickly (2005) suggest that you "play with your cards up"; that is, they encourage instructors to provide a detailed syllabus in which they are open about choices made for things like readings and assignments (p. 136). Essentially, much of the advice for adapting course materials emphasizes providing more context for students and implementing the means for documents to be networked with other documents and with relevant areas in the online course. However, adapting course materials to foster an interactive learning environment should not be limited only to replacing through text and networked documents the social and affective dynamics possible in a face-to-face class.

WHY LOOK AT COURSE MATERIALS?

As our chapter will show, a more specific concern for creating and adapting instructional materials will demonstrate that online courses can take more advantage of multimodal resources to situate and supplement print-based documents and navigational links. While Cargile Cook (2005), Rude (2005), and others argue for putting pedagogical choices before choices for materials and technology, they are not suggesting that choices about materials are unimportant or unrelated. Cargile Cook argues that pedagogy rather than technology should shape curricular policies and choices: "Pedagogically driven distance courses, as opposed to boilerplate technology-driven ones, begin with what effective instructors do best—teaching students" (p. 51). Such student-centered teaching has always been fundamentally multimodal. Similarly, Rude argues that "pedagogy is more important to the quality of the course and long-term success of the program than materials and technologies" (p. 69). Both suggest that a pedagogy-driven course calls upon instructors to examine their practice with a protocol well-defined by the scholarship of teaching and learning (e.g., "back-ward design"). In light of this concern for putting pedagogical goals, instructor values, and student needs first, when we argue for "informed practice" in online teaching we are arguing for pedagogy-driven practice.

Cargile Cook (2005) also points out that designing a pedagogy-driven course includes choices about instructional delivery models and links two models of delivery to corresponding pedagogical theories (p. 59). She explains two models of delivery—presentational and interactive—and likens the presentational delivery model to lecture-based, on-site courses and the interactive delivery model to the dialogic, on-site courses. Furthermore, she suggests that the presentational model will tend toward an objectivist pedagogy and the interactive toward a constructivist pedagogy. Rude (2005) reminds us that "the assumption of much of the literature in writing instruction is that pedagogy should be constructivist, encouraging students to take an active role in learning and performance and to work in collaboration with peers and the instructor" (p. 70). Speaking realistically, Cargile Cook makes the point that many writing courses will nevertheless contain a combination of presentational and interactive elements: "Given that most classroom activities fall somewhere between the presentational and interactive models, few actual classes will be entirely presentational or interactive in design" (p. 60). In other words, designing a pedagogy-driven course means that instructors work from a particular theory that lends itself to a particular delivery model, but they likely will have aspects of their courses that may seem (or be) more in line with a theory that does not seem to fit with their values. This practical insight frees the instructor to provide preferred approaches to assignments needed to accomplish course goals. With this in mind—that teachers may need to tend to presentational aspects of their online courses even when grounded by a constructivist theory—this chapter considers one particular presentational element of on-site and online teaching, assignment instructions. Instructional documents that guide writing assignments are significant because writing assignments customarily count for as much and sometimes more than 75% of a total grade. Given the importance of writing assignments, we believe that instructors should provide students with a written description of an assignment even if it is open-ended or based on a question in a text. According to White (2007), "many experienced teachers have learned that they must write out, distribute, and discuss their assignments if they are to be taken seriously and if a particular goal is to be made clear" (p. 5).

How to Look at Course Materials

While the advice for adapting documents is a good place to begin—providing more context and creating networked documents—we argue that in order for our course materials to be reflective of informed practice, instructors should interrogate them after they have attempted to adapt them by adding much-needed context and connectivity. To interrogate course materials, instructors can adapt a methodology from genre analysis developed by Paré and Smart (1994). Paré and Smart define "genre" in terms of patterns of regularity across four dimensions—textual features, composing processes, reading practices, and social roles—in order to "provide a lens through which researchers can examine the influence and acquisition of genres" (p. 153); similarly, instructors could look at the same dimensions of their online documents. Adjusting Paré and Smart's genre definition to suit a different purpose, we suggest that instructors begin their interrogation with the following questions:

- What textual features characterize your course materials?
- What composing practices do you use for your course materials?
- What reading practices are required with your course materials?
- What social roles do you play or need to play in course materials?

Paré and Smart's inquiry helps "researchers explore the full range of social action that constitutes an organization's repeated rhetorical strategies, or 'genres' in order to 'know more about how a genre constrains and enables writers and readers'" (p. 153). The inquiry we propose helps instructors examine course materials by asking them to consider four dimensions of their course materials: textual features, composing practices, reading practices, and social roles. Our application of "social roles" is informed by discussions about instructor roles in the online environment, particularly the work of Coppola (2005). She identifies three roles that are enacted in both on-site and online teaching: cognitive, affective, and managerial. Her research shows that these roles change when the instructor begins teaching in the online environment (pp. 97–98). Through our examination, we invite instructors to think about the ways their course materials may constrain and enable their pedagogical intentions and about ways technological choices, made by themselves or their institutions, may constrain and enable them as well. We are not proposing necessarily that there is a genre called the "online document," but that as we interrogate our courses and concern ourselves with sound pedagogy, this must include interrogating our course materials as well. Otherwise, perhaps all we have done when we teach online is provide a different way for students to access our course's content.

The method of genre analysis, as demonstrated by Paré and Smart (1994), approaches genre as social action. Such a method provides an opportunity to examine presentational documents and to attend to their inherently social qualities. While our analytical results remain conceptual, they point the way to more empirical trials. Through the process of our inquiry, we have discovered that our own assignment documents have evolved through three identifiable phases:

1. **Replacement Practice**: Posting assignment sheets directly online as word-processing documents to be printed, with a brief description that situates

them in a new environment and establishes their place within the course architecture.

2. **Sequential Learning Units**: Adapting assignment sheets to a sequential learning unit as provided by many course management systems and presenting them in a more situationally embedded and modular screen view.

3. **Multimodal Composing**: Re-creating assignment sheets and instructions with multimodal composing tools to take fuller advantage of the webbed interface.

Although we have evolved through these phases and have continued to optimize our courses, we do not intend to frame the changes strictly as a matter of linear progress. As readers will eventually see, we have begun to question the time warranted to master a proprietary course management system and would encourage fellow instructors to be wary of constraints within such systems.

As we analyze each phase of document adaptation, we will be asking a set of four questions: which textual features characterize our documents; which composing practices do we use; what reading practices do our assignment instructions require; and how do those documents serve to define the social roles of and relationships among students and teachers?

PRIOR ACTIVITY:
SCAFFOLDING THE ONLINE ENVIRONMENT

Before instructors interrogate the presentational aspect of their online courses, we would like to note one requirement for informed practice when adapting course materials: Grady and Davis (2005) point out that "Simply uploading all the course materials and handouts for a traditional course without a framework that defines how all the pieces of the course are related results in overwhelming confusion for the students" (p. 108). In other words, we must create a blueprint that includes sequenced instructional objectives and the instructional events that set up students to meet these goals, and we must also make the plan—the structure—visible to students (p. 108). According to Grady and Davis, the course syllabus can provide the necessary framework for an online course (p. 109). This instructional strategy of "scaffolding" the online environment, to use their architecture metaphor (p. 102), informs our ideas for adapting course materials to be used for the presentational aspect of our online courses. In short, scaffolding is a necessary prior activity for informed practice. Therefore, even though we consider the individual nature of course materials in this chapter, we encourage instructors to have a framework in place before they apply the method of analysis we provide, a framework that demonstrates the relationship between course goals, activities, and learning units, as presented on syllabi and within the learning units of a course management system, as illustrated in Figures 1–3.

Figure 1 illustrates the first two pages of a print-based document designed originally for an on-site course. The first page foregrounds logistical information like meeting times and places, required textbooks, and prerequisites. The document consequently relies more heavily on instructor presentation for emphasis. Not until page 2 do descriptions of learning goals and activities appear as well as a description of the online learning environment itself; and the overall presentation relies heavily on a default layout of a single column of 12pt type with one-inch margins. Figure 2, by contrast, reveals a more significant redesign that begins to reflect the second phase of adaptation to a course management system.

The page layout now resembles a web page layout. Page one contains a navigation bar to the left and a column of text occupying a more central location, and page two presents a 2-column design with greater differentiation between headings and body text, making the document easier to navigate. The document consequently relies less on instructor presentation for emphasis. The logistical information has been filtered into the bar on the left, and the course goals and activities are foregrounded on the first page. The corresponding learning units are now outlined on page 2, and considerable space is filtered and devoted to a description of the interactive online environment. More substantive descriptions of learning units have been moved up to page 2, descriptions that will correspond directly to the sequential learning units on the course web page, as illustrated in Figure 3.

We have known for a long time that the shape of text on a page differs from text on a screen. Bernhardt (1993) discusses nine key traits of on-screen text, while noting the virtues and drawbacks of both and the way they influence each other. Bernhardt's analysis helps us to recognize that screen text is situationally embedded and increasingly modular. In the first case, the screen text often calls upon readers to perform specific tasks that are part of a larger activity, and the computer is well-suited to scaffold that level of interactivity. Related to that, the higher level of modularity tends to chunk, filter, and queue text in ways that facilitate such tasks, though they may suffer from fragmentation. Print text remains better suited to longer, more complex readings that call for a linear progression.

Figure 3 illustrates the Web-based view of the Assignments area of the course management system where the learning units directly correspond to activities and units listed in the course syllabus. In sum, the redesigned syllabus and course web page depict a more visible framework in which students can observe the relationships between learning goals and individual assignments, and it becomes even more important to foreground such relationships in online courses.

Focus on the Assignment Sheet

Ideally, then, instructors use a backward design to construct the architecture of their courses, a structure focused on long-term goals and that establishes

Writing in the Social and Natural Sciences
Online ENGL 213-801: Course Syllabus — Fall 2007

Professor: Dr. Jacqueline Cason **My Office Phone:** 786-4367 **Office Fax:** 786-4383	*Office:* Professional Studies Building 208B (formerly "K") **English Dept.:** 786-4355 **Email:** <u>DrJ@uaa.alaska.edu</u>	*Contact:* e-mail; Blackboard Discussion; appointment; scheduled hours T-Th 12:00-2:00

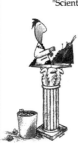

"Scientific writing, in its broadest sense, is quite likely the most triumphant, the most imitated, the most universal form of human discourse ever developed 'after Babel.' During the past 100 years, it has risen to a glorified preeminence over all other styles of written communication, having become the model of authority and presumed accuracy to which nearly all forms of expression have increasingly turned for 'advice.' As an enormous library of individual tongues that have adopted a single style of truth telling, 'the common language of science' (as Einstein called it) has evolved to a level where it seems as fully absolute, independent, self-justifying, and unassailable as the facts it claims to transmit. Indeed, it would be hard - perhaps impossible - to deny the impression that here lies the grand master narrative of modernism, ideally suited to its content. What sort of faith, then, might we say seems to beat at the heart of this discourse? Simply this: that language can be made a form of technology, a device able to contain and transfer knowledge *without touching it.*

~Scott L. Montgomery, *The Scientific Voice,* pp. 2-3

"[To] train young people in the dialectic between orthodoxy and dissent is the unique contribution which universities make to society."

~Loren Eiseley, "The Illusion of Two Cultures"

Course Description: Instruction in writing based on close analysis of readings in the social and natural sciences. This course serves as an introduction and transition into the communication styles of your chosen profession or discipline. Students will gain knowledge of disciplinary writing practices by engaging in discussion and writing about the social, rhetorical, presentational, and stylistic dimensions of published research within their fields of study.

Text & Materials:
- **Required:** *The Chicago Guide to Communicating Science* (2003), by Scott L. Montgomery.
- **Required:** *A Brief Guide to Writing From Readings* (2004), 3rd edition, by Stephen Wilhoit.
- **Required:** Mountains Beyond Mountains (2004), by Tracy Kidder
- Recommended: *Publication Manual of the American Psychological Association,* 5th ed. [APA] or the publication manual for your particular discipline, e.g. CSE, CMS, etc.

Prerequisite for Course: Prerequisites are designed to encourage student success. I will be checking Wolflink for your eligibility in the course. Methods for demonstrating eligibility include
- a grade of C or better for English 111 (You may not be enrolled in 111 and 213 simultaneously)
- a Verbal SAT score of 620 or higher OR an ACT English score of 30 or higher

1

Figure 1. Phase One: Replacement Practice.
Screen shots of the first two pages of a syllabus originally designed
for an onsite course and minimally revised for an online course.

Learning Goals:
Students will learn that

- communication is contextual and occurs at the intersection of writer, reader, and publication;
- genres evolve through practice; therefore, the rules of effective writing are descriptive rather then prescriptive;
- writing styles arise out of a discourse community's particular ways of knowing; and
- citation practices (citing sources) in academic writing are the means of joining an ongoing conversation and a way of contributing something more to that conversation.

Learning Activities:
Students will

- manipulate sentence style, such as active and passive voice, nominalizations, conciseness, etc.
- read some research abstracts in the field of discourse analysis;
- investigate the social context, rhetorical approaches, and writing genres in a specific discipline;
- read and review a book that addresses the social dimensions of scientific research and empirical ways of knowing; and
- compose such documents as syntheses, abstracts, and an experimental analysis of a peer-reviewed academic journal and research articles within.

Blackboard: We will use Blackboard as the platform for the course. Blackboard will be your access to many of the assigned readings and to subsequent writing assignments. I will ask you to use Blackboard in six primary ways in this course: 1) To check announcements at least 3-4x each week; 2) To follow the learning units for each set of assignments in the course; 3) To access readings and submit assignments; 4) To engage in collaborative projects; 5) To contact classmates and to participate in written discussions; and 3) To find links to relevant resources and websites. Occasionally, this platform will go down due to technical difficulties. It usually comes back up within a short amount of time. You will never be penalized due to Blackboard outages. If you are not sure whether it is the system or your computer, you can call the IT Services Helpdesk at (907) 786-4646, email them at callcenter@uaa.alaska.edu or check their webpage: http://technology.uaa.alaska.edu to discover the status of the system.

Virtual Participation Policy—Greater Than the Sum of its Parts

> *What life have you if you have not life together? There is no life that is not in community.*
> ~ **T.S. (Thomas Stearns) Eliot (1888–1965)**

Though you may be sitting all alone at your computer right now, you're connected to a larger group just the same as if we were all in the classroom together at this moment. I need your virtual presence in class: I need your energy, your questions, and your insights. Interacting, connecting, and engaging in the activities of a dynamic community will help you understand the course material better and remember it long after the semester is over. Because this is a 3-credit course, I expect you to **log on to the course at least 3 times a week and check your e-mail at least 3 times a week as well.** Many major assignments include specific participation activities that will earn you points. The following table describes the many ways that you can be present in the course:

English 213/ Cason/ 2

Figure 1. (Cont'd.)

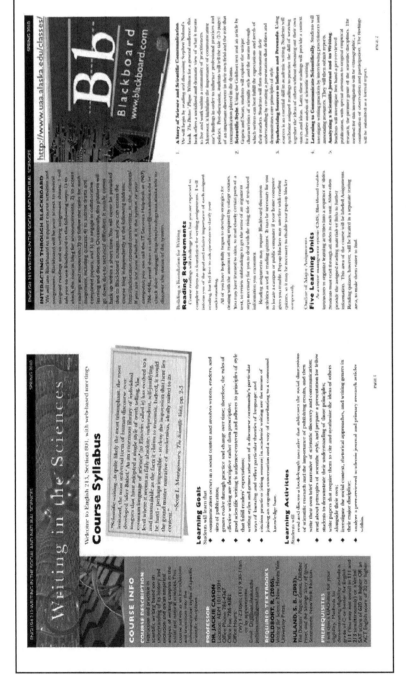

Figure 2. Phase Two: Sequential Learning Unit.
Screen shots of the first two pages of a syllabus significantly redesigned for an online course.

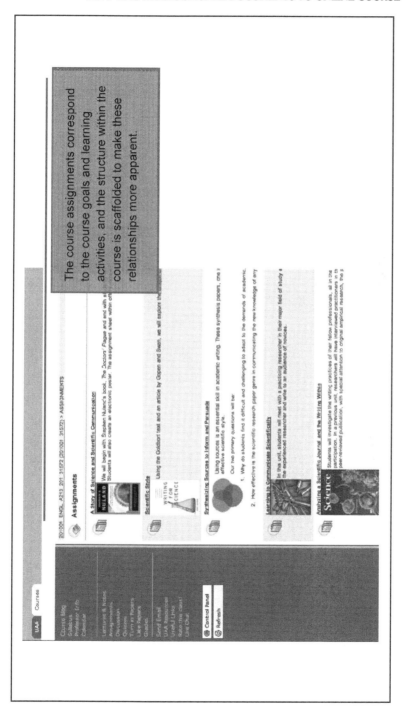

Figure 3. Phase Two: Sequential Learning Unit.
Screen shot of the Assignment Area within a course management system.

incremental activities designed to facilitate those learning goals. In other words, the backward design begins with learning goals, with the understandings that students should remember long after the course has concluded. After establishing long-term goals, instructors devise assessment strategies and learning activities that will lead to the achievement of specific goals. As Fink (2005) clearly explains, we begin first with course design and destination and then work backward from end goals to devise the student-teacher interactions that will get us to our destination. In a forward-designed course, instructors begin with individual assignments and plans for student-teacher interaction and then establish summative assessment strategies to determine whether goals have been achieved. Ideally, instructors create assessment strategies from the outset that are formative as well as summative. To that end, courses will have syllabi, policies, assigned reading documents, assignment sheets, discussion prompts, and evaluative commentary.

One type of document that stands out as pivotal in any course is the assignment sheet, a set of instructions that provide a link between course goals and assessments and that guide student performance. Moreover, the assignments occupy a significant amount of an instructor's time, and they locate instructors at their most presentational moment. Because they occupy a central role in course design, we are examining the instructional documents commonly known as the "assignment sheet" and the ways these evolve over time as instructors continually adapt them to online environments. We plan to examine textual features, composing and reading practices, and the social roles embedded within them.

The course materials we examine are from a general education course called English 213: Writing in the Social and Natural Sciences. This course uses an inquiry-based approach for teaching students to read and to write an original research report, as demonstrated in the primary scientific literature of their chosen discipline. Rather than telling students how to write a report step-by-step, the course guides students through the process of discovering empirically the way that such reports are written. In sum, students study scientific writing socially and scientifically by reading stories of discovery and by investigating and collecting data on publication contexts, article structure and design, sentence style, and citation practices. On our campus, the student cohort for the course draws heavily on the biomedical sciences, with several pre-nursing majors. Moreover, both the fields of nursing and social work have changed in the last couple of decades from a focus on clinical practice wisdom to a stronger emphasis on scholarly research and evidence-based practice, and our colleagues in other departments expect students to be familiar with the primary scientific literature, though many students have never encountered scholarly databases and journals prior to enrollment in this course.

Analysis Phase One: Replacement Practice

In phase one, we found ourselves scrambling on short notice to replace the classroom setting with an online learning space or course management system

(CMS) in which instructional assignment sheets could be posted as word-processing documents, much as they had once appeared in the on-site classroom environment as printed handouts. In other words, we began by doing some of what Grady and Davis (2005) warned against by uploading face-to-face handouts without fully enriching the online context in which they would appear to compensate sufficiently for the performance opportunities that face-to-face classrooms naturally provide. In fact, many on-site classroom instructors already post rather than print their documents (guided by formal departmental policies established to save the cost of paper copies), so these course documents may already be online at the time when instructors decide to teach online. Hence, the quickest step toward online teaching may be simply to copy course content from one CMS shell to another. This tendency toward replacement practice is often shaped by the *absence* of faculty development opportunities, workloads that acknowledge the need for time to develop online courses, and realistic timelines for going online.

Textual Features of Replacement Practice Course Materials

The textual features of online and on-site assignment sheets—margins, spacing, text size, headings, fonts—were very similar in this early phase of adaptation. Most of our documents included three levels of heading with sections on assignment overview, assignment goals in relation to course goals, and enumerated step-by-step instructions for completing the required learning activities designed to meet those goals. In other words, both on-site and online assignment sheets were designed for usability with information in discrete chunks and queued according to a deliberate hierarchy of information, each based on the conventions of printed textual communications. Moreover, the written components now included ancillary documents and online announcements that functioned to replace the synchronous oral explanation common in the on-site classroom. That is, written components had become longer and more numerous, and our assignment sheets were now accompanied by annotated models and examples for illustration, which once had been offered more dialogically during guided classroom practice. Essentially, we replaced oral communication modes with textual modes only. Additionally, our documents were distributed in multiple formats (.doc, .rtf, .pdf) to increase the ease of access.

Composing Practices for Replacement Practice Course Materials

Composing practices in the Replacement Practice phase were similar to those used for composing assignment sheets in face-to-face classes, relying heavily on word-processing technologies. However, as suggested above, a concern for document usability guided the composing process in a way that it may not have in a face-to-face classroom, and we spent more time annotating models to contextualize the documents. Usability concerns itself with the ease with which a user (student) can achieve a particular goal as a result of using a particular tool or document. Therefore, the instructor engages in the art of information design. The instructor is potentially constrained by lack of knowledge of his/her users though enabled through user and task analysis.

Reading Practices of Replacement Practice Course Materials

Reading practices required of students in Replacement Practice courses were similar to those in face-to-face courses except that interactions between instructor and student about assignments did not take place in the same way. Students needed to take the initiative as readers because the practice of posting assignment sheets online built an expectation that students would download and save those documents on their own storage device, print and annotate them as part of the critical reading process, and ask electronic questions when the written words did not suffice. They were expected to respond to instructions and models in imitative ways to produce their own technical documents offline and then upload their documents to the CMS, much as they would submit assignments in class. In fact, online and on-site classes functioned similarly in their emphasis on print-based documents composed and read from an 8.5 × 11 inch page view with a 3:4 vertical aspect ratio. To read a page-view document on the screen requires scrolling, so many readers opt to print out documents for reading offline. By contrast, screen-view documents generally offer a 4:3 horizontal aspect ratio. Content in the screen view is chunked to fit within the dimensions of a typical computer monitor (either 800 × 600 pixels or 1024 × 768 pixels), without the same need for scrolling. However, screen-view documents may require a lot more paper for printing. In replacement practice courses, both faculty and students worked primarily with word-processing documents while transferring those documents though the CMS. The CMS in this way functioned more as a site of transfer than as a site of interaction, with each party working on documents from a vertical page view and transferring them via access and submission points on the screens of their computers.

Social Roles of Instructor and Student in Replacement Practice Courses

Although both student and instructor were accessing and posting documents from the screen environment of their computers or mobile devices, with visual navigational cues, the communication and social roles remained heavily mediated by a view of the printed page. Little to no oral speech existed. When posted electronic assignment sheets were not being performed orally in a classroom setting, and when nonverbal cues that customarily invite dialogue were absent, both students and instructors relied on typed alphabetic text to achieve clarity and purpose. The social roles of instructors and students therefore tended to be somewhat fragmented in Replacement Practice courses. While print-based assignment sheets composed and read in a page view enabled a cognitive value similar in both online and on-site settings, the instructor's cognitive role in guiding learning activities was severed from the instructor's affective and performative roles. Social roles were thus constrained by our assignment sheets when mediated strictly through printed alphabetic text, a situation that restricted opportunities for instructors and students to integrate cognitive, affective, and performative roles.

Analysis Phase Two:
Sequential Learning Unit

In the second phase of adaptation, as we grew more comfortable and familiar with our course management system and the visual perspective of the online screen view, we began to adapt word-processing to a Sequential Learning Unit in the CMS.

Textual Features of Sequential Learning
Unit Course Materials

A Sequential Learning Unit, like the one provided by Blackboard's CMS, may contain any number of items and operates as a series of slides through which readers navigate one by one. Textual features of a sequential learning unit—levels of headings, spacing, text size, fonts—resembled the documents in the Replacement Practice phase. However, the slides of the Sequential Learning Unit were chunked to fill the screen with minimal scrolling. The content was oriented to a horizontal 4:3 aspect ratio and framed on the left by the course's navigational menu. As with hyperlinks in a text-based document, learning unit slides also contained links to resources outside the web page. Unlike text-based documents, however, the learning unit slides now contained embedded ancillary documents and models that popped up into a new window, offering a set of layers not available in Replacement Practice documents. Assignment sheets were situationally embedded in slides and more closely connected to online task performance. To avoid discrepancies between slides and documents, assignment instructions no longer included due dates; instead, that type of information was found only in the course calendar. The slides, then, were designed more for onscreen readability rather than usability as in the Replacement Practice phase. The result was a continued proliferation of alphabetic text, with page-view assignment sheets now embedded within the screen-view documents in an online environment.

Composing Practices for Sequential Learning Unit Course Materials

The composing processes in the Sequential Learning Unit phase were similar to those used in the Replacement Practice phase because we began with an existing print document, but we copy/pasted chunks of text directly from the document onto the CMS learning unit and gradually began to revise the text style, color, font, size, and graphics to accommodate the layout differences in the screen view. In other words, we found ourselves continuing to post word-processing assignment sheets as they already existed in the previous phase for the sake of offline reference while simultaneously chunking information slide-by-slide and adapting it visually for a screen rather than page view. The WYSIWYG (what you see is what you get) editor works with some browsers and not others, so it became almost necessary to learn html code when composing in the text boxes provided by the CMS. Our experience was that the technology was driving many of our choices in creating assignment sheets. A couple of consequences of revising directly in the CMS was that our assignment sheets no longer existed fully independent of the CMS environment, rendering them susceptible to loss or corruption unless we were sure to archive all of our courses from semester to semester. Just last semester one of our courses disappeared as our campus upgraded our CMS, and all of the revisions for that semester were lost. As we continued to revise learning units, we had to be careful to revise print-based assignment sheets to correspond accurately if we were to continue embedding them within learning unit slides. The experience of composing directly in the CMS environment was that we found ourselves constrained by its rigidity and chal-lenged by the proliferation and redundancy of slides and documents.

Reading Practices of Sequential Learning Unit Course Materials

With Sequential Learning Unit assignments, students were expected to read things online rather than from a printed page. The sequential access slowed down the process and encouraged students to pause as long as they needed to read the words. When reading on the screen rather than from a page, it is much more difficult for students to print their assignments. In fact, the CMS we used has no printer-friendly option for learning units, though some students reported that they preferred to read offline and therefore printed a series of screen views one slide at a time and thereby converted the Sequential Learning Unit into a printed text-based version of the assignment. However, because instructors can choose to either force sequential reading or allow students to navigate through chunks of materials in nonlinear ways by viewing all contents at a glance and navigating to any slide in the learning unit, students' reading practices may vary considerably. Thus, student reading practices for assignments within learning units were enabled by the opportunity to read assignment directions in discrete chunks of text with enhanced color and graphics and displayed on a screen rather than page. On the other hand, their reading practices were constrained by the fact that they may not have recognized the need to click past the overview description to enter the unit and proceed slide-by-slide with the specific instructions. Our particular courses enabled students to access a content view and read in nonlinear ways, but with that freedom came the responsibility for reading comprehensively. At a minimum, students were three clicks from the entry page of the course to the learning unit contents and had to click several times more to work through the sequence of slides. These constraints encouraged or required students to do more of their reading online. As with hyperlinks in a text document, the screen views from within the learning unit also have the capacity to link to locations within and outside the online course.

Social Roles of Instructor and Student in Sequential Learning Units Courses

The instructor's cognitive and performative roles remained distinct from one another in this phase of adaptation, not yet integrated, though we began to shift our time more toward the online screen interface rather than the printed document, and our assignment instructions were less accessible when the technology was down for repairs. The relationship and social roles of both the instructor and students were now mediated through the CMS, though students could still work with print-based documents offline, and the roles relied more on the integrity of the system to perform as promised. The instructor necessarily became more managerial in monitoring the system and had to work to help solve technological problems or direct students to the proper technology support systems in the event that they could not access items.

Analysis Phase Three: Multimodal Turn

The first two phases of adapting assignment sheets from on-site to online learning environments either relied on or began with print-based documents. However, the next phase marked a more significant shift from print-based documents to multimedia documents, from a page view to a screen view that was composed and could be accessed independently of the institutional CMS. In the process of adapting to online environments, we began turning aside from word-processing software as we provided assignment instructions to our students. The multimodal text integrated words, sounds, and images, and allowed us to merge alphabetic text with the sound of our voice and a view of ourselves and the screen that now defined our interaction. The multimodal instructions were no longer foregrounding alphabetic representations, though words clearly continued to play a role as spoken or written on the screen.

Textual Features of Multimodal Course Materials

The textual features of assignment instructions in a multimodal class included words, sounds, and images in a time-based medium. We no longer limited ourselves to documents in the traditional sense; that is, they were not limited to static, word-processed items that could be printed. Instead, they now included an integration of communication modalities. Because of this integration of modalities, "textual features" became a problematic category because it no longer referred to alphanumeric text alone but also to oral and visual modalities whose temporal sequence was not simply imposed as with a learning unit but inherent in the message modality itself. For example, a QuickTime movie created with the Screenflow authoring program will simultaneously capture screen shots of alphabetic text or web pages as well as the image and voice of the computer user guiding the screen capture. Similarly, a QuickTime movie created with a presentation program like Keynote may simultaneously include printed slides interspersed with video and voiceover. In both cases, the linear flow of information derives from the more dramatic voice and presence of the instructor rather than an imposed sequence of words on page or screen. That is, multimodal authoring tools now offered a stronger performative platform that was inclined toward narrative, where we could better establish storylines and subject positions. Redundancy remained in the sense that print-based assignment sheets still existed alongside the multimodal texts, but the multimodal texts now functioned more like a classroom performance.

Composing Practices for Multimodal Course Materials

The composing process in this phase called for a variety of practices, ranging from assembling multimodal assets (images, sounds, words) to mapping a storyboard and script, to recording, editing, and exporting the performance. Composing was guided less by usability and readability in a traditional sense and more by our sense of performing for a remote audience. Therefore, this was by far the more difficult transition for us because it required us to move outside our comfort zones and familiar composing environments and closer to a screen-based medium with which many students are already familiar. Composing in multimedia was like learning to do everything over again, opposite-handed. It was very different to work with voice-overs, music, still images, and video and to learn to layer it onto a timeline.

Multimodal composing was much less likely to serve as a form of replacement practice for text-based communications, and it was more in accord with students' use of technology in their personal lives. It is worth noting that both of us came to teaching with a strong orientation toward print-based composing. Our status was linked to the primacy of alphabetic print-based literacies. We were familiar with words—how to generate them, organize them, and present them to an audience in a specific context for a specific purpose. In spite of the challenges that rapid change in communication technologies has presented, we were able to watch our composing practices adapt to the new medium. It has been a gradual process of letting go and learning new strategies. Some of the skills of sequencing and transition transferred to an extent, as do notions of coherence, but it truly was a new experience in juxtaposition. Alphabetic texts have long had an audiovisual aspect, but even a term like "transition" became more complex than a sentence or two between paragraphs when we thought about moving between frames.

The composing process for multimedia texts was transformed from the print-based page-view environment to a timeline screen-view environment that was more compatible with online learning. Instead of working exclusively from a page-oriented view, we began to work within a screen view and timeline. Figure 4 illustrates the multimedia composing environment as distinct from the multimedia viewing environment for the presentation program Keynote and the screen-capture program Screenflow. The viewing environment appeared the same for both because each was exported as a QuickTime movie. But the composing environment was quite different: Keynote looks more like the slides of a PowerPoint program, while Screenflow has a more apparent timeline that allows authors to edit vertical layers as well as horizontal sequencing.

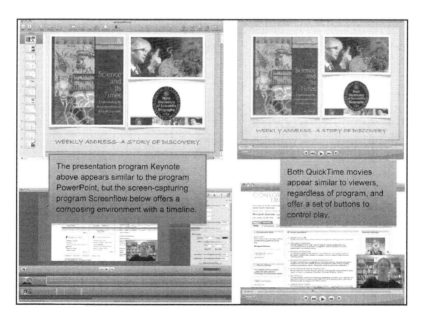

Figure 4. Screen shots of composing environments in contrast with viewing perspectives.

Both sets of images depict an assignment demonstration: the top level a narrative of scientific discovery and the bottom level a method for researching library databases and periodical literature. The top images show the slide presentation program Keynote, and the bottom images show the screen-capturing program Screenflow, capable of simultaneously capturing the screen and the computer user in the frame. From the viewers' QuickTime perspective, the movies play the same, but from the composers' view, the authoring experience is quite different.

Consequently, we were now more conscious of time elapsing for our students because we could quantify the duration of each movie and even more conscious of the time it took to compose effectively because we had to script our oral presentations, compose them, and then spend further time editing before posting to our courses.

Reading Practices of Multimodal Course Materials

Students were able to view assignment instructions online, perhaps from a laptop or even from a mobile computing device on a small screen. They could access our multimedia documents through a free movie player like QuickTime or Windows Media Player, which could be embedded in the CMS, posted on a course blog, or distributed through a designated YouTube channel. They were not able to navigate as easily through different parts of the document, so it became necessary for us to chunk our information into clips of shorter duration that could easily be viewed several times.

Students were able not only to view us speaking to them but to view the assignment instructions or web pages that became part of the assignment. As the Screenflow images in Figure 4 above demonstrate, students could witness directly what it was like to visit and conduct research within the electronic library as they worked on their assignments instead of relying exclusively on written alphabetic instructions, which they had then to imagine as an image of the screen. At the same time, they could see our face and listen to our voice as we guided them through the process of completing an assignment.

It is also worth noting at this point that as we analyzed the textual, composing, and reading practices through each phase of our own online teaching development, it became apparent that the phases were not exclusive. As Figure 5 demonstrates, all three types of documents coexisted within a course—print-based documents, Sequential Learning Units, and multimodal texts. We therefore wish to underscore the co-presence of all three phases; a co-presence analogous to the enriched environment of an on-site classroom where instructors observe and listen to students and engage in dialogue, where they perform their assignment instructions and guide students through incremental practice that leads to increasing independence. The print-based document at the top of the figure is

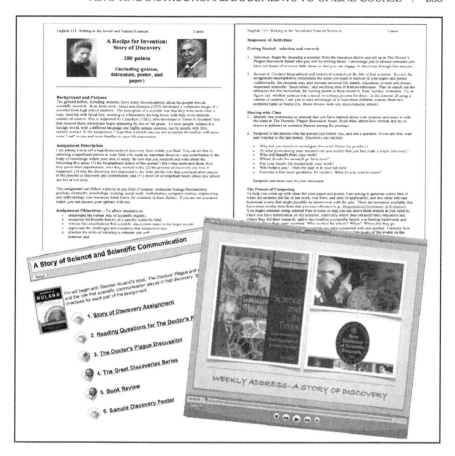

Figure 5. Screen shots demonstrating a progression and layering
of print-based documents, learning units, and multimedia
texts for a single assignment.

designed for printing or physical distribution. The Sequential Learning Unit in the bottom left serves to distribute documents, chunk instructions, and provide supplemental resources. The multimodal text performs and demonstrates the assignment. This level of integration shaped the variety of roles that we as instructors were playing as we discuss in the next section.

Social Roles of Instructor and Student in Multimodal Courses

This third phase we have identified—the turn toward multimodal texts—is still in process in our courses, but we began to see that it offered us the possibility of integrating our roles as we instructed students on the steps for completing learning activities and producing their own documents. While alphabetic text lends itself to the development of complex rational arguments, it does not do full justice to nonverbal modes of thought. The more abstract nature of print privileges the cognitive and rational over the affective and emotional, and this is likely the reason we experienced a fragmentation of our cognitive, affective, and performative roles. In a multimedia environment, our cognitive and performative roles were reunited when we composed our assignment instructions. We became a voice and an actor upon the screen, where we could unite our managerial and facilitator roles with our cognitive and performative roles. The next step for us is to provide students with similar authoring tools and to incorporate more interactive programs (VOIP, Voice Over Internet Protocol) like Skype or iChat. To date, our CMS software, Elluminate Live, has presented too many barriers across operating systems and browsers to be fully functional for real-time interaction.

CONCLUSION

The method of genre analysis of Paré and Smart (1994) has provided a heuristic that helped us answer the questions with which we began and to identify three distinct phases of adaptation that could inform further faculty development. It is important to answer these questions because they will enable instructors to make choices informed by pedagogy and to be less constrained by institutional decisions about technology. These questions lead instructors to become more conscious of the textual properties of not only their assignment instructions but also their other course documents, their composing practices, and the way these shape student reading practices; they make it more likely that instructors can integrate their various roles within the classroom instead of being fragmented persons forever trying to put the pieces back together in a coherent fashion.

So what does it mean to adapt materials so that they are suitable for an online course, and how do instructors adapt these materials over time? One thing our examination has revealed is that we are going to continue to exist in a world of alphabetic text, building on that familiar terrain while venturing into new territory. Skills we have developed over the course of our teaching careers will remain vital and will transfer as we develop new skills for communicating in an online environment. It will take patience to adapt our materials incrementally, beginning with what we know and building upon that foundation. Many of our skills will transfer, yet inevitably we will spend time in both worlds, working to make old documents fit the new environment. As we continue to inhabit an emerging online environment and to compose from within that context, we have begun to see that online spaces present a multimodal environment in which alphabetic texts remain a meaningful part, and we can glimpse the possibilities that other modalities afford. Though our institutions may invest heavily in training us to use a centralized course management system to recapitulate what we do in the on-site classroom, adapting our documents to the online environment does not necessarily mean that we must subscribe to such a system. The time spent learning a complex CMS might be better spent learning to aggregate and organize our materials in other ways and to select the software programs appropriate to our disciplines, those that enable us to merge word, sound, and image in a time-based medium. The choices we make should ultimately be guided by our course goals and content and not by centralized decisions, and we can use these arguments to persuade our institutions to invest in training that is more discipline specific.

When teaching online and creating instructional materials for an online environment, instructors should be informed by the notion that we have the composing tools to integrate our roles, even in the online classroom. The online classroom need not be "a neutralized version of the real time, real space" of the on-site classroom (Farber, 2008, p. 217). We can instead reinvent our classroom persona in ways that allow us to create documents rich with our presence, our voice, and our passion. Multimedia composing is both performative and affective. Moreover, we should be informed by an awareness of the reading and composing practices of students themselves. We must be tuned into their developing literacies as we develop our own. The multimedia language of the screen has become the current vernacular; and it can communicate thoughts and complex meanings that are different from and independent of alphabetic text. In sum, to teach online, or in the classroom, is to inhabit the multimedia spaces our students take for granted and to grow familiar and more comfortable with the means and tools for accessing and creating content in that environment.

REFERENCES

Bernhardt, S. (1993). The shape of text to come: The texture of print on screens. *College Composition and Communication, 44*(2), 151–175.

Cargile Cook, K. (2005). An argument for pedagogy-driven online education. In K. Cargile Cook & K. Grant-Davie (Eds.), *Online education: Global questions, local answers* (pp. 49–66). Amityville, NY: Baywood.

Carr, S. (2000). As distance education comes of age, the challenge is keeping the students. *The Chronicle of Higher Education, 46*(23), A39–A41.

Carter, L., & Rickly, R. (2005). Mind the gap(s): Modeling space in online education. In K. Cargile Cook & K. Grant-Davie (Eds.), *Online education: Global questions, local answers* (pp. 123–139). Amityville, NY: Baywood.

Coppola, N. W. (2005). Changing roles for online teachers of technical communication. In K. Cargile Cook & K. Grant-Davie (Eds.), *Online education: Global questions, local answers* (pp. 89–99). Amityville, NY: Baywood.

Farber, J. (2008). Teaching and presence. *Pedagogy: Critical Approaches to Teaching Literature, Language, Composition, and Culture, 8*(2), 215–225.

Fink, L. D. (2005). A self-directed guide to designing courses for significant learning. Retrieved from http://www.deefinkandassociates.com/GuidetoCourseDesign Aug05.pdf

Grady, H. M., & Davis, M. (2005). Teaching well online with instructional and procedural scaffolding. In K. Cargile Cook & K. Grant-Davie (Eds.), *Online education: Global questions, local answers* (pp. 101–122). Amityville, NY: Baywood.

Paré, A., & Smart, G. (1994). Observing genres in action: Towards a research methodology. In A. Freedman & P. Medway (Eds.), *Genre and the new rhetoric* (pp. 146–154). London, England: Taylor & Francis.

Rude, C. (2005). Strategic planning for online education: Sustaining students, faculty, and programs. In K. Cargile Cook & K. Grant-Davie (Eds.), *Online education: Global questions, local answers* (pp. 67–85). Amityville, NY: Baywood.

White, E. (2007). *Assigning, responding, evaluating: A writing teacher's guide* (4th ed.). Boston, MA: St. Martin's.

Winters, K. (2010). Quilts of authorship: A literature review of multimodal assemblage in the field of literacy education. *Canadian Journal for New Scholars in Education, 3*(1), 1–12. Retrieved from http://www.cjnse-rcjce.ca/ojs2/index.php/cjnse/article/view/161/106

http://dx.doi.org/10.2190/OE2C12

CHAPTER 12

Expanding the Scaffolding of the Online Undergraduate Technical Communication Course

Dan Jones

One of the most widely used learning management systems in American colleges and universities, Webcourses or WebVista, has compounded the challenges for both online instructors and their students because it allows numerous options for developers, instructors, students, and administrators. To illustrate the complexity and variety of available tools, Figure 1 overviews the common tools associated with Webcourses.

On our campus (both the main campus and our many regional campuses), instructors differ widely in the online tools they use, and of course, this is the same practice at many other college campuses. Many instructors supplement their courses with tools not offered by Webcourses, for example, using PowerPoint accompanied by video and audio, screen-capture video, wikis, podcasts, social networking sites such as Facebook and MySpace, YouTube, and iTunes U, to mention only some of the more popular ones. Blogging and journal features were recently added to the discussions area of Webcourses and offer additional options for instructors on our campus. I have used YouTube as part of discussion topics requiring students, for example, to find and discuss various video accounts of Exxon Valdez, Three Mile Island, the two space shuttle disasters, and Apollo 13. Podcasts have been used by others to replace handwritten comments on student assignments.

As a whole, these additional tools offer limitless possibilities for the online environment, and the future for teaching online courses looks more promising

237

Organization Tools

- Calendar: Enter important events and deadlines, and allow students to enter their own events.
- Search: Search for content in the course.
- Syllabus: Provide course requirements, objectives, and policies.

Communication Tools

- Announcements: Post important information in a central location.
- Chat: Chat with other users in the course in real time, or use the Whiteboard to display images.
- Discussions: Post and respond to messages on specific topics.
- Mail: Send messages to other users.
- Roster: List students enrolled and group members for any groups.
- Who's Online: Chat with other users who are logged in to the Learning System.

Student Learning Activities

- Assessments: Create quizzes, self-tests, and surveys.
- Assignments: Create assignments for students to submit online.
- Goals: Create goals that list the qualitative and quantitative performance expected in the course.

Content Tools

- Learning Modules: Organize and present content and activities to students.
- Local Content: Allow students to easily access large files from a portable medium, such as CD-ROM.
- Media Library: Create a glossary or image collection.
- Web Links: Create links to Internet resources.

Student Tools

- My Files: Allow students to store their own files.
- My Grades: Allow students to check their grades.
- My Progress: Allow students to track their own progress.
- Notes: Allow students to take notes.

Figure 1. Common tools in Webcourses.
Source: Faculty Center for Teaching & Learning, University of Central Florida.

than ever before; however, limitless tool options can also result in excessively complicated and sometimes confusing course environments. Based on my 15 years of experience in teaching online courses, my advice, especially for first-time instructors of online courses, is to make the structure of their online courses clear and simple for the students. The important goal is to make all of this structure as transparent as possible so that even students new to learning online will have little difficulty in finding what they need to find to learn what they need to learn using the tools provided.

Others have commented on this need for transparency. In "Teaching Well Online with Instructional and Procedural Scaffolding," Helen Grady and Marjorie Davis (2005) define scaffolding "as those strategies that a teacher uses to help learners span a cognitive gap or leap a learning hurdle" (p. 103). They discuss the scaffolding metaphor, noting that the scaffolding used to help construct a building is removed when the work is completed. It is not an essential part of the building itself. The scaffolding metaphor is an apt one for developing online classes because, as Grady and Davis suggest, "It's this image of a structural support system that provides help, strength, assistance, protection, guidance, and capability to the learning community as it works to build the shared knowledge that is the online course" (pp. 103–104).

They suggest that a different type of scaffolding must be constructed for the online course consisting of two elements: instructional scaffolding and procedural scaffolding; the former involving strategies for increasing the interactive nature of teaching and learning, and the latter helping students manage the online learning environment. Or, as Grady and Davis (2005) state from the point of the view of the student, for instructional scaffolding, students "want to know explicitly what they will be learning as well as the benefits of learning activities" (p. 108), and for procedural scaffolding the focus is on "*how* students will interact and learn the course content" (p. 115, italics in original quote).

The authors discuss helpful strategies for both types of scaffolding. Topics they discuss for instructional scaffolding include effective use of the Web in links in a syllabus, dividing the course into the appropriate number of units for covering the content, creating appropriate assignments and deliverables, creating the learning space or "the look, feel, and usability of the course" (Grady & Davis, 2005, p. 113). And importantly, they discuss assessment and evaluation as part of this same scaffolding, including a brief mention of grading rubrics.

Concerning procedural scaffolding, they cover various strategies for creating a sense of community in the online classroom. They suggest that students create personal home pages, and they suggest that instructors maintain a class listserv, schedule online chats (preferably synchronous), have moderated discussions, follow interaction protocols, use discussion boards, and use teams whenever possible and create these teams carefully for aiding new students or for effective peer review. In sum, the authors provide a useful framework for further discussion.

In "Students in the Online Technical Communication Classroom," Angela Eaton (2005) also provides a useful framework for further discussion, one tied to establishing an effective ethos in online courses. She comments on advice students have for current and future instructors. The advice includes respecting the students' time by being careful about the time demands of course features, being explicit about the benefits of the course activities, and structuring due dates fairly; further, being involved in the online class through providing regular feedback and being personable; and structuring courses carefully, including choosing technology to serve pedagogy instead of the other way around by using multiple delivery methods within the course to support sound pedagogical purposes, being careful with hybrid courses, and being aware of departmental advertising and student expectations.

Eaton (2005) provides a good beginning list to building ethos in an online course. She reminds us that as we develop our online courses, we should always keep in mind how what we design will be perceived and used. Her advice on being personable is particularly telling: "To become more personable, instructors can use student names and give explicit compliments. Good online instructors will use every technique good traditional classroom instructors use but will use them more frequently and perhaps more consciously" (p. 40).

In this chapter, I make a case for three additional ways the scaffolding of the typical online undergraduate technical communication course can be expanded to improve the online learning experience for instructors and students. In the first part of this chapter, I suggest that a system of folders can work just as effectively as the more commonly used linear walk-through learning modules. In the second part, I show how well-designed evaluation rubrics can be a helpful element for any good online learning space. In the third or final part, I show that instructors must continually work on establishing and maintaining a strong ethos throughout the duration of their online courses.

USING A SYSTEM OF FOLDERS

In this section, after discussing some of the reasons learning modules are widely used, I discuss an alternative of a system of folders and its advantages.

Learning Modules

Many instructors choose to use learning modules to help students walk through a particular assignment or group of assignments on one module for one week, several weeks, or even more. Individual modules can be as simple or as complex as instructors have the skill to make them. At their simplest, modules might provide brief overviews of each weekly topic and include a link to a quiz on the reading, for example. At a more complex level, modules might provide a detailed overview or introduction for the particular topic, a list discussing specific objectives for the module, at least several subtopics for the larger module topic, a review of the key points or activities, an overview of issues to be discussed in the separate discussions area, specific assignments, and separate reading assignments—all easily accessible in one place, typically, in the main menu of the course. See Figure 2 for a typical structure for an online course with learning modules.

When learning modules are well-designed, they are an excellent way to walk students through the course subject matter whether the content is broken into weekly, biweekly, monthly, or other combinations. For some, modules are the best substitute for the classroom lectures.

Standard learning modules have their advantages. Instructors can build on what they typically do in the traditional classroom with their lectures, they can control what students see and when they see it as well as control the pace of the course, and they can minimize confusion for students by simply requiring them to work their way through the modules. Students also typically appreciate the clear structure provided by a series of well-designed modules (when they are well-designed), they often feel a greater sense of progression as they work their way from module to module, and they can often see how they are meeting various course objectives as they complete each module.

A System of Folders

Although the learning modules tool in Webcourses makes it relatively easy to design and deliver standard learning modules, instructors can cover the course content using effective alternatives. Over the past 5 years, I have provided a system of easily accessible folders in the course content or main page area. I prefer using a system of folders over modules for a variety of reasons. I find it easier to build a system of folders than to build traditional modules (mapping out a series of detailed modules can require a great deal of time); folders can be easily maintained once built, they work easily and well with other features of Webcourses (for example, announcements, the calendar, reminders sent through e-mail, the Web Links feature), and they work easily with any of the many non-Webcourses tools mentioned earlier. As with the traditional modules approach, with a system of folders and sub-folders, instructors can cover material the way they would in course lectures, and they can control the pace of the course by releasing folders only when they are needed.

Additionally, as with traditional learning modules, relying on a system of folders requires keeping matters as simple as possible. To keep matters simple, I provide only two visible folders on the main page, one titled Course Information and one titled Class Assignments (see Figure 3).

The Course Information folder provides information about the course, while the Class Assignments folder provides handouts and other files concerning specific

```
                Introduction
                 Welcome
                 Syllabus
                Modules
                   Module 1 – Topic 1
                                Overview
                                Objectives
                                Readings
                                  Read Chapters 1 and 2
                                Discussions
                                  Post responses to prompts
                                Assignments
                                  Task 1 – Post Exercise 1
                                  Task 2 – Begin project draft
                                Resources

                   Module 2 – Topic 2
                                Overview
                                Objectives
                                Readings
                                Discussions
                                Assignments
                                  Task 1
                                  Task 2
                                Resources

                   Module 3 – Topic 3
                                Overview
                                Objectives
                                Readings
                                Discussions
                                Assignments
                                  Task 1
                                  Task 2
                                Resources

                   Module 4, etc.
                Discussions
                   Week 1 Topics
                   Week 2 Topics
                Course Resources
                   Web links
                   Articles, etc.
```

Figure 2. Typical structure for an online course with learning modules.

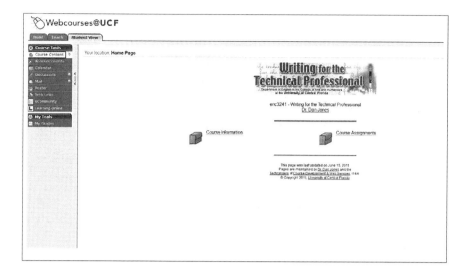

Figure 3. Two major folders on main page.
Source: Faculty Center for Teaching & Learning,
University of Central Florida.

assignments. In the Course Information folder, I provide the same kinds of handouts for all of the online classes I teach: the course syllabus, the weekly schedule, grading criteria, a blank worksheet for students to use for determining their course grade, a sample completed worksheet, an overview of the purpose of the discussions threads, the rubric I use for grading the discussion postings for the course, and protocols concerning online courses and good computer practices. In effect, all of these handouts concern the policies for the course. The second major folder, Class Assignments, consists of subfolders, and these vary depending on the course, but all concern work students will complete in the course. For my introductory technical communication course, for example, I provide one subfolder for each major class assignment: the Letter and Résumé, Instructions, the Report Option, and the Proposal Option (allowing students to choose to complete either a report or a proposal for their final assignment). Each of these subfolders contains other subfolders; for instance, Assignment Requirements, Sample Student Documents, and Sample Professional Documents.

For my more advanced undergraduate technical communication courses, I provide many more subfolders in the Class Assignments area: subfolders containing PowerPoint files highlighting important points from the reading, exercises concerning the reading, and handouts on research, to mention only a few.

This system of folders works well. Using a system of folders, instructors will find that online courses can be easily updated from semester to semester or year to year, revisions to any files can be made quickly during a particular semester, and folders and files can be easily available or hidden at particular points in the semester at least as readily as any can be in any modular approach. As for students, they can quickly find what they need, quickly download any necessary files and follow up with questions about specific handouts, and readily see an overall well-structured plan for the course.

Folders Combined With Other Course Tools

With folders, instructors can also easily build redundancy into the course. For example, the announcements tool can be used to let students know when any new handout is available or any due date is pending, and the calendars tool can be used to remind them what is due each week (in addition to the weekly schedule provided in a folder). I use the calendar tool extensively in my online courses, providing details concerning the reading assignments and other requirements by the day, week, and month. Students consulting the calendar regularly are able to see what they need to do each day of the course throughout the semester. The assignment handouts can also provide various due dates, including due dates for any drafts, peer reviews, and final versions. Students can also receive reminders about due dates through Webcourses mail.

Another way of looking at using a system of folders as discussed here is to recognize the folders as a different way to provide the content of the course. They provide less emphasis on detailed, linear modules, but still provide the content in an easily accessible and understandable way. If an instructor prefers, the content in these folders and subfolders can be built in the same fashion as traditional modules: introductions, objectives, subtopics, activities, and so on. So the two approaches are certainly not different online pedagogies, and importantly, the two can be combined to work together effectively. For example, students can access the basic modules in the main menu part of the course and access much of the same information or additional information through a clear and well-organized system of folders.

Folders and File Management

An ongoing problem for using a standard module approach or a system of folders approach or a combination of the two is file management. As even experienced instructors of online courses will admit, it can sometimes be difficult and time-consuming to keep track of the many different files that are typically uploaded by the instructor or instructional designer for an online course each semester. And the problem can be compounded if instructors are teaching several online courses each semester, as many do at our university. Also, using a system of folders and subfolders can generate quite a few files to keep organized.

A variety of approaches can be used to address this problem. Many instructors keep files generic and easily import all or most of the files unrevised with each new semester, and these are good approaches for those who prefer to use them. However, like many instructors, I constantly update most of my handouts from semester to semester and quite often while I am teaching the courses. For those who do the same, I recommend clearly naming each file with the course prefix and number, semester and year the handout is used, and a brief handout title. (For example, ENC 3241 Spring 2010 Syllabus or a slightly more abbreviated version for those who prefer simpler file titles: ENC3241Sp2010Syllabus.) As I make my updates, I just make sure I include the new semester and year as part of the file title so I know I am working with the latest copy of that particular handout. (This approach works better than relying on the date of the file.) I also backup these files in several ways offline (in addition to the backup features provided by Webcourses) so that I always have access to this important data.

A system of files, combined with a variety of helpful course tools, is only one way to make the online learning experience easier for both instructors and students. For those who need to find ways to make the grading easier, at least the grading of the online discussions, and more importantly, to help students learn from the assessment of their work, rubrics of various kinds can also be quite helpful.

USING EVALUATION RUBRICS

As I mentioned earlier, folders are one way to map out the virtual learning space for students. Evaluation rubrics are another. In this section, I briefly summarize some of the background concerning rubrics, discuss some of the major advantages and disadvantages of using them, discuss the typical applications of rubrics for assessing online discussion, provide some additional strategies for using rubrics for online courses, and discuss typical student reactions to rubrics.

History of Evaluation Rubrics

Evaluation rubrics have a long history for use at the K–12 and college levels. Maha Wilson's *Rethinking Rubrics in Writing Assessment* (2006) is the most recent controversial book-length study. Chapter 2 of her study, "There is a Cow in Our Classroom: How Rubrics Became Writing Assessment's Sacred Cow," offers a brief but helpful history of the rubric's gradual development. She cites Adams Sherman Hill, Harvard Professor of Rhetoric and Oratory, and the English Composition Card he developed around 1900 as one of the earliest examples. It seems Professor Hill was "annoyed by the increase in incorrect English usage he saw in new students," so he created "a list of stan-dardized abbreviations focusing almost exclusively on surface errors" (p. 16).

As Wilson observes, "With one broad stroke, Hill's English Composition Card answered the three urgent questions in writing assessment: how does one assess and rank students' writing fairly, quickly, and easily?" (p. 17) Of course, Wilson points out that "good writing is not simply grammatically correct" (p. 17) while also expressing her understanding of why such a rubric would be adopted.

Advantages and Disadvantages of Rubrics

The literature both in support of rubrics and critical of rubrics is plentiful. In Audrey Quinlan's (2006) helpful study, she points to five major advantages for using rubrics. They "provide students with expectations about what will be assessed"; "provide students with information on the standards that need to be met"; "provide students with indications of where they are in relation to goals"; "increase consistency in teacher ratings of performance, products, or understanding"; and "provide teachers with data to support grades" (p. 26). Other common advantages are that they can improve student performance, help students become more thoughtful about their work, reduce the amount of time instructors spend evaluating work, and are easy to use and explain.

Negative views of rubrics are easy to find too. While providing her helpful history of rubrics, Wilson is highly critical of their shortcomings, commenting that they "stripped . . . the complexity that breathes life into writing" (Wilson, 2006, p. 23). Alfie Kohn (2006) comments, "some observers criticize rubrics because they can never deliver the promised precision; judgments ultimately turn on adjectives that are murky and end up being left to the teacher's discretion" (p. 13). Kohn's larger concern is that the increased use of rubrics, especially in earlier levels of education than the college level, can lead to students more focused on the superficial in their writing and to teachers, if they agree to apply the same rubrics, who "check [their] judgment at the door" if they are "willing to accept and apply someone else's narrow criteria for what merits that rating" (p. 13).

While the debate about rubrics continues, their popularity continues to increase, and although they have their shortcomings, especially concerning assessing complex pieces of writing, they can be and have been used with some accuracy to assess other assignments. Rubrics are increasingly used online by many instructors as one of many ways of assessing performance for various assignments and activities for many courses in numerous disciplines. Resources concerning how to create rubrics for many purposes are widely available. In addition to Quinlan's (2006) book, Dannelle Stevens' *Introduction to Rubrics* (2005) and Judy Arter's *Creating and Recognizing Quality Rubrics* (2009) are especially helpful. Accessing good rubric Web sites, downloading and improving upon rubric templates, learning rubric-creating software, and becoming familiar with sample rubrics commonly used by others are just some of the many ways instructors can develop this particular tool. One of the better Web sites on rubrics in general is Rubrician.com available at http://www.rubrician.com/general.htm. Much of the content here is aimed at creating rubrics for K–12 education, but many of the ideas can be useful at the college level too.

One useful rubric software tool is Rubric Builder, available at http://www. rubricbuilder.on.ca/, a site that also provides other good resources on rubrics. Helpful rubrics are even available for determining the quality of online courses. The Web site Rubric for Online Instruction provides one particularly appealing model (see California, n.d.). Good cautionary advice is also available concerning the limitations of a variety of web resources and rubric creating software (Dornisch & McLoughlin, 2006).

Rubrics and Online Discussions

Rubrics can be used effectively for grading online discussion posts, and good research is available to support this point. In "Assessment and Collaboration in Online Learning," Karen Swan, Jia Shen, and Starr Roxanne Hiltz (2005) cite numerous sources, published over the past two decades, showing how students find online discussions more fair and democratic than traditional classroom discussions, how asynchronous discussions create "a certain mindfulness and reflection among students," how the ongoing discussions create a sense of community, and how "asynchronous online discussion is a particularly rich vehicle for supporting collaborative learning" (p. 47). The authors recommend creating rubrics, first, by "establishing the goal or goals of the discussion," second, by identifying "characteristics of messages that would support the established goal," and, third, "by taking each characteristic and specifying differing levels of performance for each and assigning scores for these" (pp. 48–49). They confirm that individual student discussion performance will be improved, but they express their concern that rubrics "may not ensure collaborative performance" (p. 50). They recommend developing rubrics that reward collaboration and suggest that instructors can reward students for extending or refuting other students' postings, for creating new and active discussion threads, and for smaller group discussions reward not only for individual contributions but also average the grade for the group contributions.

Of course, assessment of discussion posts can be done without rubrics by, for example, simply grading the number, frequency, and length of the posts. Webcourses will easily generate student reports on each student concerning the number and frequency of posts for each posting assignment. But many instructors want more quality from the posts and more value in posting them for the students. Well-designed rubrics are not only helpful for assessment purposes, but they are also good learning tools for students. Creating substantial rubrics takes time and can be a challenge, even though Webcourses provides a convenient tool for creating these grade forms, as many as are needed for various kinds of discussion posts, both individual and team discussions. Still, individual instructors in a variety of disciplines typically want to measure different things in the posts, and instructors often will want to measure different things for different posts within one course.

Strategies for Using Rubrics for Online Courses

As I mentioned earlier, numerous resources are available for designing good rubrics, and the topic is too complex to do it justice here. Still, I have found the following four strategies helpful for my purposes.

First, make students aware of the rubrics used in the course before using the rubrics to assess their work. One way to make students aware of the rubrics upfront is to make them available for the students to review before the first discussion posts are graded. (Some instructors require students to sign and return a form stating that they have carefully reviewed and understand all course policies and the general layout of the course, a requirement in addition to taking a student orientation quiz often used by instructors of online courses.) I post the rubric I use for the semester as a Word document in the Course Information folder so students can become familiar with my criteria before they make their first posting. This approach lets them know up front what is expected before they post and makes them be more careful about their postings from the outset. If necessary, I modify the discussion post rubric as the semester progresses.

Second, avoid using too many different rubrics. As I mentioned, I currently use only one rubric for the discussion posts in my online courses, and this rubric has served my purposes well (see Figure 4). I have expanded this particular rubric over the past few years, and now it is more specific than ever before, but my students seem to appreciate the additional details. Other instructors may prefer using a simpler rubric for their purposes. Students typically respond well to a rubric whether it is simple or more complex, as long as it is clear.

Third, make the rubrics fair. One way to make rubrics fair is to avoid deducting too many points for relatively minor weaknesses. Design the point system for the rubric so that it is possible to receive 90 to 100 points for each group of discussion postings. But of course, create a system that also awards far fewer points for those who are providing much less effort, and remember to create a rubric awarding a "0" for late or missed discussion posts.

Fourth, make sure each rubric accurately reflects the objectives of the assignment. As with the challenges of creating fair rubrics, creating rubrics that reflect the objectives of the assignment is a matter of experience and good judgment and can take considerable time during the course planning process. For my students' discussion posts throughout the semester, my objectives are for the students to demonstrate a good understanding of the assigned reading and the topic covered, demonstrate strong writing skills, demonstrate they have done the reading carefully, and interact meaningfully with the other students in their posts. So my

Grading Rubric for Discussion Postings

	Unsatisfactory	Average	Good	Excellent	Late or missed
Complete and on topic	Content does not address one or more required topics in adequate detail or strays from topic in one or more responses 15 pts	Content addresses all of the required topics with adequate details and is on topic for all responses 18 pts	Content effectively addresses all of the required topics with good details and is on topic for all responses 22 pts	Content impressively addresses all of the required topics with unusual thoroughness and is on topic for all responses 25 pts	Response not posted by deadline or missed 0 pts
Well written	Contains more than two errors in grammar or mechanics or organization or prose style 15 pts	Contains two errors in grammar or mechanics or organization or prose style 18 pts	Contains one error in grammar or mechanics or organization or prose style 22 pts	Contains no errors in grammar or mechanics or organization or prose style 25 pts	Response not posted by deadline or missed 0 pts
Reflects on reading	Content does not adequately reflect on reading missing quoting a passage from the reading for one or more responses to one or more prompts 15 pts	Content adequately reflects on reading quoting at least one helpful passage from the reading for each response to a prompt 18 pts	Content effectively reflects on reading quoting at least one helpful passage from the reading for each response to a prompt 20 pts	Content impressively reflects on reading quoting at least two passages from the reading for each response to a prompt 25 pts	Response not posted by deadline or missed 0 pts
Posts follow-up responses	Does not meet minimum requirement of responding to at least four other posts 0 pts	Meets minimum requirement of responding to at least four other posts, and responses are adequately detailed 16 pts	Meets minimum requirement of responding to at least four other posts, and responses are effectively detailed 20 pts	Meets minimum requirements of responding to at least four other posts, and responses are unusually detailed or helpful or significant 25 pts	Response not posted by deadline or missed 0 pts
Total possible points	45 pts	70 pts	84 pts	100 pts	0 pts

Figure 4. Rubric for discussions.

discussion rubric assesses their posts based on completeness and staying on topic, the quality of the writing, use of support from the reading, and the quality of their follow-up posts. Of course, objectives and performance criteria are a subjective matter, and it is important to recognize that while these objectives and criteria are useful for me, they may not be for another instructor. Additionally, while it takes some time to create meaningful rubrics, some students will appreciate the effort and the clarity, and the posts or other assignments they create will be better because of the extra help.

Student Reactions to Rubrics

Student reactions to the rubrics I have used have been positive (Jones, 2010). They appreciate knowing the specific areas for which they did well and the areas in need of improvement. When asked if they thought the current rubrics for the brief bio and the discussion posts were too detailed or about right, students' typical responses were "About right." When asked if the rubrics provided a good idea of what did or did not need improvement, one student responded, "Yes. I don't often get points off, but when I do, I know exactly why and what to remember for the next assignment." Another student commented, "I think a mixture of the rubric and your explanation of what you expect gave me the complete picture. If you had only used the rubric and never explained your expectations I think I would have needed clarification." A third student commented, "The rubrics have definitely provided me a good idea of what did or did not need improvement. They are both broken down very precisely and according to the grade received, it's extremely easy to see whether a response was complete and on topic for instance or whether it needs to be improved in future posts." And when asked to comment on the rubrics as a tool to help them learn the course material more effectively, a typical response was "I think so, yes. The rubric requirements help me to focus more on the details of the text (rather than skimming) so that I'm sure I have crafted a complete response."

Rubrics perhaps work best for smaller online classes, those with 35 or fewer students. Those who teach larger online classes (sections with 100 or more students) have more difficulties largely because of the time involved. Or at least this is what some of my colleagues teaching larger classes have told me. Still, many instructors even with these large class sizes have used rubrics successfully depending, of course, on the nature of the assignment and whether or not teaching assistants are available to help with the grading. As for rubrics for assessing discussion posts, instructors should keep in mind that rubrics will be easier to create and easier to apply if the discussion posts themselves are carefully created. Resources for creating good discussion questions are available too.

Using a system of folders and using rubrics help enhance the online learning experience for everyone involved in the course. However, going even further by strengthening the instructor's ethos is at least as important.

USING ADDITIONAL TECHNIQUES
TO ESTABLISH ETHOS ONLINE

As I mentioned earlier, the importance of building and projecting ethos in online classes should not be underestimated. The ethos of instructors in the traditional classroom is built from the moment they enter the classroom, if not earlier (for example, what former students tell others about their instructors). The quality of the syllabus and the course texts, the demands of the course, the confidence and demeanor of instructors, their command of the course content, their personality as it is viewed by the students, their receptiveness to student questions, and their ability to answer these questions clearly—through these and countless other ways, instructors establish their ethos in the classroom as students carefully observe them in action. Similarly, an online ethos is a matter of the instructor's online presence or persona—the authority and credibility established by demonstrating many of the same elements mentioned above but in an online environment.

Of course, teaching online also presents some different and some more demanding challenges for building authority and credibility. In addition to using the strategies covered by Eaton (2005) and summarized earlier, the following have proven useful for my online courses.

Understanding and Controlling
the Online Tools

Two major ways instructors enhance ethos are first to make sure they understand the tools used in this online environment, both their advantages and disadvantages, and second, to show their students their control over these tools. (Similarly, instructors who take the time to create and provide a good system of folders as well as one or more well-designed and fairly applied rubrics also enhance their ethos in this online learning space.) In addition to being knowledgeable about Webcourses or any other online learning system used by the university and the tools provided, a good understanding of effective web design and effective online course design is essential. Fortunately, most colleges and universities offering online courses today provide some kind of support for faculty and typically provide many online resources for faculty to continue improving their skills.

Knowing how to integrate non-Webcourse tools (or tools not part of whatever learning management system an instructor is using) if they are selected is essential too. If instructors are going to use PowerPoint with video or podcasts, they need to make sure they work well and as seamlessly as possible within the course. And it further helps if instructors know what assignments and materials to include that make the best use of the online medium. Focusing on the Web as a means of communication and including materials available on the Web as well as providing interactivity all help in this regard.

In sum, instructors should know how to use the online learning environment for their purposes and its advantages. This concern has been a focus for many in technical communication since the inception of online courses and online programs. Emily Thrush and Necie Elizabeth Young (1999) provided a good overview of the challenges as did Mary F. O'Sullivan (1999), in a special issue of *Technical Communication Quarterly* over a decade ago. In a subsequent more recent special issue of *Technical Communication Quarterly*, guest editors Beth Hewett and Christa Ehmann Powers (2007) summarized some key themes, reminding us that those who teach online courses "need instructional approaches that address distinctive qualities of teaching and learning online" and "need adequate orientation about online teaching and learning approaches" (p. 2).

Contacting Students Before the Online Course Begins

Instructors can focus on other strategies for enhancing ethos too. Contacting students before the first day of class is essential. Waiting to contact them until the first day of the class is often too late. Many students want to know in advance what texts they are using because increasingly, many order their texts through resources other than university book stores. In addition, many students want to get a head start on the first week. Contacting students several weeks in advance is a good start to building ethos. My first effort for establishing ethos is to e-mail everyone enrolled in my online courses 2 or 3 weeks before the beginning of the semester. I have developed an effective pre-semester message I send to all of the students enrolled at their non-Webcourses e-mail address on our Knights server. (Our university now contacts students only through their Knights e-mail address, an address all registered students are required to have and to access regularly for privacy and other reasons.) This e-mail is fairly lengthy and has multiple headings. After informing the students of the purpose for my message, I cover details concerning the course objectives, discuss the class as a mediated (partially online) or online (completely online) course, remind them about the first day of class beginning promptly on the first day of the semester, remind them that complete details about the course will be available once they have access to the course, provide them the required textbook titles and ISBN with a reminder that they must have the books by the first day of class, and inform them of the assignments for the first week. I also remind them that although the course will be challenging, I have structured it in such a way that they will find it easy to navigate and to learn. This preliminary message provides a lot of information that students would otherwise write to me about and request if I did not provide this message. So it saves me time, and establishes that although I have high expectations I am more than willing to help all of those who show up prepared and ready to begin.

Of course, instructors experienced in teaching online courses also use a variety of other strategies for the first week of classes, during the semester, and at the end of the semester. Our instructional designers refer to these strategies, as well as the strategies of tasks to perform before each semester begins, as online course logistics. See "Teaching Online: Online Course Logistics" (http://teach.ucf.edu/resources/online-course-logistics/) for helpful summaries for what to do for all of these phases of an online course (Center, 2009a).

Setting a Professional Tone in Class Announcements

Establishing a supportive and professional tone in the announcements area on the first day of class is also helpful for enhancing ethos. For the first day of class, I post an overview message that essentially walks everyone through all of the tools used in the course and what their purposes are. (Webcourses also makes a student orientation quiz available, and many instructors prefer to use this quiz to make sure students have become familiar with the structure of the course.) As with the pre-semester message to the class, this announcement is a big time-saver for me. I seldom receive questions concerning the environment of the course, and I set many students at ease—students new to online learning who might otherwise be anxious about their online learning experience.

Creating a Separate Brief Bios Thread and Participating

Creating a separate brief bios thread in the Discussions area of the course is a significant way to establish ethos and a sense of community. Of course, there are other ways to achieve similar results. As I mentioned earlier, Grady and Davis (2005) commented on requiring students to provide personal home pages, with photos and some personal information, stating that "Students universally evaluate these personal homepages as very helpful as they engage with one another" (p. 116). Webcourses offers the tool of e-community, a link through which students can find out details about each other and see photos or other representations—if they choose to make the photos or other representations available. However, I have found a brief bios thread more helpful. Students are required to post their bio in response to very specific questions: questions concerning their major and reasons for choosing their major, reasons for selecting this university, the most challenging college course they have taken, their writing background, their computer skills, and their hobbies and subject interests outside of their major. Of course, the topics required here can vary depending on the course and especially for graduate courses. For undergraduates, I have also found it helpful to have them discuss where they see themselves professionally 5 years from now. Many typically have not given the matter much thought yet, and the topic leads to many interesting speculations. It also showcases the relevance of college courses to their career goals. Making a brief bios thread or area available for easy access for everyone with detailed bios will make the course more personable and will prove useful for group work throughout the course.

Importantly, instructors should post their own brief bio and post it first in a brief bios thread to set a certain tone for the course and to establish a strong ethos. I address all of the same questions I ask my students to address and at the same time provide a narrative or my story, so to speak, beginning with summarizing my career path, discussing my hobbies and interests, and looking ahead to the future. By leading with my story, I can be more certain that those responding have first read my brief bio, and by posting my brief bio first I also set a courteous and professional tone. This brief bio is a serious assignment and one that all of the students will find helpful. The brief bios play the additional role of becoming especially helpful during the peer reviews and later during teamwork on various projects. Students can consult these bios rather than post information about themselves within their groups. The brief bios are a good tool not only for building ethos both for the instructor and the students (many students have impressive backgrounds and credentials), but the bios are also a good tool for helping with collaborative work and building a sense of community.

Contributing Often to Online Discussions

Contributing to the online discussions as often as possible is another effective way for instructors to develop ethos. Not every discussion will require instructors to contribute, but depending on the discussion topic, instructors can further build ethos by posting respectful, informed, and well-reasoned contributions to the class discussions. Complimenting particular posts by students and following up with additional insights will help build both ethos and a sense of community for the course. Participating sets the tone that the discussions are important in other ways, and instructors, of course, can and do learn from their students in the online discussions just as they do in the traditional classroom. And, as mentioned earlier concerning rubrics, well-designed discussion posts—those that meet course objectives, are clear, are doable, and so on—give the students confidence that instructors are in charge of the subject matter and the course as a whole.

Showing Sensitivity to the Needs of the Students

Returning to a point made earlier by Eaton (2005) in "Students in the Online Technical Communication Classroom," one of the strongest or best ways to build ethos is to be aware of and sensitive to the needs of the students and to their lives as students. Like faculty, they lead busy and hectic lives. They typically take five classes a semester. Many work at least part-time, and many have other demands on their time with volunteer work or with extracurricular activities. Of course, it must be made clear that once they sign on to the course—make a commitment to take the course instead of dropping it during the first week of class—they have made a commitment to do all of the work required regardless of what is going on in their lives elsewhere. Still, conveying a caring attitude about their many other commitments helps build ethos in ways that none of the others strategies mentioned above can. Cultivate a supportive environment in other ways, including providing prompt responses to any e-mails and using supportive language in the responses and in announcements throughout the course will also enhance the course.

Developing Authenticity

Grady and Davis (2005) suggest that "what is most challenging is developing an authentic interactive learning environment online" (p. 101). The importance of the point cannot be emphasized enough. In other words, develop and provide a genuine, college-level, demanding online learning space. Most students can recognize a sham when they see one. And of course, another dimension of the authentic interactive learning environment online is the authenticity of the instructor. An instructor's online persona can be well-crafted but must also be genuine. Just do what most experienced instructors do for their courses, whether they are taught face-to-face or taught entirely online: use clear language when addressing the students, use clear language in all of the class handouts for the course, set high standards in the grading criteria for rubrics, provide clear grading criteria either as part of the syllabus or in a separate handout, spell out specific protocols for online behavior and qualities necessary for succeeding in online courses, and so on.

FULFILLING BEST PRACTICES

Rapid and constant developments in tools for developing and extending online courses make knowledge about structure and ways to expand and improve it all the more essential. As mentioned earlier, the tools available within a course management system as well as all of the additional tools that can supplement one learning system or another are increasing dramatically. Some of the biggest challenges facing those who teach online courses include keeping up with the trends and deciding which new tools might be most helpful, and then learning how to use them effectively. As the building of online courses becomes more complex, the structure must be more sophisticated while also meeting widely accepted best practices for institutions offering online programs and online courses. (Our university provides a good summary of these practices at http://teach.ucf.edu/pedagogy/best-practices/ (Center, 2009b)). The additional suggestions covered here—using a system of folders and combining these effectively with other online course tools; focusing more on creating quality evaluation rubrics, particularly for online discussions; and strengthening the instructor's ethos in the online environment—all fulfill common best practices. Like so many other practices, these strategies contribute significantly to developing the interactive environment students need and want for this kind of learning experience.

REFERENCES

Arter, J. (2009). *Creating & recognizing quality rubrics: A study guide.* Princeton, NJ: Educational Testing Service.

California State University, Chico. (n.d.). What does a high quality online course look like? *Rubric for online instruction.* Retrieved March 9, 2010, from http://www.csuchico.edu/celt/roi/index.shtml

Center for Distributed Learning. (2009a). *Teaching online: Online teaching logistics.* Retrieved July 9, 2012 from http://teach.ucf.edu/resources/online-course-logistics/before-the-course-starts/

Center for Distributed Learning. (2009b). *Teaching online: Pedagogy.* Retrieved July 9, 2012 from http://teach.ucf.edu/pedagogy/best-practices/

Dornisch, M. M., & McLoughlin, A. S. (2006). Limitations of Web-based rubric resources: Addressing the challenges [Electronic version]. *Practical Assessment Research & Evaluation, 11*(3), 1–8. Retrieved May 2, 2010, from http://pareonline.net/getvn.asp?v=11&n=3

Eaton, A. (2005). Students in the online technical communication classroom. In K. Cargile Cook & K. Grant-Davie (Eds.), *Online education: Global questions, local answers* (pp. 31–48). Amityville, NY: Baywood.

Faculty Center for Teaching & Learning. (n.d.). Teaching online: Deciding which course tools to use. *University of Central Florida.* Retrieved March 8, 2010, from http://www.fctl.ucf.edu/TeachingAndLearningResources/LearningEnvironments/TeachingOnline/index.php

Grady, H. M., & Davis, M. T. (2005). Teaching online with instructional and procedural scaffolding. In K. Cargile Cook & K. Grant-Davie (Eds.), *Online education: Global questions, local answers* (pp. 101–122). Amityville, NY: Baywood.

Hewett, B. L., & Powers, C. E. (2007). Guest editors' introduction: Online teaching and learning: Preparation, development, and organizational communication. *Technical Communication Quarterly, 16*(1), 1–11.

Jones, D. (2010). Personal communications. Anonymous student survey.

Kohn, A. (2006). The trouble with rubrics. *English Journal, 95*(4), 12–15.

O'Sullivan, M. F. (1999). Worlds within which we teach: Issues for designing World Wide Web course material. *Technical Communication Quarterly, 8*(1), 61–72.

Quinlan, A. M. (2006). *A complete guide to rubrics: Assessment made easy for teachers, K-college.* Lanham, MD: Rowman & Littlefield Education.

Stevens, D. D. (2005). *Introduction to rubrics: An assessment tool to save grading time, convey effective feedback, and promote student learning.* Sterling, VA: Stylus.

Swan, K., Shen, J., & Hiltz, S. R. (2005). *Assessment and collaboration in online learning.* Retrieved March 2, 2010, from http://74.125.155.132/scholar?q=cache:UNSM4SAsCTcJ:scholar.google.com/+%E2%80%9CAssessment+and+Collaboration+in+Online%22&hl=en&as_sdt=40000

Thrush, E. A., & Young, N. E. (1999). Hither, thither, and yon: Process in putting courses on the Web. *Technical Communication Quarterly, 8*(1), 49–59.

Wilson, M. (2006). *Rethinking rubrics in writing assessment.* Portsmouth, NH: Heinemann.

http://dx.doi.org/10.2190/OE2C13

CHAPTER 13

Innovation in the Distributed Technical Communication Classroom

Lee S. Tesdell

When I first started teaching technical communication courses online in 2004 at my university, I was primarily concerned with the software, hardware, and ways to "convert" course content to online delivery (Tesdell, 2004). I approached online teaching from a technology-driven perspective rather than a pedagogy-driven perspective (Cargile Cook, 2005). As I look back on that time now, however, I see that in my online courses, I had in place the components for an activity system: students; an instructor; tools that included texts, computer technology, and the Internet; and a shared purpose with my students—creating technical documents. According to Russell (2003), activity theory

> understands learning not as the internalization of discrete information or skills by individuals, but rather as expanding involvement over time, social as well as intellectual, with some other people and the tools available in their culture. These networks of people and their shared tools, acting together for some shared purpose (such as learning to write in a composition class) are called *"activity systems."* (italics in original)

Although I did not think of them that way initially, the actors in our system are my students and me; our shared tools are the technologies we use to connect across time and distance.

Today, in addition to the activity system perspective, I see a clear connection to distributed work as discussed by Spinuzzi (2007):

Work is becoming more distributed: distributed across time, space, disciplines, fields, and trade; distributed across a multiplicity of stakeholders; distributed through telecommunication and digital technologies. Technical communication researchers have been investigating these separate aspects of distributed work for some time, although often not in connection with each other. (p. 272)

Combining these two perspectives, this chapter argues that learning has also become more distributed when conducted online. Out of this distributed learning activity system, then, to both students and instructors come benefits and challenges. Most important among them is the opportunity for us to innovate and engage in creative pedagogy. Innovation, as I define it, refers to changes wrought by online instruction's distributed activities, such as those that occur between instructor and student, in assignments, and in the opportunities for cooperative learning. In this chapter, I argue that distributed learning provides an opportunity for teachers of technical communication to innovate their pedagogy. Online instruction allows for a distributed student population—a population distributed not only geographically but also culturally and experientially. Innovations made possible by the online medium and by these kinds of distribution include providing cross-cultural collaborations, drawing on distributed online resources rather than a single textbook, and decentering pedagogy from instructor to students. This decentering recognizes that in an online class, expertise may be more distributed, and therefore authority may need to be more distributed too, making lecture-based instruction less viable.

I use online learning, e-learning, and distributed learning as essentially synonymous. I discuss distributed learning in the light of activity theory as a way to detail the relationship among the human actors, the goals of the teaching/learning, and the technology in the online classroom, and I consider the benefits and challenges that instructors (myself included) have discovered teaching online. Throughout, I frame this discussion as an argument for innovative teaching and learning in the online technical communication classroom.

THE DISTRIBUTED LEARNING ACTIVITY SYSTEM

It may be tempting to look at online pedagogy as conventional teaching that simply features the addition of new software that allows distance learning. This is not the real story of distributed learning, however, since that is too narrow a definition of what we do in online classrooms. Instead, if we consider online classrooms as activity systems that take place at distributed learning sites, we are able to take a fresh look at our pedagogy. To do so may yield insights that help us to develop and improve our students' educational experiences.

A distributed learning activity system is centered in the participants and their learning goals; the software and hardware are necessary ingredients, though not the center of the system. In a distributed classroom, the activity system is made up of the teacher, the students, the tools, and, importantly, the purpose of the activity. Depending on the type of online learning—synchronous, asynchronous, or both—the system itself is distributed over distance and, potentially, time. While tools are not the center of the enterprise, they offer both teachers and learners the technology that allows us to be distributed but also connected in our learning and teaching. Learning, according to activity theorists, involves not only taking in discrete pieces of information but also, as Russell (2002) suggests, instantiating an activity system such as "a course of study or a distributed learning design group . . . . [Such] a functional system of social/cultural interactions . . . constitutes behavior and produces that kind of change called learning" (p. 5). Russell helps us to understand that online "construction zones" are the places where students in distributed learning situations learn to do these kinds of writing and learning. In an online technical communication class, the distributed learning activity system brings the students and teacher together to use their software programs and ideas to act for the "shared purpose" of learning to write technical documents such as instructions, technical reports, and usability tests (Russell, 2002).

My experiences in the online technical communication classroom have allowed me to recognize the elements that make up the distributed activity system in an online course. For example, I hold synchronous (real-time) meetings with my students. My goal within these meetings is to bring as much of the interaction of a face-to-face class as possible to my online synchronous classes. For example, below are some of the interactions that I observed in a weekly synchronous class meeting that included student presentations:

- **Warming up.** As a kind of preliminary to the topic, we often have conversations on nonclass topics to get warmed up. For example, recently the outdoor temperature in Mankato in the morning was –8F (weather is a big topic of conversation in the Midwest). I commented on that extremely cold temperature and a student in Florida replied that it was 70F where he lives. Another student in Taiwan remarked that it was warm where he was as well. This kind of conversation "warmed" us up for the more serious topics at hand. While such interactions may seem trivial and are not necessarily topical to the course, they do seem to help establish a genial atmosphere that is conducive to easy discussion and trust within an activity system in which the actors are widely distributed and may not be able to see each other.
- **Back-channeling and chatting in teams.** Students work together online in their teams to make their team presentations without the intervention of the teacher. Side conversations in the chat room are always related to the current student's presentation topic but may help the presenters, when they read the comments, to explain their topics more fully. This kind of backchannel

allows student presenters to multitask by watching the roll of the chat conversation as they present their topics and refer to those questions in the run of their presentation, from time to time. Their teammates may then use the chat window to guide the discussion without disrupting the presentation. For example, my students this semester in a course on international technical communication, while one team summarized a chapter in Lovitt and Goswami's text *Exploring the Rhetoric of International Professional Communication: An Agenda for Teachers and Researchers*, the responding team used an assigned chapter in Samovar, Porter, and McDaniel's *Intercultural Communication: A Reader* to critique the Lovitt and Goswami text. Sometimes the chat conversation would go off onto related tangents, such as a topical URL; these two threads became branches of the same tree. While this parallel conversation could be potentially disruptive to the ongoing student presentation, in this case, it was informative.

- **Facilitating.** Students sometimes take over the function of facilitator when I, as the instructor, am having technology problems. Or conversely, I advance the slides for a student who has technology problems. In one specific case, the student's audio continued to work so that he could continue his presentation even though he could not see his own slides in the online meeting software. He, however, did have a copy of his slides at home and could continue speaking about them as I advanced the slides on his behalf.

Identifying and learning the technologies that make these interactions possible is another important key to creating an effective distributed activity system. When I first began teaching online, I used software that offered only chat. Students would prepare a topic for class, and we would discuss it in a chat window in UCompass Educator. Soon after that first experience, my university began using Desire2Learn (D2L), a statewide-sponsored learning management system. The next step I took was to use a synchronous meeting software tool called Macromedia Breeze. Later, when the Adobe company purchased Macromedia, Adobe renamed the product Connect Pro. With Connect, students can prepare their presentations on slides and use the audio feature to talk the rest of us through their presentation. I also use the chat window for asking questions during the presentation so that the students' audio presentation will not be interrupted. Then, because there is a video feature in D2L, I began using the webcam feature. I quickly learned that the video required much more Internet bandwidth than the audio, and there seemed to be very little pedagogical gain from looking at the students' heads when they spoke or were listening to other students. Alternatively, we turned on the webcam to "freeze" a still photo in order to preserve bandwidth. Later I dispensed with video altogether, not finding it pedagogically beneficial. As this example illustrates, instructors need to keep pace with technological advances, but they also need to watch for instances when more is not necessarily better—when the situation calls for simpler technology. (For a more detailed discussion of this point, see Gibson and Martinez's chapter in the previous section of this volume.)

Considering both the activities we engage in and the tools that allow us to engage, I have found that the essence of interactivity in online classes are the negotiations that take place among students and between students and instructors. I use the word "negotiations" advisedly. To negotiate implies two-way communication and the possibility of both sides critically examining their assumptions, shifting positions, and learning from each other. This willingness to learn and adapt is an important part of the activity in a distributed learning system. Negotiation through online discussion helps the actors in the system develop online personas, and it may lead to trust, which is another important element in distributed learning. We trust each other to be committed to the shared purpose of the course: to become technical communicators. This trust develops from the following activities:

- We get to know each other's voices in all meanings of the word "voices."
- We get to know each other's audio mannerisms.
- We get to know chat patterns and level of personal information that we are willing to produce about ourselves.

Through these activities, we develop trust that, even though we are lacking body language cues of our interlocutors, allows us to depend on each other during the important business of learning within the classroom activity system.

INNOVATION AND THE ONLINE
CLASSROOM

When viewed as distributed activity systems, online courses encourage innovative pedagogy. According to practitioners like Marwan Tarazi at Birzeit University, e-learning lends itself to innovation:

> Essentially, e-learning is about improving the quality of learning through using interactive technology and online communication and information systems in ways that other teaching methods cannot match. . . . Hence, proper adoptions of e-learning will inherently bring about qualitative improvements in education and efficiency of processes. (Tarazi, 2006, p. 6)

Tarazi here is referring to the Palestinian university educational context in which the accepted pedagogical approach in the universities is the formal lecture. Those of us who prefer participatory and interactive pedagogies can easily understand his optimism for e-learning. At the same time, it is possible, as

St.Amant has pointed out, that there may be some resistance from instructors who are used to the lecture format and may not be prepared for the switch to online delivery of their courses (St.Amant, 2007). Furthermore, although online delivery facilitates interactive teaching, it does not prevent anyone from lecturing. Teachers who prefer that format can find ways to deliver their lectures online using technologies, using podcasts, videocasts, and other streaming applications.

Starke-Meyerring and Wilson (2008) concur with Tarazi (2006) that distributed learning (in their case called *globally networked learning environments*) is a location for pedagogical innovation:

> They are learning environments that represent new visions of globally networked learning and extend well beyond the confines of traditional local classrooms. To realize their visions, they pursue innovative pedagogies; instead of being limited to local classrooms, these learning environments link students to peers, instructors, professionals, experts, and communities from diverse contexts; challenge students to negotiate and build shared learning knowledge cultures across diverse boundaries; and provide students with new opportunities for civic engagement in a global context. (Starke-Meyerring & Wilson, 2008, p. 2)

Rosemarie Park of the University of Minnesota's Adult Education & Human Resource Development program, writes with her colleagues about a change in pedagogy that occurs in a blended learning (conventional classroom teaching blended with some online components) classroom.

> Because of the very nature of this environment, learners must both actively engage in the material and communicate with the facilitator and other learners. Instead of waiting for the teaching professional to manage the learner, the learner is called to engage with the content and self-determine what they understand and what they might need help with. Some have described the computer-mediated environment as being managed by the student learner. (Park, Digby, & Conroy, 2008, p. 6)

Here we see the learner being empowered in ways that are less likely in a conventional classroom.

Building on these descriptions of online pedagogy, in the next section, I illustrate how online instruction can become creative and innovative, especially when faced with linguistic, cultural, temporal, and technological challenges. Online classrooms provide an excellent situation in which to teach our students that innovation can be an appropriate response to such challenges.

Language and Culture

Distributed learning gives students access to partners in cultures outside their own: students find themselves working across geographic boundaries ranging from across campus to across international borders. My current online class roster, for example, includes a full-time technical writer from western Pennsylvania, a United States citizen who is teaching English in Taiwan, and a full-time master's student on campus in Mankato, Minnesota. In addition, for one project I have partnered my students with students at the University of Applied Science in Karlsruhe, Germany; Xiamen University of Technology, Xiamen, Fujian Province, China; and Birzeit University in the Palestinian Territories; and I have, in the past, completed cooperative assignments with students at the Writers Block in Bangalore, India. These are cross-cultural connections that bring pedagogical benefits to all students. They learn to negotiate in a way that helps them to understand communication (to some degree) with their partners in the United States, China, the Palestinian Territories, Germany, or India. Indian students, for instance, have a good command of English but use vocabulary that Minnesota students may not have heard before like "lorry" for "truck," "motorway" for "highway," or "football" for "soccer." In one recent correspondence I received from an Indian colleague, he used the term "we can engage further," whereas I would have used the phrase "we can continue to work together." Likewise, it may be an eye-opening experience for my U.S. students to learn from their German interlocutors that the German students can work in multiple languages, whereas even though many Minnesota students have studied a second language (usually Spanish) for 4 years in high school, they are not able to use the language in any meaningful way. (For a more detailed discussion of the cross-cultural advantages and challenges of online learning, see Thrush and Popham's chapter in the previous section in this volume.)

While these cultural negotiations promote understanding, they can also create challenges. Even as students interact with international interlocutors online, there is room for failure of communication. While this is a desirable outcome as a step on the way to intercultural competence, it can also prevent understanding. When we work across cultures, we negotiate language, accent, national holidays, differences in semester calendars, and personality. Lack of communication due to a lack of body language and other face-to-face communication features can be another challenge.

Distributed Online Resources

A second innovation that online teaching brings to the table is distributed online resources. Online delivery of courses allows for not only the use of conventional resources such as textbooks and articles but also for guest speakers who would not otherwise be able to attend my classes. I have recently taught and delivered online a course in online documentation. In that course, I used a textbook by Dr. Thomas Barker and another book by Anne Gentle. At a certain point in the semester, after my students had read and discussed most of the material in both texts, I contacted the authors by e-mail to ask if they would be willing to attend an online class meeting and speak to my students. They both agreed and a lively discussion resulted. The feedback from my students was positive. In this case, the online course delivery allowed for guest speakers in a way that would not be feasible in a face-to-face course. Another advantage I have found is that I can record the class meetings and post the links to those recordings in Adobe Connect Pro. This means that unlike a face-to-face class meeting, the instructor and student can review the class meeting at any time. This recorded meeting becomes another distributed online resource available to students and instructors alike.

The availability of international students to partner with my students in virtual work teams is an important addition to my online and face-to-face courses. Currently my students are conducting a digital writing survey with partners in three overseas universities (see above). They are using Skype, Facebook, and an e-mailed questionnaire as communication tools to collect data on the digital writing habits of students in all four universities. Electronic communication tools are obviously critical to this kind of student work, and these distributed online resources are available to both face-to-face and online students.

De-Centered Pedagogy

A third innovation that has emerged in my online classes is the possibility of a de-centered pedagogy. On April 21, 2010, at 6:55 p.m., a fire alarm went off in my building on campus. I had just logged in to Adobe Connect to begin the 7 p.m. class. Clearly I was required by the university safety rules to leave the building. I gave control of the online meeting in Adobe Connect Pro to two students and left the building. I returned 20 minutes later to find the students doing just fine in class discussion. In this case the technology allowed the synchronous class to continue meeting. If we had been meeting in a classroom in that affected building, class would have been disrupted for the entire 20 minutes. I see this last outcome as beneficial in two ways: software allowed us to continue class without the instructor for 20 minutes, and the authority in the classroom was passed easily from the instructor to two students. What this experience shows is that while students do need some direction, if the syllabus clearly lays out the tasks to be completed and there is a clear agenda for each meeting, students are capable of running their own class meetings online is such emergencies.

Another example of de-centered pedagogy concerns private communication between students during class. In Adobe Connect Pro, students can send private chat messages to any member of the class. While this capability could be regarded as a way to undermine the authority of the instructor, I would also see it as a way for students to arrange virtual team meetings, send comments about presentations, and to make needed changes to the management of team projects. Clearly the electronic communication tools make private conversations between students easier since they are already all "in class" together in the synchronous class meeting room.

In my online classes then, several interesting and useful elements have emerged that make the online pedagogy experience creative and innovative for both the instructor and the students.

Time

Scheduling courses conveniently for students is important, but such scheduling can bring challenges for both students and instructors. In our own program we offer or are planning to offer courses at mutually acceptable times, including Saturday mornings and workday evenings. We are even contemplating early mornings to catch students in time zones 8–12 hours earlier than ours. Such flexibility in scheduling may be necessary to accommodate students in distant time zones (as in the case of Central Time Zone and India), but it is important locally as well. Our evening class meeting times are popular with students who are full-time employees.

Even with our efforts to provide convenient meeting times, students must often negotiate time zones to participate in my university's online courses. A student in Jerusalem gets up in the wee hours of the morning to participate at 7 p.m. Central Standard Time (CST). Our students in India are 11½ hours ahead of CST and Taiwan, 13 hours ahead. In another recent example, while on a trip in June 2010, I spent the night in transit in Dubai. In order to teach my 7 p.m. CST class in Minnesota, I had to wake up at 3 a.m. Dubai time. This is not convenient, but it is preferable to a face-to-face class, which would have given me only two options: cancel the class or don't travel.

Scheduling across time zones is clearly a difficult challenge, especially complicated when semesters, holidays, or weekends don't match up. In another recent example, the weeklong Easter holiday in Germany coincided with the week that we had planned to collaborate with German students on our usability project.

Technology

Distributed learning environments require some students to use unfamiliar software and hardware while, in the same class, other students may know more about the software and hardware than the teacher does. Meloncon (2007), in her discussion of the things that technical communication instructors should be prepared for in teaching online, asks the question, "Am I prepared for the possibility that some students will know more about the technology than I do?" Ironically, this situation can well be an advantage in any classroom, online or face-to-face. For example, as I described previously, there have been instances when I have to hand over the meeting software to a student; my student's software experience allowed us to prevent a difficult situation. In contrast, technologies are not always as reliable as I'd like them to be. Thunderstorms can knock out the electricity and with it the Internet access. Even if students' laptops can continue on batteries, the Internet hubs are dependent on electricity to function, and class ends abruptly. Even without weather intervention, a number of times Connect has ground to a halt during class. This may be due to the server being overloaded or to bandwidth problems. In any case, the hardware and software are not perfect and will certainly malfunction sometimes.

One of the most persistent hardware problems I encounter at the beginning of a semester is to encourage students to use headsets in synchronous meetings and to get their microphones working properly. Students commonly use headsets but rarely as online learning tools, so I often need to remind them that audio feedback is a problem in class. To nip some of those software/hardware use problems in the bud, I hold a test meeting with my online students in Connect before the semester begins. To address the problem of audio settings, I put a note on the introductory slide for every class with instructions for completing the Audio Setup Wizard. For the beginner online student and instructor, another important hurdle to clear is mastery of the software that is necessary for the online course to function. Hewitt and Ehmann (2004) write that though technology is indeed a hurdle for some instructors and students, "the train has left the station and is powering down the tracks. Educators cannot halt its journey, and that may, indeed, be a positive development" (p. xv). And we have to accept that online teaching requires new software, and we must learn to use it effectively.

On a less serious note, synchronous online classes can experience unexpected audio distractions. I have witnessed several interesting ones: pets at home bothering student owners, roommates interfering, and children needing attention. In the distributed learning environment, instructors must learn to accept the possibility that the student is not only participating in class but also is eating supper and watching a game on television.

Online instructors may also need to address challenges that result from students and sometimes their own lack of access to high-speed Internet. Recently, I experienced the rural-urban accessibility digital divide personally as I drove home from my university campus in Mankato, Minnesota. As I drove, I needed to find Internet access in order to attend the online student chapter meeting of the Society for Technical Communication. I stopped in Wells, Minnesota, at a convenience store and a restaurant. No luck. I stopped again 10 miles farther down the road at a truckstop in Alden. Again, no luck. Another 10 miles down the road I found the Internet at a McDonald's in Albert Lea, Minnesota, but it was conditional. I had to sit near the window facing the east since the motel next door actually provided the wireless Internet. Clearly small-town Minnesota is less wired to the Internet than the cities and the universities where we are indeed spoiled with fast reliable bandwidth.

Online instructors should realize that their students might live with or occasionally experience the same connectivity challenges, especially if they connect from rural settings in the United States or other parts of the world. St.Amant

(2007) points to several examples of this divide between haves and have-nots both in bandwidth and reliability of electrical power. In addition, data I gathered in the Palestinian areas in April, 2009, showed that for some poor students, just getting connected would be out of financial reach. In Ramallah, one of the main towns in Palestine, the cost for an Internet connection ranged from $16 to $53 per month depending on the connection speed. One of my colleagues paid $32 for a 512 Kb connection per month, an acceptable connection speed for using Moodle, the e-learning platform in use at Birzeit University. For residents of Jerusalem, there were both Israeli and Palestinian vendors available. One additional consideration is that for Palestinians who do not have a landline, installation of a line would be a prerequisite for Internet at home since Internet access usually comes over the landlines. For a wireless option, Cellcom, an Israeli phone company, offered a 2Mb connection device for $53 a month. Locally, a new laptop costs between $800 and $1,000. For low-income families in many places in the world, these prices may put distributed learning out of reach. One effort to bridge the economic digital divide is the One Laptop Per Child program that aims to distribute economical, childproof, low-maintenance laptops in schools around the world that cannot afford to provide computers to their students. The jury is still out as to as to the effectiveness of this program, but it is clearly an interesting attempt to connect students with their peers around the world in the service of education (Madden, 2009).

THE CONSEQUENCES OF INNOVATION

While our online classes encourage innovative pedagogy, we may also be opening the door to some pedagogical chaos as well. This kind of pedagogy is not necessarily neat and clean but rather a little messy and chaotic around the edges. In the international online teaching environment, Herrington and Tretyakov recognize the reality and the necessity of "confusion, chaos, and disarray" when they turn their students loose in their Global Classroom Project (GCP). "Because efficient collaboration is difficult to develop when crossing cultural, technological, temporal and linguistic boundaries, confusion and chaos are natural results. The chaos may be uncomfortable, but it is real and it is necessary (in the sense of both "unavoidable" and "beneficial") when struggling to reach cooperative goals" (Herrington & Tretyakov, 2005, p. 276). I have found this to be true in my own online teaching. Various kinds of "confusion, chaos, and disarray" have found their way into my synchronous classroom. Just last week a student's laptop died. She was on a trip to San Antonio, Texas, and was attending class from the computer in the hotel lobby. She was not familiar with the computer and at one point when something didn't work correctly, we all heard "Oh s _ _ t" in our synchronous meeting. As I mentioned earlier, now and then I hear dogs barking in the background, a Minnesota Twins baseball game on the television, or a child asking a parent for something. These are by and large problems that do not happen in a face-to-face classroom.

Innovative online instruction can also be time-consuming. In recent research, Worley and Tesdell (2009) found that teachers spent more time with their online students than they did with their face-to-face students.

> This research study compares the instructional time and effort it took the authors to teach the same course online and FTF in their respective universities. The results of the two-semester study show that both authors spent more time per student, approximately 20% more, in the online courses. The authors speculate a number of factors contributed to this difference and the perception that teaching in an online environment takes more time and effort than teaching in a FTF environment. (p. 138)

Clearly, then, the distributed learning activity system yields benefits and its own set of challenges for its participants. Benefits of the system include opportunities for students to work across cultural and language differences to gain cross-cultural competence, to learn new technologies that may be useful on the job, to work with other students they would not otherwise be able to work with, and to cooperate across time and distance on assignments. Accompanying these benefits are challenges, such as cultural and language differences, technology that doesn't always work, time zone differences, a sometimes heavier workload for instructors, and the gap between the haves and the have-nots for access to online courses.

While any classroom may be theorized as an activity system, the distributed nature of online classes adds complexity and complications that require instructors to be quick witted and innovative, responding on the fly to unforeseen situations that arise when any part of the system unexpectedly changes. My experiences have taught me to see online teaching as a type of creative work that takes place within a distributed activity system—shared pedagogical goals, my students, myself, the course materials, and the tools we use to connect across time and distance. Within this system, we work together to accomplish a common goal as we learn to innovate—both as teachers and as learners. In so doing, we help prepare students to be innovative, resourceful thinkers in workplaces that may well turn out to be distributed activity systems too.

REFERENCES

Cargile Cook, K. (2005). An argument for pedagogy-driven online education. In K. Cargile Cook & K. Grant-Davie (Eds.), *Online education: Global questions, local answers* (pp. 49–66). Amityville, NY: Baywood.

Herrington, T., & Tretyakov, Y. (2005). The global classroom project: Troublemaking and troubleshooting. In K. Cargile Cook & K. Grant-Davie (Eds.), *Online education: Global questions, local answers* (pp. 267–283). Amityville, NY: Baywood.

Hewitt, B., & Ehmann, C. (2004). *Preparing educators for online writing instruction.* Urbana, IL: National Council of Teachers of English.

Madden, J. (2009). CALL and the "$100 laptop." *CALL-EJ Online.* Retrieved July, 2009, from http://callej.org/journal/11-1/madden.html,11:1

Meloncon, L. (2007). Exploring electronic landscapes: Technical communication, online learning, and instructor preparedness. *Technical Communication Quarterly, 16*(1), 31–53.

Park, R., Digby, C., & Conroy, A. (2008, November). *Blended learning as a tool for human resource development in a global context.* Paper presented at the 6th Asian Conference of the Academy of HRD, Bangkok, Thailand.

Russell, D. (2002). Looking beyond the interface: Activity theory and distributed learning. In M. Lea & K. Nicoll (Eds.), *Distributed learning: Social and cultural approaches to practice* (pp. 64–82). London, England: Routledge. Retrieved from http://www.public.iastate.edu/~drrussel/drresume.html

Russell, D. (2003). *Activity theory and composition.* Retrieved from http://www.mhhe.com/socscience/english/tc/russell/RussellModule2.htm

Spinuzzi, C. (2007). Guest editor's introduction: Technical communication in the age of distributed work. *Technical Communication Quarterly, 16*(3), 256–277.

St.Amant, K. (2007). Online education in an age of globalization: Foundational perspectives and practices for technical communication instructors and trainers. *Technical Communication Quarterly, 16*(1), 13–30.

Starke-Meyerring, D., & Wilson, M. (2008). Learning environments for a globally networked world. In D. Starke-Meyerring & M. Wilson (Eds.), *Designing globally networked learning environments: Visionary partnerships, policies, and pedagogies* (pp. 2–17). Rotterdam, The Netherlands: Sense.

Tarazi, M. (2006, October). *E-learning prospects in Palestine.* Retrieved from http://www.thisweekinpalestine.com/details.php?id=1924&ed=132&edid=132, 102

Tesdell, L. (2004). Converting technical communication courses to online delivery: Learning objects, software tools, and delivery media in an e-learning environment. In J. Williams (Ed.), *IPCC Proceedings* (pp. 210–214). 2004 International Professional Communication Conference.

Worley, W., & Tesdell, L. (2009). Instructor time and effort in online and face-to-face teaching: Lesson learned. *IEEE Transactions on Professional Communication, 52*(2), 138–151.

http://dx.doi.org/10.2190/OE2C14

CHAPTER 14

Library Services for Online Students

Britt Fagerheim

With the rise of distance education and changing student research habits, teaching faculty and librarians are faced with new challenges with students working on class research projects. The ways in which students are using, or not using, library resources and conducting secondary research is changing in the modern digital age. Studies show many students are using free Web sources instead of library databases and scholarly articles, which presents a challenge for both librarians and instructors seeking to help students learn the literature of their majors and future professions. One study found that students at all undergraduate levels indicated free Web resources were their first choice for conducting secondary research (van Scoyoc & Cason, 2006). Another study finds that younger students (the Millennial Generation) tend to use free Web resources rather than subscription library resources (Holliday & Li, 2004). Students' familiarity with Google and proclivity for searching the free Web is a factor that librarians and instructors must take into account with all students but especially with distance education students. A survey of distance education business students in Ireland showed that students' first choice for information was either Blackboard or a Web search engine, depending on their information need, following by the library's online resources (Byrne & Bates, 2009). Another study has shown that distance students use the Internet for research more than on-campus students (Brouse, McKnight, Basch, & LeBlanc, 2010).

The challenge doesn't end with access to quality library resources. A recent national study has shown that many students find research more challenging in the current electronic environment due to the sheer volume of information available and the difficulty of identifying the most useful or relevant information (Head & Eisenberg, 2009a). A companion study also found that many students develop a research strategy reliant on a small collection of information sources that they turn to regardless of their information need (Head & Eisenberg, 2009b). According to a Pew Internet and American Life Project report, "A great challenge for today's colleges is how to teach students search techniques that will get them to the information they want and how to evaluate it. . . . Although academic resources are offered online, it may be that students have not been taught, or have not yet figured out, how to locate these resources" (Jones, 2002, p. 13). For many students, whether on the main campus or studying via distance education, access to resources is only one piece of the research puzzle; effectively finding and using information is another challenge. Some of the ways faculty can address these issues in distance education courses, which are explored further in this chapter, are by including a librarian in their online class and working with a subject librarian or distance education librarian to incorporate resources and tutorials into a course. Faculty can also work with librarians to navigate the increasingly challenging copyright environment with distance education and help distance education students know about the library resources available to them.

In response to these challenges presented by distance education, libraries are adapting both the resources and services traditionally provided by librarians and the methods by which librarians work with faculty and students. This chapter will discuss how libraries are working with distance education faculty to help students find and use information for their research projects and how faculty and instructors can take advantage of evolving library resources and services for their students. Librarians are working with faculty more closely in online and distance education courses, developing embedded librarian programs; creating Web sites with information and resources for distance learners; using new technology to create online tutorials and learning modules; purchasing electronic books, e-journals, and online databases to provide access to the library's resources from any location; creating online research guides; helping faculty navigate copyright issues; and incorporating library resources into content management systems (Figa, Bone, & Macpherson, 2009; Gandhi, 2003; Tang, 2009).

INTEGRATING LIBRARY RESOURCES AND INSTRUCTION INTO ONLINE COURSES

A key issue for reaching students is to integrate library resources into their courses and for librarians and faculty to work together to make library resources accessible to students. Librarians see a need to inform both students and faculty about the library resources and services available and market those resources so they are understood and used. The literature shows that many faculty and students in distance education are not aware of the library resources available to them, and, at the same time, faculty and instructors' guidance plays a major role in the resources students seek out for their research projects (Shelton, 2009). According to several studies, many faculty members acknowledge the importance of library resources to online courses, but many do not require any library research or actively encourage interaction with a librarian (Thomsett-Scott & May, 2009). At some institutions, studies show that faculty often do not know about the resources available from the library and sometimes do not expect much interaction from the library, while other studies show a high level of library resources being incorporated into online courses (Coahoy & Moyo, 2005). Inclusion of a librarian in online classes is a method for bringing research expertise and assistance to the students. Librarians often refer to this as an embedded librarian program. Librarians with subject-specialist skills interact with students within the course management system (CMS), posting in discussion forums, answering individual questions, posting links and information about relevant resources, and in some cases, providing instruction on specific aspects of research related to the course (Figa et al., 2009). At an exclusively online university, the embedded librarian program focused on a required course taken early in the students' academic careers (Veal & Bennett, 2009). In addition to monitoring an Ask Your Librarian discussion forum, the activities of the embedded librarian included posting information about resources and benefits at strategic points in the semester, monitoring course discussion lists, and creating custom research guides (Veal & Bennett, 2009). At another university, librarians are given the status of Teaching Assistant within Blackboard (Herring, Burkhardt, & Wolfe, 2009). With this access to the class, their activities include posting instructional materials related to general library use such as accessing electronic books as well as materials specific to the research projects in the class (Herring et al., 2009). The librarians also created video tutorials explaining effective research techniques. In most of these instances of librarians embedded within the CMS, support and advocacy by the faculty is vital to the success of the program and for students to utilize the expertise of the librarian (Figa et al., 2009).

Course management systems are a common element of most distance education programs. While increasing amounts of information, resources, and student interaction takes place within the campus CMS such as Blackboard, Desire2Learn, or Moodle, there is rarely any built-in library component to many of these systems, and they are often run by the campus IT department without library involvement (Jackson, 2007). Consequently, library resources are often not well-represented in course management systems. Some libraries have taken a proactive approach, working with campus and library IT departments to incorporate selections of library electronic resources into courses in the CMS. At the University of Texas at Austin, librarians worked with the Blackboard administrators to include a link on each course page leading to research tips and a selection of library electronic resources relevant to the course or subject area, as well as a link to the contact information for the relevant subject librarian (M. Ostrow, personal communication, December 9, 2008). Another example of course-specific library materials automatically integrated into courses in a CMS is Duke University's system to include a course-specific library research guide, if available, in each course (Daly, 2010). If a course-specific guide is not available, the system will automatically create a link to a subject-specific research guide.

If there is no system in place to automatically include library resources, instructors might need to take a more active role in ensuring that links to library resources or library help guides are available to students at the location in the CMS in which assignments to conduct secondary research are introduced. Faculty often have a range of options for working with librarians at their university. Librarians at many universities are assigned to specific departments and work with faculty in those departments on library instruction or incorporating subject-specific resources into assignments or course pages. Many libraries with extensive distance learning programs also have a position of distance education librarian (Gandhi, 2003; Hines, 2008). This person works partly or exclusively with distance education students, faculty, and programs to create resources and policies for distance education library services and advocates for incorporating library resources into distance and off-campus courses. At some institutions, librarians work with faculty from the beginning of the course development process to incorporate library resources into new courses and are able to propose relevant library materials for inclusion in the course (Leong, 2007; Veal & Bennett, 2009). Depending on the assistance available at a particular library, Technical Communication faculty can seek out their subject librarian or a distance education librarian.

LibGuides is an increasingly popular Web-based program for creating online resource guides to highlight a selection of sources and research tips. There are currently over 1,100 academic and school libraries using the LibGuides software to create subject and course-specific guides (Springshare, 2010). The guides provide a fairly simple format for librarians to link to electronic databases, books, Web sites, and general research-related information. Each guide has its own Web address, making it easy for a faculty member to link to the guide from within a CMS or course Web site. Librarians at Utah State University create LibGuides at the request of the instructor or faculty member and typically gear the content toward a specific research assignment. These research guides often include specific databases and e-journals as well as general research tips such as citing sources and for distance education courses, information about specific policies geared toward helping distance learners access library resources. For example, the English studies librarian worked with a faculty member to create a LibGuide for a graduate level distance education Technical Communication course, which includes article databases specific to research in technical communication, search tips, resources for finding relevant books at USU and other universities, information about finding dissertations, and conducting a literature review. While library research guides often augment face-to-face library instruction sessions, they can be the sole bridge for distance students needing quality information resources. In light of the research about students' inclination to turn to free Web resources for course-related research and difficulties with filtering the amount of information they retrieve, these course research guides can both narrow the field to specific, relevant resources as well as point students to high-quality resources they might not be familiar with.

Another option for faculty is asking their librarians to create screencasts (short screen-capture videos) or other tutorials to demonstrate searching techniques in article databases and other techniques for using library resources. Screencasts are short, usually modular videos that help re-create some of the elements of a demonstration common in face-to-face library instruction (Betty, 2008). For example, librarians have created screencasts to demonstrate search strategies for databases such as Web of Science or videos demonstrating how to find the full text of an article within the library collections. Studies have shown that graphical and interactive online tutorials can be effective for communicating information about conducting research and are a useful method for librarians to provide instruction to students without access to face-to-face library instruction (Brumfield, 2008; Markey, Armstrong, & De Groote, 2005; Oehrli, Piacentine, Peters, & Nanamaker, 2011). At the University of Florida, a subject librarian working with an online engineering program created instructions and tutorials for using collections of subject-specific databases and also included techniques for conducting research such as brainstorming topics and keywords; the collection of tutorials was titled the "Library Lounge" and was available to all courses in a particular program (Kennedy, 2007).

In addition to video tutorials, faculty teaching synchronous courses through an interactive broadcast system have an additional option. As with face-to-face instruction sessions, faculty might invite the distance education librarian or their subject librarian to "meet" with the class virtually and present a selection of resources or discuss research issues and answer questions as they arise, similar to the subject-based sessions in face-to-face classes.

DIGITAL LIBRARIES

The above sections described some of the options for collaboration between teaching faculty and librarians seeking to help students develop research skills. The following sections will highlight the changing library collections and how faculty can take advantage of these resources in their online classes. Faculty do not need to have lower expectations for their online students' research projects. Electronic journals and electronic databases are popular at academic libraries, giving students and faculty ubiquitous access to scholarly materials. For the average member library of the Association for Research Libraries, 51% of all the money spent on library collections goes toward electronic materials (Kyrillidou & Bland, 2009). As an even more acute example, in the 2006–2007 academic year, health sciences libraries, which serve schools of medicine and allied health, report that a median of 70% of the funds spent on library collections goes toward electronic materials (Kyrillidou & Bland, 2008).

Databases relevant to technical communication available at many university libraries include the ACM Digital Library and IEEE Electronic Library, containing articles and proceedings related to software development and documentation and human-computer interaction. The MLA International Bibliography, ComAbstracts, and Web of Science databases contain article citations on communications research, business communication, education, software development, and many other aspects of technical communication. In addition, Digital Dissertations provides access to the full text of recent doctoral dissertations and a selection of masters' theses in Technical Communication and most other academic subjects. Key technical communication journals available electronically include the Society for Technical Communication's journal, *Technical Communication*, as well as *Technical Communication Quarterly*, *Journal of Business and Technical Communication*, and the *Journal of Technical Writing and Communication*, among others. These databases and e-journals are popular with faculty and students both on the main campus as well as those studying via distance education for the immediate access to information and journal articles. Faculty can also use these online resources to create electronic reading lists in the campus course management system, much like traditional print course packs or library e-reserves.

Another option for integrating library materials directly into a CMS or online course is through e-books, which provide another avenue for access to scholarly materials. Electronic books have proven slower to catch on than electronic journals and databases, but they are beginning to grow in popularity (Hernon, Hopper, & Leach, 2007; Shelburne, 2009). Some studies have shown that library users prefer print books over electronic books (Levine-Clark, 2006), while respondents in another study stated that e-books were difficult to read on the screen and e-books were difficult to navigate (Shelburne, 2009). Other studies have found that undergraduates are mainly interested in reading short sections of texts online, indicating that e-books might be ideal for reference collections in which students typically are using only a short section or chapter of a book (Hernon et al., 2007). However, library users do indicate they are attracted to the 24/7 access independent of the library building and features such as searching within the text (Levine-Clark, 2006). One study has shown that distance education students use e-books at a higher rate than on-campus students when the e-book collections were specifically geared toward distance education programs (Grudzien & Casey, 2008). At Utah State University, the librarians responsible for purchasing books within their subject areas focus e-book purchases in the disciplines in which print books are most commonly requested by distance education students.

E-books range from electronic versions of individual scholarly titles to groups of e-books such as Safari Books Online. Safari Books Online contains a rotating collection of e-books focused on technology and computers, potentially relevant to technical communication students. Libraries also have the option to purchase current e-books from aggregators such as NetLibrary. This enables students to access a large number of e-books with one subscription through the library. NetLibrary currently has a respectable number of technical communication e-books available full-text. Many libraries put the records for their e-books in the library catalog, so a search for books brings up both print and electronic material, with the electronic books available instantly. Again, students might need reminders or instructions from faculty or librarians in order make full use of these e-resources.

A potentially more groundbreaking development regarding e-books is the Google Books project. Google is digitizing the print collections of a group of U.S. and international libraries, with 7 million books digitized as of summer 2011 (Google, 2011). About 2 million books are out of copyright (in the public domain) and can be read online in their entirety. The bulk of the material, about 75% of the digitized books, are out-of-print (not available commercially) but in copyright. Currently, all records are searchable from Google Books, but only short snippets are available for the in-copyright but out-of-print material. The American Institute of Publishers and the Authors Guild brought a class-action lawsuit against Google in 2005 over issues involving copyright, user privacy, absent rights holders, and competition (American Library Association, 2009). The proposed settlement called for nonprofit academic institutions such as academic libraries to have the option of purchasing institutional subscriptions to the Google Books database (American Library Association, 2009). This has the potential to greatly enhance the availability of online books previously available only in print. However, the settlement was rejected in court on March 22, 2011, diminishing the likelihood of institutional subscriptions to the Google Books full-text (Band, 2011). For the foreseeable future, full-text searching of the Google Books database is allowed, but only short snippets of retrieved material are displayed if the materials are in-copyright.

One element regarding distance education and electronic library resources is the importance for academic institutions and libraries to provide straightforward methods for students and instructors to access library resources off-campus. Whereas on-campus students expect the convenience of accessing library elec- tronic resources from their home or office, for distance education students, this is an absolute necessity. At the same time, vendors typically require that all users of the databases first "prove" that they are affiliated with the university. Students, faculty, and staff at a particular institution can typically access online resources by EZ Proxy, Shibboleth, virtual private network (VPN), or another method of authenticating users off-campus based on the computer IP address. A tradi- tional proxy or VPN authentication requires users to configure their computer to connect to a server on campus; the difficulty for some to configure their computers along with the problems raised by firewalls makes these methods less than ideal (Eggleston & Ginanni, 2009). Methods of off-campus access include EZ proxy or single-password authentication systems such as Shibboleth, which require campus-affiliated users to authenticate with a username and password assigned to them by the library or campus IT and do not require anything to be downloaded or installed on their computer (Lawrence, 2009). One issue for faculty members is to ensure that any links placed within an online reading list or the course management system are accessible to off-campus students. If library resources are authenticated via EZ Proxy, a proxy prepend or short URL must be added at the beginning of the Web address for each e-journal, database or other subscription resource. This prepend redirects off-campus users to a login page where they enter their university or library credentials. While a library might have an automated system for adding the prepend (NCSU Libraries, 2011), most often the faculty member must consult with a librarian for advice or assistance on properly creating links for off-campus access to library resources.

Access to Physical Resources

To help faculty and students access physical resources, many libraries send books and videos to distance learners at their homes and will scan print articles and e-mail them to the student or instructor (Hines, 2008). Some useful books related to technical communication, including core reference texts, are not yet available electronically or only affordable in print. Shipping print materials does not address the time constraints students often operate under, but it does enable students and faculty to access the physical resources available through their library. Some libraries pay both the cost of shipping books to students and also the cost of returning the book. At Utah State University, the library pays the cost of sending out materials and also includes a prepaid mailing label for sending the book back to the library. Other libraries pay only the cost of sending the materials to the distance education students and faculty but not the cost of shipping the materials back to the library (Hammill, 2008). If students are pressed for time, this will not be a viable option, but for upper-division or longer-term projects typically carried out by graduate students and faculty, requesting print materials can be a useful option.

Reciprocal borrowing agreements are another way distance education students and faculty can access print resources. Academic libraries in some states form consortiums that, among other purposes, coordinate agreements to allow students to borrow materials in person from any other academic institution in the state (Tang, 2009). For example, in the state of Utah, an agreement among members of the Utah Academic Library Consortium allows students at any Utah academic library and several academic libraries in Nevada to check out books from any member library (Resorce Sharing Committee, 2000). In Illinois, an agreement among the members of a library consortium enables students or member institutions to borrow materials from any member library; this provides the libraries with a vast collection of materials to ship to their distance education students (Consortium of Academic & Research Libraries in Illinois, 2010). A far-reaching agreement of the Greater Western Library Alliance enables students and faculty to check out materials, in person, from a group of 32 research libraries located in 17 states in the West and Midwest (Greater Western Library Alliance, n.d.).

Depending on the local situation, faculty and students might have access to traditional interlibrary loan services. At Utah State University, there is an increasing number of tenure-track faculty and graduate students working and studying at three regional campuses and via distance education. The specialized nature of their research requires that they have access to specific print books and other material not available electronically. However, the regional campuses rely entirely on the main campus library. In 2009, the USU Library implemented a policy to provide interlibrary loan to distance education faculty and graduate students and subsequently modified the program to include "Purchase on Demand." When a book is requested by a distance education faculty or graduate student that the library does not own, the interlibrary loan office will attempt to purchase the book from Amazon.com or another rush order service. The shipping and the library cataloging process is expedited and the book is sent to the patron, usually arriving within 1 week of the request. The benefit of the Purchase On Demand program is that faculty and graduate students can then check out the materials for the 16 weeks, according to their borrowing privileges from USU, instead of the much shorter loan period set by the lending library when the material is borrowed via interlibrary loan. When the item is returned, it is placed in the general collection and available for other library patrons. If the material requested is not available via Purchase On Demand either because it is out of print or too expensive, the library will borrow the material through interlibrary loan. Other academic libraries also provide interlibrary loan to distance education student, although this service is far from universal (Michigan State University Libraries, n.d.; Oregon State University, 2010).

Even with the rise of electronic materials, there is still a large amount of material, books in particular, available only in print. For the foreseeable future, distance education students and faculty will therefore need to continue using print material in order to access the full range of resources for their research projects.

Online Reference Services

Another challenge for distance learners and faculty is not having access to a physical library building and therefore not knowing that librarians are available to help with individual research questions (Gandhi, 2003). In recent years, librarians have increasingly been utilizing electronic means to connect with distance students and adapting reference services to the communication styles of the students. Many academic libraries have been providing e-mail reference for many years, and more recently have added instant messaging reference services and text reference services (Online Reference, 2010). A difficulty that librarians face, however, is making sure that students know librarians are available to help them and that they know how to reach a librarian. This is another instance in which faculty members can take advantage of methods for students to remotely contact a librarian by placing this information within easy reach of students in the CMS or course Web site. In addition, some libraries are taking the initiative to be more accessible to the students at their point of need and in the locations where the students are online. At Utah State University and other campuses that provide research guides for specific classes, students can find the e-mail address, telephone numbers, and text messaging numbers for the library or their subject librarian within each course research guide, along with a chat box where they can send an instant message directly to the reference desk or in some cases to their subject librarian. Some librarians are making this chat box available within library databases, such as the popular EbscoHOST article databases (Pival, 2010). In this way, students and faculty will be able to get help at the point of need, and the librarians will be more visible to off-campus students.

Copyright

Copyright laws are another challenge growing in complexity for faculty and librarians alike; an online teaching environment presents new challenges for incorporating resources into a class. Distance education librarians have seen a concern among faculty about what materials they can legally use in online classes and how they are permitted to use the materials (Hines, 2006). Under copyright law, all works are automatically granted copyright protection at the time a new work is created, including literature, music, photography, images, and other creative works (U.S. Copyright Office, 2008). Registration or attaching a copyright notice to a work is not required, which might cause confusion about what is under copyright protection, particularly on the Internet. Fortunately, higher education faculty and instructors can apply principles of fair use and in some cases with distance education—the TEACH Act—in order to use some copyrighted materials in their teaching without paying copyright fees for each use.

Section 107 of the Copyright Act established that use of a copyrighted work is permitted if the use meets certain criteria of "fair use" (Copyright at USU, 2010). Fair use typically allows including selections of copyrighted material in the classroom for educational purposes, under certain conditions (NOLO, 2007). The four factors to consider when deciding whether materials can be used under fair use are

- Purpose and character of the use, i.e., commercial use or nonprofit/ educational use;
- Nature of the copyrighted work, i.e., fiction or nonfiction, published or unpublished;

- Amount and substantiality of the portion of the work used in relation to the work as a whole; and
- Effect of the use upon the potential market for or the value of the copyrighted work (NOLO, 2007).

There are many "checklists" available on the Internet for evaluating a fair use argument (Brigham Young University Copyright Licensing Office, 2006). However, each fair use judgment is unique, and the criteria must be weighed by the faculty member planning to use a copyrighted work.

The TEACH Act of 2002 (Technology, Education, and Copyright Harmonization Act) provided an update to copyright law to address issues with transmission and displays of copyrighted material in distance learning (Copyright Clearance Center, 2005b). There are, however, significant stipulations within the TEACH Act. Among other requirements, materials must be an integral part of the class experience (not supplemental materials such as textbooks or course readings); controlled by or under the supervision of the instructor; and analogous to the type of performance or display that would take place in a live classroom setting (University of Texas Libraries, 2007). Specific requirements of the TEACH Act include specifications that "reasonable" efforts must be made to prevent retention and dissemination of copyrighted works, materials should be available only to currently enrolled students, students must be informed that the materials they access are protected by copyright, and the educational institution, in addition to being a nonprofit institution, must have a policy on the use of copyrighted materials and provide copyright resources for faculty (Copyright Clearance Center, 2005a). Considering these constraints, fair use is often used for distance learning courses if the TEACH Act does not provide the necessary permissions (University of Texas Libraries, 2007).

One area of the TEACH Act that might be of interest to distance education instructors are the stipulations covering digitizing and displaying videos in an online course. The TEACH Act specifically addresses transmitting films and other audiovisual materials for educational purposes within a distance education setting under the direction of the instructor and as an integral part of a class session (Band, Butler, Crews, & Jaszi, 2010). While the TEACH Act specifies the transmission of a film must be in reasonable and limited portions, some legal experts argue the TEACH Act could permit the streaming of significant portions of a film "in light of the overarching purpose of the TEACH Act, which is to allow the use of all copyrighted materials in distance education in ways that are analogous to their use in a physical classroom" (Band et al., 2010). Faculty members will likely need to seek out experts at their university for assistance with interpreting these regulations. At Utah State University, the Media Production group and the Distance Education office handle the process of securing copyright and streaming films, with help from the instructional designers at the Faculty Assistance Center for Teaching. These groups work together to make sure that copyright laws are followed, while still enabling faculty to include the materials they need in their classes.

Faculty who would like to include resources from the library's online article databases and electronic journals need to be aware of copyright issues and licensing restrictions. Licensing agreements often specify that instructors can link to full-text articles within a database but cannot save a file, such as a pdf, into the course management system. Most online subscription databases and e-journals provide a durable, or permanent, link to each full-text article within the database or e-journal. As noted above, faculty members might need to seek help from a librarian for details about a particular library's licensing agreements and locating or creating durable URLs.

Incorporating images into a Web site or course page and providing course packs to students are two other issues related to copyright that distance faculty might face. Creators of Web sites or online courses should assume all images are under copyright. It is not always sufficient to merely provide an acknowledgment for a photo or image; a safer option is to look for a "terms of use" or copyright information for the image to find out exactly how and where the image is allowed to be displayed. For classroom use, such as creating print handouts, fair use rules typically apply, but the situation is not always so straightforward with online displays or transmittal of images. Fortunately, there are many images in the public domain and images that have been given creative commons licensing. Creative Commons enables creators or authors to specify the copyright restrictions for their work, often allowing use with attribution for noncommercial purposes (Creative Commons, 2010). Using images with appropriate creative commons licensing prevents faculty from needing to obtain written permission. Course packs are also an area in which faculty can unknowingly violate copyright. If the campus bookstore traditionally supplies packets of supplement materials to students and sells the course packs to cover the cost of the copyright permissions, this same process applies to distance courses.

Libraries and other university departments ideally will provide Web sites and other information for faculty to inform them of copyright issues and the methods by which they can use materials within their online courses (Copyright Licensing Office, 2006; MLibrary, 2007). Given the issues that arise around online teaching and learning, it is safe to assert that copyright is likely to be an actively discussed and debated topic in the future.

Virtual Online Environments

Regardless of the institution or situation, "Where educators and students go, librarians must follow" (Davis & Smith, 2009). One of the more innovative realms in which faculty and librarians are interacting with students is in Second Life and other virtual online environments. Second Life is a 3-D virtual environment wherein users interact in real time using self-created personas; these spaces are sometimes referred to as multiuser virtual environments (Greenhill, 2008). Within Second Life, universities and other entities can purchase space and set up a virtual university, which can also be accompanied by a virtual library building (Kattelman, 2008). At one university that offered classes in Second Life, librarians presented library-related minilectures to students within Second Life, and librarians "attended" class sessions and answered questions about library resources, while another library developed a space in Second Life to provide access to a selection of the library's digital collections (Davis & Smith, 2009; Swanson, 2007). Other librarians have utilized space in Second Life to collaborate with campus faculty members (Buckland & Godfrey, 2010).

Despite the initial success of Second Life, activity and membership has leveled off (Little, 2011). Publication of related journal articles in the library literature are concentrated around the years 2007–2008, and more recent authors are raising doubts about the future of academic institutions in virtual online environments, particularly in light of a decision by the company that owns Second Life to eliminate educational discounts (Little, 2011; Sanchez, 2009). Other academics are arguing that new virtual online worlds will replace Second Life, particularly for distance education (Little, 2011). Open Cobalt is a large-scale open-source workspace currently under development, and OpenSimulator is another nascent open-source system with some similarities to Second Life (Young, 2010). The EDUCAUSE Virtual Worlds Constituent Group is continuing the conversation around the role of academia in multiuser virtual environments, and the San Jose State University School of Library and Information Science is developing SLOODLE (Simulation Linked Object Oriented Dynamic Learning Environment), an open-source system integrating the virtual worlds of Second Life and OpenSimulator with the Moodle course management system (EDUCAUSE, 2011; SLOODLE, 2011). What is the future of these virtual worlds for higher education? That remains to be seen, but if an academic institution is involved in one of the 3-D environments currently available, faculty will likely have an opportunity to collaborate with the librarians in this space.

Information Literacy and Online Education

Information literacy involves the ability to effectively select, retrieve, use, and evaluate information (Association of College and Research Libraries, 2010), and this concept forms the core of many library instruction programs. Librarians are creating online services and products, such as interactive tutorials, to help students acquire these skills and then working with faculty to incorporate these library tutorials and instructions into online classes at the correct time and sequence. Opportunities abound for collaboration between teaching faculty and librarians, and indeed, a closer collaboration might be more imperative in an online learning context than with traditional face-to-face courses. Together, teaching faculty and librarians can help to address the seeming contradiction that due to the proliferation of electronic resources and the abundance of readily available information, students report that they perceive completing course-related research to be more difficult than in the days of predominately print resources (Head & Eisenberg, 2009a). The specifics may vary based on library and institution, but faculty members and instructors can work with their librarians to help students navigate the information landscape and access the best resources for their needs. Faculty members can invite librarians to provide expertise and instruction from within the course management system, interacting directly with students through online discussion groups or via interactive broadcasts, or through help guides and tutorials. In addition, faculty members and students can take advantage of online libraries and electronic resources to access scholarly materials, such as databases, e-journals, and e-books, while remembering that students might need additional help to find and search these resources and interpret and filter the sources they retrieve. At the same time, librarians are developing procedures to ensure that distance students have access to the physical resources of the library through reciprocal borrowing programs and free mailing services. Faculty can also initiate collaborative efforts and push librarians in the directions they need to go in order to best serve distance education students.

As online education programs expand, the library will follow the lead of the institution and reach out to students and faculty. Through innovative policies and procedures, electronic collections, and online instructional materials, faculty and librarians can work together to help their students in the realm of online education, just as they do with on-campus students.

REFERENCES

American Library Association. (2009). *Google Books settlement.* Retrieved September 8, 2009, from http://wo.ala.org/gbs/

Association of College and Research Libraries. (2010). *Introduction to information literacy.* Retrieved March 18, 2010, from http://www.ala.org/ala/mgrps/divs/acrl/issues/infolit/overview/intro/index.cfm

Band, J. (2011). A guide for the perplexed, part IV: The rejection of the Google Books settlement. *Library Copyright Alliance.* Retrieved from http://www.librarycopyright alliance.org/bm~doc/guideiv-final-1.pdf

Band, J., Butler, B., Crews, K., & Jaszi, P. (2010). *Issue brief: Streaming of films for educational purposes.* Retrieved May 13, 2010, from http://www.librarycopyright alliance.org/bm~doc/ibstreamingfilms_021810.pdf

Betty, P. (2008). Creation, management, and assessment of library screencasts: The Regis Libraries animated tutorials project. *Journal of Library Administration, 48*(¾), 295–315.

Brigham Young University Copyright Licensing Office. (2006). *Checklist for fair use.* Retrieved May 9, 2010, from http://www.lib.byu.edu/departs/copyright/overview/Checklist_for_Fair_Use.pdf

Brouse, C. H., McKnight, K. R., Basch, C. E., & LeBlanc, M. (2010). A pilot study of instructor factors and student preferences. *Journal of Educational Technology Systems, 38*(1), 51–62.

Brumfield, E. J. (2008). Using online tutorials to reduce uncertainty in information seeking behavior. *Journal of Library Administration, 48*(3), 365–377.

Buckland, A., & Godfrey, K. (2010). Save the time of the avatar: Canadian academic libraries using chat reference in multi-user virtual environments. *Reference Librarian, 51*(1), 12–30. doi: 10.1080/02763870903389319

Byrne, S., & Bates, J. (2009). Use of the university library, elibrary, VLE, and other information sources by distance learning students in University College Dublin: Implications for academic librarianship. *New Review of Academic Librarianship, 15*(1), 120–141. doi: 10.1080/13614530903143169

Cahoy, E. S., & Moyo, L. M. (2005). Faculty perspectives on e-learners' library research needs. *Journal of Library & Information Services in Distance Learning, 2*(4), 1–17.

Consortium of Academic & Research Libraries in Illinois. (2010). *What is I-Share?* Retrieved March 9, 2010, from http://www.carli.illinois.edu/mem-prod/I-Share.html

Copyright at USU. (2010). *Fair use: The ins and outs.* Retrieved July 18, 2011, from http://usu.edu/copyrightatusu/materials/fairuse-ins-outs.cfm

Copyright Clearance Center. (2005a). Copyright basics: The TEACH Act. *The Campus Guide to Copyright Compliance.* Retrieved November 23, 2010, from http://www.copyright.com/Services/copyrightoncampus/basics/teach.html

Copyright Clearance Center. (2005b). *The TEACH Act: New roles, rules and responsibilities for academic institutions.* Retrieved March 5, 2010, from http://www.copyright.com/media/pdfs/CR-Teach-Act.pdf

Copyright Licensing Office. (2006). *BYU copyright licensing office.* Retrieved March 5, 2010, from http://www.lib.byu.edu/departs/copyright/

Creative Commons. (2010). *Creative commons.* Retrieved May 14, 2010, from http://creativecommons.org/

Daly, E. (2010). Embedding library resources into learning management systems: A way to reach Duke undergrads at their points of need. *College & Research Libraries News, 71*(4), 208–212.

Davis, M. G., & Smith, C. E. (2009). Virtually embedded: Library instruction within Second Life. *Journal of Library & Information Services in Distance Learning, 3*(¾), 120–137. doi: 10.1080/15332900903375465

EDUCAUSE. (2011). *Virtual worlds constituent group.* Retrieved July 13, 2011, from http://www.educause.edu/groups/VW

Eggleston, H., & Ginanni, K. (2009). Simplifying licensed resource access through Shibboleth. *The Serials Librarian, 56,* 209–214.

Figa, E., Bone, T., & Macpherson, J. R. (2009). Faculty-librarian collaboration for library services in the online classroom: Student evaluation results and recommended practices for implementation. *Journal of Library & Information Services in Distance Learning, 3*(2), 67–102. doi: 10.1080/15332900902979119

Gandhi, S. (2003). Academic librarians and distance education: Challenges and opportunities. *Reference & User Services Quarterly, 43*(2), 138–154.

Google. (2009). *Google Books settlement agreement.* Retrieved September 9, 2009, from http://books.google.com/agreement

Google. (2011). *Google Books settlement agreement.* Retrieved July 19, 2011, from http://books.google.com/googlebooks/agreement/

Greater Western Library Alliance. (n.d.). *Agreements & licenses.* Retrieved July 19, 2011, from http://www.gwla.org/agreements-and-licenses

Greenhill, K. (2008). Do we remove all the walls? Second Life librarianship. *Australian Library Journal, 57*(4), 377–393.

Grudzien, P., & Casey, A. M. (2008). Do off-campus students use e-books? *Journal of Library Administration, 48*(3), 455–466.

Hammill, S. J. (2008). Tallying the chad marks in the ballot box: A survey of distance learning library services in Florida's state universities. *E-JASL: The Electronic Journal of Academic and Special Librarianship, 9*(2).

Head, A. J., & Eisenberg, M. B. (2009a, February 9). Finding context: What today's college students say about conducting research in the digital age. Project Information Literacy progress report. *The Information School, University of Washington.* Retrieved from http://projectinfolit.org/pdfs/PIL_ProgressReport_2_2009.pdf

Head, A. J., & Eisenberg, M. B. (2009b, December 1). Lessons learned: How college students seek information in the digital age. Project Information Literacy progress report. *The Information School, University of Washington.* Retrieved from http://projectinfolit.org/pdfs/PIL_Fall2009_finalv_YR1_12_2009v2.pdf

Hernon, P., Hopper, R., & Leach, M. R. (2007). E-book use by students: Undergraduates in economics, literature, and nursing. *The Journal of Academic Librarianship, 33*(1), 3–13.

Herring, S. D., Burkhardt, R. R., & Wolfe, J. L. (2009). Reaching remote students. *College & Research Libraries News, 70*(11), 630–633.

Hines, S. S. (2006). What do distance education faculty want from the library? *Journal of Library Administration, 45*(1), 215–227.

Hines, S. S. (2008). How it's done: Examining distance education library instruction and assessment. *Journal of Library Administration, 48*(3), 467–478.

Holliday, W., & Li, Q. (2004). Understanding the millennials: Updating our knowledge about students. *Reference Services Review, 32*(4), 356–366.

Jackson, P. A. (2007). Integrating information literacy into Blackboard: Building campus partnerships for successful student learning. *The Journal of Academic Librarianship, 33*(4), 454–461.

Jones, S. (2002). The Internet goes to college: How students are living in the future with today's technology. *Pew Internet and American Life Project.* Retrieved from http://www.pewinternet.org/~/media//Files/Reports/2002/PIP_College_Report.pdf.pdf

Kattelman, B. (2008). It's time for a Second Life. *College & Research Libraries News, 69*(10), 614–617.

Kennedy, K. (2007). Providing online information literacy instruction to nontraditional distance education engineering students. In A. Daugherty & M. F. Russo (Eds.), *Information literacy programs in the digital age: Educating college and university students online* (pp. 115–125). Chicago, IL: Association of College and Research Libraries.

Kyrillidou, M., & Bland, L. (2008). ARL Academic Health Sciences Library statistics 2006–2007. *Association of Research Libraries.* Retrieved March 1, 2010, from http://search.ebscohost.com/

Kyrillidou, M., & Bland, L. (2009). ARL Statistics 2007–2008. *Association of Research Libraries*. Retrieved March 1, 2010, from http://www.arl.org/bm~doc/arlstat08.pdf

Lawrence, P. (2009). Access when and where they want it: Using EZproxy to serve our remote users. *Computers in Libraries, 29*(1), 6.

Leong, J. (2007). Marketing electronic resources to distance students: A multipronged approach. *Serials Librarian, 53*(3), 77–93.

Levine-Clark, M. (2006). Electronic book usage: A survey at the university of Denver. *portal: Libraries & the Academy, 6*(3), 285–299.

Little, G. (2011). Managing technology: Should I stay or should I go? Academic libraries and Second Life. *Journal of Academic Librarianship, 37*(2), 171–173.

Markey, K., Armstrong, A., & De Groote, S. (2005). Testing the effectiveness of interactive multimedia for library-user education. *portal: Libraries & the Academy, 5*(4), 527–544.

Michigan State University Libraries. (n.d.). *Off campus users*. Retrieved September 3, 2009, from http://www.lib.msu.edu/about/ils/offcampus50.jsp

MLibrary. (2007). *Copyright basics*. Retrieved March 5, 2010, from http://www.copyright.umich.edu/basics.html

NCSU Libraries. (2011). *Library article linker*. Retrieved July 13, 2011, from http://www.lib.ncsu.edu/librarylinker/

NOLO. (2007). *Copyright and fair use*. Retrieved 5 March, 2010, from http://fairuse.stanford.edu/Copyright_and_Fair_Use_Overview/chapter9/index.html

Oehrli, J. A., Piacentine, J., Peters, A., & Nanamaker, B. (2011, March 30–April 2). *Do screencasts really work? Assessing student learning through instructional screencasts*. Paper presented at the ACRL National Conference, Philadelphia, PA.

Online Reference. (2010). Retrieved 13 March, 2010, from http://www.libsuccess.org/index.php?title=Online_Reference

Oregon State University. (2010). *Services for OSU extended campus students and faculty— Policies and procedures*. Retrieved December 2, 2009, from http://osulibrary.oregon state.edu/offcampus/policies.htm

Pival, P. (2010, February 18). *Embedding chat widgets within EBSCO databases*. Retrieved from http://distlib.blogs.com/distlib/2010/02/embedding-chat-widgets-within-ebsco-databases.html

Resource Sharing Committee. (2000). *Reciprocal borrowing agreement*. Retrieved from http://aaa.usu.edu/Assessment/Standard_Five/UALC_Reciporcal.pdf

Sanchez, J. (2009). Facing realities. *Library Technology Reports, 45*(2), 5–8.

Shelburne, W. A. (2009). E-book usage in an academic library: User attitudes and behaviors. *Library Collections, Acquisitions, & Technical Services, 33*(2/3), 59–72. doi: 10.1016/j.lcats.2009.04.002

Shelton, K. (2009). Library outreach to part-time and distance education instructors. *Community & Junior College Libraries, 15*(1), 3–8.

SLOODLE. (2011). Retrieved July 13, 2011, from http://slisweb.sjsu.edu/sl/index.php/SLOODLE

Springshare. (2010). *LibGuides community*. Retrieved March 19, 2010, from http://libguides.com/community.php

Swanson, K. (2007). Second Life: A science library presence in virtual reality. *Science & Technology Libraries, 27*(3), 79–86. doi: 10.1300/J122v27n0306

Tang, Y. (2009). Placing theory into practice: An exploration of library services to distance learners at Jacksonville State University. *Journal of Library & Information Services in Distance Learning, 3*(¾), 173–181. doi: 10.1080/15332900903375432

Thomsett-Scott, B., & May, F. (2009). How may we help you? Online education faculty tell us what they need from libraries and librarians. *Journal of Library Administration, 49*(1), 111–135.

University of Texas Libraries. (2007). *Copyright crash course: The TEACH Act.* Retrieved May 13, 2010, from http://copyright.lib.utexas.edu/teachact.html

U.S. Copyright Office. (2008). *Copyright basics.* Retrieved from http://www.copyright.gov/circs/circ1.pdf

van Scoyoc, A. M., & Cason, C. (2006). The electronic academic library: Undergraduate research behavior in a library without books. *portal: Libraries & the Academy, 6*(1), 47–58.

Veal, R., & Bennett, E. (2009). The virtual library liaison: A case study at an online university. *Journal of Library Administration, 49*(1), 161–170.

Young, J. R. (2010). After frustrations in Second Life, colleges look to new virtual worlds. *The Chronicle of Higher Education.* Retrieved from http://chronicle.com/article/After-Frustrations-in-Second/64137/

http://dx.doi.org/10.2190/OE2C15

CHAPTER 15

"Keeping it Real": Contextualizing Intellectual Property and Privacy in the Online Technical Communication Course

Natalie Stillman-Webb

Teaching technical communication online can bring new pedagogical strategies and with them different forms of communication, collaboration, and information distribution. Yet with the potential for easier distribution of information online come questions of ownership of that information and ethics in its digital transfer. What happens, for instance, when an image of a bone density scan used as a figure in a proposal for a new machine includes patient identifying information? Or an email list of past donors for a nonprofit fundraising campaign is accidentally sent to individuals outside the organization? There is a need to address the limits of textual sharing—legal, ethical, and practical. How have interpretations or conceptions of intellectual property and privacy changed with the proliferation of digital texts and online education? How can instructors of such courses negotiate intellectual property issues while taking advantage of communication technologies that support effective teaching of technical writing? What aspects of intellectual property beyond "fair use" or the educational context need to be considered in light of the types of work done in technical writing courses? This chapter presents strategies for negotiating between "keeping it real"—encouraging students to gain technical writing experience by composing for outside organizations—and addressing intellectual property and privacy issues in theory and practice within the online technical communication course.

ACADEMIC-ORGANIZATIONAL
PARTNERSHIPS

Technical communication instructors in both on-campus and online settings have recognized the student benefits of writing for external audiences. In preparing students for work as technical communicators or for writing within their chosen professions, tying course assignments to real-world contexts and purposes can be an effective strategy for combining theory and practice, introducing students to professional writing contexts and genres, motivating them as they see tangible results of their work, and helping them make the transition to the workplace. Compared with responding to case studies or to hypothetical situations and audiences, such assignments can help students shape their communication for an audience they can interact with and learn from. Students may write course documents that draw upon the context of an organization they are already affiliated with as an employee, member, or volunteer, or they may be assigned an organization through an academic-corporate partnership. They can complete client-based projects as groups or individuals, projects that may involve communication problem solving, desktop publishing, or research and report writing. Alternately termed "project-based learning" (Dubinsky, 2004), "client-based learning" (Hansen, 2004), "experiential learning" (Cooke & Williams, 2004), "classroom-workplace collaborations" (Blakeslee, 2001), or "workplace activity network" participation (Spinuzzi, 1996), client-based project pedagogy has long been employed by technical communication instructors and can be a practical, course-based alternative to more intensive, programmatic technical writing internships.

Real-world writing experience is also gained through service-learning, a practice that has grown rapidly over the last decade and is now well-established within technical communication. With a service-learning project, students are paired with a local nonprofit organization to create documents the organization needs but lacks the personnel or resources to create. Like client-based projects, service-learning partnerships allow students to see the rhetorical effects of their writing—from grant proposals to newsletters or Web sites—in the public sphere. Such projects have the additional advantage of engaging students where writing and social issues meet and expanding their sense of civic awareness, with reflection on these larger social issues an important component of the learning process (Henson & Sutliff, 1998; Huckin, 1997; Matthews & Zimmerman, 1999).

The online technical communication class can be a fertile space for such student-organization partnerships. Online communication resources can help facilitate "real world" learning by foregrounding the textual production process in an environment in which most communication takes place in writing. Such an environment, wherein students frequently communicate with the instructor, fellow students, and the organization via various writing technologies, can help reinforce the importance of workplace writing skills and of using the writing process to plan and revise even routine messages for professional communication.

Employing technology for synchronous or asynchronous communication, online technical communication courses incorporating organizational or corporate partnerships can facilitate collaborative text production, peer review of texts, and communication with partner organizations. Whereas it can be difficult during busy daily operations for nonprofit employees or volunteers to take time to meet with students in person, communication technology can free conversation participants from time and space constraints. If working in groups, students can coordinate writing tasks via electronic communication as well as manage and share drafts of documents created for the organization. And students can receive electronic feedback (often in a more timely manner than in face-to-face courses) from the organization, instructor and peers.

Yet ease of textual distribution also brings potential pitfalls. Unless it is a Web-based text that is password protected, each time a document file is viewed it is downloaded and a new copy created, which can lead to a proliferation of copies. This can be problematic when content of the digital text comes from the client company or organization and may potentially include information not intended for public release. While large corporations have developed policies and procedures when it comes to proprietary or confidential information, with smaller companies and nonprofits this may not be the case. The benefits of communication and collaboration in the online technical communication class are thus complicated by issues of intellectual property and privacy that can arise when working with off-campus entities.

Such issues of intellectual property and privacy, however, remain largely unaddressed in the client-based learning or service-learning literature. One exception is Thomas Huckin's (1997, p. 7) articulation of the connection between service-learning and technical communication, in which he includes as the third of four criteria for selecting service-learning writing projects the need to choose projects that do not involve confidential information. Nevertheless, a careful determination at the outset of a project may not always rule out students coming in contact with confidential information, throughout several weeks of research and conversations within the partner relationship. Even seemingly straightforward projects involving composition of routine documents can involve information—customer lists, financial statements, company policies—not meant for audiences beyond a specific context and group of readers, and even carefully screened projects can yield questions regarding proprietary or confidential information once underway.

Although these issues regarding sensitive information within the context of a client project or service-learning project may also emerge in the face-to-face classroom, they are intensified online: relying on electronic transmission of texts, the online environment makes the facility, speed, and breadth of distribution both a benefit and a potential drawback. While an unintentional disclosure of proprietary information might be a problem in the face-to-face course, it can become an exponentially bigger problem online. Consider, for example, a peer review scenario in which a student inadvertently includes protected information in a document draft. In an on-ground class peer review session, only two or three fellow students might briefly view the particular information as part of a hard copy document that is returned to the writer at the end of the session. In an online class, this same text posted to a peer review group—even within a password-protected site—is now available for multiple views, downloading and storage on peers' hard drives, and from there potentially wide distribution, as the document may now be read on a shared computer, saved on a flash drive that goes missing, transferred along with a hacked email account, or accidentally emailed to the wrong user.

Building community and sharing writing within the online class can thus be at odds with protecting proprietary or confidential information of partner organizations and their clients. Creating assignments in which students draw on course content to create technical communication for an organization can be problematic as these projects are inflected by the organization's proprietary processes or its customers' privacy. Even with careful choice of topics these issues can arise, partly out of the growth of various legal contexts—in particular intellectual property and privacy law—that have evolved to address electronic dissemination of information in an attempt to keep up with new production technologies and digital practices. Just as composition scholars have advocated foregrounding legal issues of ownership and authorship in teaching students to avoid plagiarism or what has also been termed "patchwriting" (Howard, 1995), I believe it is useful to critically examine with students legal conceptions of intellectual property and privacy—not in order to legislate writing practice but in order to emphasize ethics and enable student agency within textual decision-making processes.

Intellectual Property

In theorizing relationships between writing instruction and intellectual property, scholars have focused primarily on questions of authorship within an academic context, addressing fair use of teaching materials (Logie, 2005; Lunsford & West, 1996; Woodmansee & Jasci, 1995); potential problems of student plagiarism (Haviland & Mullin, 2009; Howard & Robillard, 2008; Warnock, 2009); copyright or licensing of online course materials (Faber & Johnson-Eilola, 2005; Throne, 2000), or ownership of texts in peer writing groups (Spigelman, 2000). Engaging in debates about the legal aspects of intellectual property, compositionists have critiqued the trend toward greater copyright restriction, discussing the ways in which Congress and the judicial branch have responded to new technologies for digital reproduction with legislation (such as the Copyright Term Extension Act [CTEA] of 1998, Digital Millennium

Copyright Act [DMCA] of 1998, and the Technology, Education, and Copyright Harmonization [TEACH] Act of 2002) or court decisions (such as in Basic Books v. Kinko's or MGM v. Grokster) that have favored content producers or copyright owners over individual users. Such discussions have effectively advocated for the preservation of instructors' ability to use multimodal texts in the classroom and students' ability to draw upon existing texts to create their own compositions; however, they do not consider intellectual property issues that can arise specifically in technical communication classes, the role of outside organizations as student writing partners or potential student employers, or the ways in which students will encounter intellectual property issues once they have left the university and entered the workplace.

In a technical communication context, consideration needs be given to the ways in which conceptions of workplace intellectual property (both legal and practical) are different from academic ones. Authorship functions differently in the technical writing workplace from ideas of individual authorship embedded in copyright fair-use guidelines, for example. This is seen in the common workplace practices of collaboration, boilerplate, template use and single sourcing. Locke Carter notes of single sourcing, "As a practice, single sourcing puts pressure on the seemingly stable constructs of the writer and the document in ways that many previous innovations have not" (2003, p. 318).

Another difference in workplace authorship as defined legally is the "work-for-hire" clause within U.S. copyright law, which attributes ownership of a document to the organization and not the individual:

> In the case of a work made for hire, the employer or other person for whom the work was prepared is considered the author for purposes of this title, and, unless the parties have expressly agreed otherwise in a written instrument signed by them, owns all of the rights comprised in the copyright.
> (U.S. Copyright Act, 1976)

In Jessica Reyman's discussion of plagiarism, she cites "work-for-hire" as one example of "how the 'legal author' differs from the original, solitary individualized author construct of the academy" noting that "this shift of authorship from the individual to the organization no doubt supports acts of copying and re-use common in [workplace] settings" (2008, p. 65). In other words, company ownership of documents—whether individually or collaboratively produced—makes possible the reuse of texts composed within the organization. Authorship is thus different in workplace contexts students will encounter in service-learning projects and after graduation. Although students working on a client or service-learning project aren't subject to the work-for-hire clause (unless there is a specific agreement made in advance) since they are not contracted employees or paid interns, teaching such differences in authorship is useful in preparing students for the different treatment of textual ownership in the workplace context. Like work-for-hire, other provisions within copyright law and the larger umbrella of intellectual property law are useful in examining the differences of workplace authorship.

Intellectual property law regarding digital texts, which students may associate most readily with personal use and press coverage of peer-to-peer media exchange, has different implications in the workplace, not simply in the sense of an obligation to dutifully protect the intellectual property of a project partner, but in terms of ethical choices in textual use. Not only can laws governing intellectual property be different from those in an educational context but so can the stakes and ethical dimensions. In addressing ethics, it is helpful to draw on McKee and Porter's assertion (based on the work of Jonsen and Toulmin) that "ethical decision-making requires attentiveness to people's lives—and to the complexities, differences, and nuances of human experience" (2009, p. 27); "general principles alone," they insist, are not sufficient; instead, "ethical reasoning has to proceed through some kind of analytic consideration of the particular circumstances of the case" (p. 28). As instructors we can facilitate this consideration of circumstances and individual implications by presenting a diversity of approaches in the classroom in the form of legal cases and organizational case studies, discussing the ways in which human lives are affected. Although every technical communication textbook addresses ethical issues and notes the importance of considering multiple audiences and stakeholders for documents (offering examples such as the Challenger shuttle disaster or Three Mile Island accident as instructive communication failures), such textbook discussions of ethics aren't brought into connection with workplace intellectual property.

A compelling illustration of the importance of attention to copyright and ethics in software programming practice is offered by Brian Ballantine, who begins his analysis of the rhetoric of advocates of open-source programming by discussing the consequences of ignoring intellectual property (2009). Ballantine relates his experience working as a software engineer for a medical company, beta testing a software application allowing doctors to view via the Web patient MRI and CT scans:

> In this instance, a software engineer working for the hospital had modified, or hacked, the application's code in order to provide an additional feature for the software. All of the software in use came with strict warnings about not tampering with an application's code. In addition, companies went out of their way to deliberately obfuscate their code. That is, we wrote code to try and protect our code. The unfortunate side-effect of the hospital engineer's alterations was that it caused some of the images under review to be in a mirrored or reversed format. Consequently, in a procedure to remove a brain tumor, a surgeon actually started an operation on the wrong side of a patient's head. (2009, pp. 68–69)

Ballantine goes on to point out that, while an "isolated incident," "I believe the flagrant disregard and disrespect for the obfuscation techniques employed in the hospital software point to a larger cultural, legal, and ethical disconnect regarding copyrighted works in digital form" (p. 69). Some information is not meant to be "free and open," as Ballantine argues, emphasizing that responsibility comes with digital access (p. 76). Ballantine's remarks point to contexts in which corporate intellectual property needs to be considered. Though our students will likely not meet with such a dramatic situation, we can use such examples to help bring awareness of where ethics come into play with proprietary information, particularly in digital form. Whatever our sense of corporations, it is important to consider how choices involving digital proprietary information may affect individual stakeholders.

One factor that may have contributed to the decision in the example above to hack the code—aside from the likely belief that the hack was in the greater good of improving the software—is a sense that digital information seems less fixed, less authoritative, and more malleable. Digitally, then, it may be easier for individuals to disregard copyright. It is useful to talk in the classroom about terms of authorship and when texts are clearly not meant to be treated as boiler-plate. Cases in which sensitive or proprietary information is involved are fine places to consider digital choices in terms of copyright, the limits of authorship, and effects on stakeholders.

In the workplace such proprietary information can fall under the larger umbrella of intellectual property law that is "idea protection" and what Siva Vaidhyanathan terms "a complex web of trade secret laws, unfair competition laws, contractual obligations, and industry traditions" (2001, p. 33). Organizations may have proprietary information, from simply confidential information to trade secrets, that includes "lists of customers or potential clients, 'source code' for computer programs, and corporate policies" (p. 19). Note that some of these types of texts are rather routine items that students might work on or incorporate as they complete a client project: using a list of potential clients to create marketing documents, employing existing Web source code as a template for a new page linked to the company homepage, or reviewing existing organizational policies in order to create a document such as a volunteer handbook. While it is unlikely that students will in the course of a school project come into possession of the recipe for Coca-Cola or be accused of economic espionage, off-campus partners that are smaller organizations or nonprofits with only a few employees and flatter hierarchies may allow more access to information than will larger organizations. It is thus useful to discuss in the classroom the ways that intellectual property functions in the workplace—perhaps looking at trade-secret laws, which are primarily governed by state statutes—and encourage in students a sensitivity to information and a critical awareness of when actions have been taken (in warnings, nondisclosure statements, or in Ballantine's case, obfuscation of code) to protect it.

Privacy

In the context of the classroom-workplace partnership, students may encounter not only organizational intellectual property but also potentially individual intellectual property and privacy. Privacy laws, while separate from intellectual property legally, function to protect individual confidential information. And, as with intellectual property, composition scholars have looked at privacy as it pertains within an academic setting, for instance examining student privacy on campus wireless networks (Poe & Garfinkel, 2009) and student legal challenges of requirements to submit their texts to Turnitin and other online plagiarism-detection services, invoking the Family Educational Rights and Privacy Act (FERPA) (Purdy, 2005). There is also substantial recent work on the ethics of writing research and privacy rights of research subjects (Anderson, 1998; Lamos, 2009), especially as this research involves digital texts (McIntire-Strasberg, 2007; McKee & Porter, 2008). Yet unaddressed are situations in which students may come into contact with the privacy rights of others within within a class project or in a future workplace.

As more information is rendered digitally through company innovations as well as (in some industries) federal mandates, there is increased availability of data about individuals through organizational databases and embedded in multiple workplace processes. This includes not only confidential information about employees but also that of customers or patients. Legally, individual privacy is written into such statutes as the Final Rule on Privacy of Consumer Financial Information (the Gramm-Leach-Bliley Act) of 1999, which prohibits financial institutions and real estate agencies from disclosing individuals' financial information, and the Video Privacy Protection Act (VPPA) of 1988, which protects customer audiovisual rental and sale records. As a specific example here, however, I would like to focus on the health professions and those companies and organizations that service them, for which privacy law takes the form of the Privacy Rule portion of the Health Information Privacy Accountability Act (HIPAA). Issued in 2002, six years after HIPAA, the Privacy Rule reflected a recognition by Congress that health information privacy was threatened by technological advances. The rule protects individually identifiable health information, which is to be accessed only by those authorized to provide treatment. Information security is addressed specifically in the "Privacy of Individually Identifiable Health Information" section:

(a) *General requirements.* Covered entities must do the following:
   (1) Ensure the confidentiality, integrity, and availability of all electronic protected health information the covered entity creates, receives, maintains, or transmits.
   (2) Protect against any reasonably anticipated threats or hazards to the security or integrity of such information.

(3) Protect against any reasonably anticipated uses or disclosures of such information that are not permitted or required under subpart E of this part.

(4) Ensure compliance with this subpart by its workforce. (HIPAA, 1996)

In addition to protecting "health information the covered entity creates, receives, maintains or transmits" requiring diligence on the part of personnel as well as information technology security, the HIPAA Privacy Act charges healthcare organizations with ensuring that third parties or business associates also comply with the privacy and security standards. Recently, this direct responsibility for protecting private health information of individuals was expanded beyond health care organizations to contractors working with them, by the HITECH privacy provisions of the American Recovery and Reinvestment Act that President Obama signed into law on February 17, 2009. This law expands the protection of HIPAA by requiring entities that work with healthcare organizations and come in contact with personal health information to secure that information, answerable not just to the healthcare organization but to the federal government. Currently, many companies are in transition with their digital records as they work to comply with the law. Companies were given funding as part of the economic stimulus in recognition that this transition to confidential data protection is not a simple process, especially as small companies are asked to rapidly implement sophisticated, expensive database software. Preserving data security can be further complicated when company work is outsourced internationally and affected by different countries' laws (St.Amant, 2008).

As such legal privacy developments can inflect the sharing of student documents created within a healthcare-related organizational context, they are issues for instructors to be aware of as we work in partnership with those in the health professions. For technical writers, use of "deidentified" information is appropriate as long as identifiers have been removed. Yet deidentification of private health information does not mean simply removing a name or a social security number but involves either omitting 18 different identifiers or using a statistical method to render the individual's information de-identifiable. Students working in partnership with health organizations should be made aware of the Privacy Rule so that patient privacy isn't inadvertently compromised. This is important not only with textual but also with visual rhetoric: for instance, a student writing documentation for a hospital procedure that involves a software program must ensure that screen captures intended to illustrate complex portions of the procedure omit or obscure any patient identifying information, or substitute pseudonyms for actual patient names. Similarly, documentation that includes approved photographs of a fluid-sample analysis process must avoid including in the frame any identifying information on a vial label. I must point out that these legal privacy provisions such as HIPAA and HITECH are intended to address and prevent willful misuse of individuals' protected information, more so than the inadvertent disclosure that is more likely to occur in the course of an academic-workplace partnership. However, it is nevertheless important for instructors of technical communication to be able to discuss issues of privacy associated with workplace contexts. In non–healthcare-related fields, this might involve scenarios such as the need for a student working on a project for a human resources office to protect employee information, or a student writing for an attorney to protect personal information of clients. Technical communicators act ethically as they consider stakeholders while composing and distributing digital texts.

As with Ballantine's software copyright example, in which a decision to flout copyright nearly resulted in a wrong-site surgery, the ethical issues involved in proprietary or confidential digital information are most compelling when they are invoked not on an organizational level but on an individual level. This shifts the debate from property in terms of the organization or corporation (the latter term from the Latin *corpus* or body) to the relationship of such organizations with the individual body and with individuals' bodily property and privacy. The legal privacy provisions I've discussed thus govern not just *intellectual* property but *bodily* property, as information grounded in the corporeal. These issues involving the individual and the body can be framed within larger, more public debates over genome sequencing, DNA ownership and privacy, and genetic information made available to employers and insurers. Battles for discursive control over the body are manifested in human genome debates, as individuals have lost lawsuits over rights to their own particular gene sequences while companies patent genetic knowledge and specific treatments based on that knowledge. Such legal debates, as well as the movement toward health data protection in acts such as HIPAA (1996), might be seen as at odds with new digital possibilities for public extension of the body, through photo and video self-revelation in personal blogs/vlogs, social media, image and video hosting/sharing sites, as well as virtual worlds. Foregrounding such tensions between personal, organizational, and public texts, and discussing concepts such as informed consent can be useful in emphasizing ethical agency.

CONCLUSIONS

I have overviewed here some areas for consideration in assisting students in negotiating workplace writing environments. However, attending to issues of intellectual property and privacy in educational and organizational partnerships does not equal buying into a corporate concept of knowledge as property that ignores poststructuralist critiques of subjectivity and textual ownership, the model of the university as a place for conversation and the free exchange of ideas, or the potential of Web 2.0 for interaction and collaboration. Nor should such awareness necessitate taking on a role of surveillance as instructors or promoting, as Sean Zwagerman (2008) argues (invoking Foucault in a critique of plagiarism detection software) "academia's anxious embrace of panoptic technologies" (p. 692). Instead, the strategy of drawing on legal constructions is not one of anxiety but one of purposeful pedagogy, in offering students critical thinking skills that can come to bear on digital composition and distribution of texts.

What I am arguing for is an attention to workplace intellectual property and privacy issues in the technical communication classroom, one that foregrounds ethics in critically considering different choices and their potential effects on stakeholders. Examination of workplace laws, policies, debates, and case studies may not replace discussions of academic ones but may be used in dialog with them. Instructors can foreground for students the differences between academic and workplace concepts of authorship and intellectual property through discussing debates about intellectual property and privacy. Useful resources include the Conference on College Composition and Communication's Intellectual Property Committee/Caucus online reports of the Yearly "Top Intellectual Property Developments" (n.d.), as well as monthly intellectual property reports, which provide useful information on new developments in law and policy that affect writing instruction and research. Instructors can also reference the "Ethical Principles" adopted by the Society for Technical Communication (1998), where the section on "Honesty" addresses issues of intellectual property and the "Confidentiality" section those of privacy, or the "Code of Ethics" adopted by the Association for Teachers of Technical Writing (2011), which touches on responsibilities involved in information sharing, for not only technical writing instructors but also professional technical writers. Through discussing legal and practical implications of various communication choices, students can learn of different perspectives—in addition to the commonly discussed "fair use" guidelines—that affect workplace information distribution. Instructors can precede client projects with discussions of such issues, encouraging students to read about intellectual property and privacy, and work through case studies in ethics and digital writing. Just as we don't want to be trapped in a position of scrutinizing every sentence for plagiarism, so we don't want the role of teaching students to blindly uphold company policies that may not be legal or in the public good but instead seek a position that emphasizes agency in ethical practices.

On a practical level, a useful strategy is to aim for open communication between instructor and organization, and between student and organization. Effective communication between instructor and organization can include, as some have advocated, keeping in contact throughout the project (Matthews & Zimmerman, 1999, p. 400) and working to build long-term relationships with service-learning or client partners (Grabill, 2004, p. 90). Being aware of intellectual property or privacy concerns voiced by a particular partner can help instructors address issues of sensitive information that emerge in projects and help students make ethical decisions about digital sharing.

It is also important for client and student to have from the beginning of the project a common understanding of not only project scope and timeline and academic requirements of students, but also about peer-review activities and textual sharing that will be part of the composition process. A student-authored project proposal can help to begin a project with a mutual awareness of project goals, expectations, and time commitment, and some service-learning scholars advocate a contract between students and the service-learning or project partner (an Internet search yields numerous examples). Yet it is not likely to be useful to write a confidentiality clause into such documents as a matter of course. As I have discussed these intellectual property and privacy issues with attorneys, they have emphasized that the responsibility for confidentiality and information security ultimately rests with the organization or company. In fact, a trade secret is not legally defined as a trade secret unless clear efforts have been made to protect the information. In a service-learning or client project, the partner will have a clearer sense of the responsibilities regarding data protection than will the students or instructor. Thus, if the organization finds that the project it has assigned a group of students involves confidential information, it is that organization's duty to protect the information or, if it deems necessary, to ask the students to sign a confidentiality agreement. Once again, as instructors our job should be one of teaching critical thinking and ethical practices, and not one of surveillance.

Nevertheless, from our classroom side, we can indeed work to secure digital information within student projects. It is useful to talk with students about where digital project content will be stored, discussing steps they can take to keep information secure. Instructors can also create a private space for electronic conversations and document sharing between group members and instructor, on a password-protected online learning management system, wiki, or Web-based data-storage service rather than a publicly-accessible space. Many students like to share completed client project or service-learning project texts with employment contacts or include them in an employment portfolio, and this is appropriate once the organization has made the text public or explicitly approved its use.

In preparing our students for workplace practices, genres, and technologies, client-based and service-learning projects are excellent methods. Within online spaces we can discuss issues of ownership and privacy critically, interrogating legal changes as they reflect emerging technologies. And as we work with digital texts, we can yet retain emphases important to technical communication on context, ethics, and agency.

REFERENCES

Anderson, P. V. (1998). Simple gifts: Ethical issues in the conduct of person-based composition research. *College Composition and Communication, 49*(1), 63-89. Retrieved from http://www.jstor.org/stable/358560

Association for Teachers of Technical Writing. (2011). *Code of ethics.* Retrieved June 1, 2012, from http://www.attw.org/?q=node/107

Ballantine, B. D. (2009). In defense of obfuscation: Questioning open source and a new perspective on teaching digital literacy in the writing classroom. In S. Westbrook (Ed.), *Composition and copyright* (pp. 68-89). Albany, NY: SUNY Press.

Blakeslee, A. (2001). Bridging the workplace and the academy: Teaching professional genres through classroom-workplace collaboration. *Technical Communication Quarterly, 10,* 169-192.

Carter, L. (2003). The implications of single sourcing for writers and writing. *Technical Communication, 50*(3), 317-320.

Conference on College Composition and Communication Intellectual Property Committee/Caucus. (n.d.). *Yearly top intellectual property developments.* Retrieved June 1, 2012 from http://www.ncte.org/cccc/committees/ip/ipreports

Cooke, L., & Williams, S. (2004). Two approaches to using client projects in the college classroom. *Business Communication Quarterly, 67*(2), 139-152. doi: 10.1177/1080569904265321

Dubinsky, J. (2004). The status of service in learning. In T. Bridgeford, K. S. Kitalong, & D. Selfe (Eds.), *Innovative approaches to teaching technical communication* (pp. 15-30). Logan, UT: Utah State University Press.

Faber, B., & Johnson-Eilola, J. (2005). Knowledge politics: Open sourcing education. In K. Cargile Cook & K. Grant-Davie (Eds.), *Online education: Global questions, local answers* (pp. 285-300). Amityville, NY: Baywood.

Grabill, J. T. (2004). Technical writing, service-learning, and a rearticulation of research, teaching, and service. In T. Bridgeford, K. S. Kitalong, & D. Selfe (Eds.), *Innovative approaches to teaching technical communication* (pp. 81-92). Logan, UT: Utah State University Press.

Hansen, C. (2004). At the nexus of theory and practice: Guided, critical reflection for learning beyond the classroom in technical communication. In T. Bridgeford, K. S. Kitalong, & D. Selfe (Eds.), *Innovative approaches to teaching technical communication* (pp. 15-30). Logan, UT: Utah State University Press.

Haviland, C. P., & Mullin, J. A. (Eds.). (2009). *Who owns this text? Plagiarism, authorship, and disciplinary cultures.* Logan, UT: Utah State University Press.

Health Information Privacy Accountability Act of 1996, 45 C.F.R. § 164.306. (2007). Retrieved from http://www.gpo.gov/fdsys/pkg/CFR-2007-title45-vol1/content-detail.html

Henson, L., & Sutliff, K. (1998). A service learning approach to business and technical writing instruction. *Journal of Technical Writing and Communication, 28*(2), 189-205.

Howard, R. M. (1995). Plagiarisms, authorships, and the academic death penalty. *College English, 57,* 788-806.

Howard, R. M., & Robillard, A. (2008). *Pluralizing plagiarism: Identities, contexts, pedagogies.* Portsmouth, NH: Boynton/Cook.

Huckin, T. (1997). Technical writing and community service. *Journal of Business and Technical Communication, 11*(1), 49-59.

Lamos, S. (2009). Texts of our institutional lives: What's in a name? Institutional critique, writing program archives, and the problem of administrator identity. *College English, 71*(4), 389-414.

Logie, J. (2005). Parsing codes: Intellectual property, technical communication, and the World Wide Web. In C. Lipson & M. Day (Eds.), *Technical communication and the World Wide Web* (pp. 223-241). Mahwah, NJ: Lawrence Erlbaum Associates.

Lunsford, A. A., & West, S. (1996). Intellectual property and composition studies. *College Composition and Communication, 47*(3), 383-411. Retrieved from http://www.jstor.org/stable/358295

Matthews, C., & Zimmerman, B. B. (1999). Integrating service-learning and technical communication: Benefits and challenges. *Technical Communication Quarterly, 8*(4), 383-404.

McIntire-Strasburg, J. (2007). Multimedia research: Difficult questions with indefinite answers. In H. A. McKee & D. N. DeVoss (Eds.), *Digital writing research: Technologies, methodologies, and ethical issues* (pp. 287-300). Cresskill, NJ: Hampton.

McKee, H., & Porter, J. E. (2008). The ethics of digital writing research: A rhetorical approach. *College Composition and Communication, 59*(4), 711-749.

McKee, H., & Porter, J. E. (2009). *The ethics of internet research: A rhetorical, case-based process.* New York: Peter Lang.

Poe, M., & Garfinkel, S. (2009). Security and privacy in the wireless classroom. In A. C. Kimme Hea (Ed.), *Going wireless: A critical exploration of wireless and mobile technologies for composition teachers* (pp. 179-195). Cresskill, NJ: Hampton.

Purdy, J. (2005). Calling off the hounds: Technology and the visibility of plagiarism. *Pedagogy: Critical Approaches to Teaching Literature, Language, Composition, and Culture, 5*(2), 275-295.

Reyman, J. (2008). Rethinking plagiarism for technical communication. *Technical Communication 55*(1), 61-67.

Society for Technical Communication (1998). Ethical principles. Retrieved June 1, 2012 from http://www.stc.org/about-stc/the-profession-all-about-technical-communication/ethical-principles

Spigelman, C. (2000). *Across property lines: Textual ownership in writing groups.* Carbondale, IL: Southern Illinois University Press.

Spinuzzi, C. (1996). Pseudotransactionality, activity theory, and professional writing instruction. *Technical Communication Quarterly, 5*(3), 295-308.

St.Amant, K. (2008). The privacy problems related to international outsourcing: A perspective for technical communicators. In B. Thatcher & C. Evia (Eds.), *Outsourcing technical communication: Issues policies and practices* (pp. 165-184). Amityville, NY: Baywood.

Throne, D. W. (2000). Copyright and Web-based education: What all faculty should know. In R. A. Cole (Ed.), *Issues in Web-based pedagogy: A critical primer* (pp. 247-259). Westport, CT: Greenwood.

United States Copyright Act of 1976, 17 U.S.C. § 201. (2011). Retrieved from http://www.copyright.gov/title17/circ92.pdf

Vaidhyanathan, S. (2001). *Copyrights and copywrongs: The rise of intellectual property and how it threatens creativity.* New York: New York University Press.

Warnock, S. (2009). *Teaching writing online: How and why.* Urbana, IL: National Council of Teachers of English.

Woodmansee, M., & Janszi, P. (1995). The law of texts: Copyright in the academy. *College English, 57*(7), 769-787.

Zwagerman, S. (2008). The scarlet P: Plagiarism, panopticism, and the rhetoric of academic integrity. *College Composition and Communication, 59*(4), 676-710.

Afterword

Kelli Cargile Cook and Keith Grant-Davie

The idea for *Online Education 2.0: Evolving, Adapting, and Reinventing Online Technical Communication* came to us as we discussed how our online work had changed since our first collection was published. Over the years, we had not only taught online, but we had also trained graduate students to teach writing online and mentored both junior and senior colleagues as they began their online teaching experiences. At Utah State and Texas Tech where we work, our graduate programs have experienced healthy growth, and many of our graduate students came to us as both experienced online learners and teachers. We found that our online teaching experiences were enriched as these students shared their experiences with us.

At the same time, more of our colleagues across the country were talking with us about the online programs they were teaching and developing. Online education, which seemed novel when we started our first collection, has become almost ubiquitous, although its manifestations are still quite varied. As we noted in our first collection, the forces behind this growth in online education were many: a financial crisis that gripped many institutions in the United States, expanded opportunities to reach untapped student populations, and competition from private and for-profit institutions of higher education combined to bring online education into the forefront of educational innovation.

This changing educational climate and the variety of online educational experiences it sparked prompted us to begin this new collection. As we noted in the introduction, we wanted this collection to move beyond the exploratory questions and answers of the first collection, so we developed three sets of questions as prompts. In this Afterword, we offer our answers to these questions, based on our reading of the chapters in this volume and our conversations with its contributors. We do not assume that our answers are complete or the only answers to these questions, but we hope that our final thoughts will serve as discussion springboards for those individuals and groups who read this collection.

Fiscal Questions: The recession of the last few years has had a profound impact on higher education, bringing reduced funding and staff cutbacks from which we are given little hope of relief in the near future. How is online education responding to what we call this "new austerity"?

In some instances, the budget crunch of the past 5 years appears to have driven programs to teach more online courses and to innovate, doing more with less. Chapters such as Maid and D'Angelo's as well as Tillery and Nagelhout's describe fiscally stretched institutions that reconfigure programs, departments, and colleges in lean years. We suspect that the increase in contingent and temporary faculty results from salary budget reductions, as these individuals are less expensive to employ and can be used on an "as-needed" basis. This increase has had both positive and negative effects. For example, moving courses online allows institutions, such as Arizona State University and Davenport University, to hire contingent faculty from a professional pool that is more geographically dispersed. These hires can be beneficial to online technical communication programs because often they are professionals or practitioners who bring a wealth of work experience to the classroom. Across-distance collaborations are another benefit. As Tesdell notes, online learning not only allows students to be dispersed geographically, but it also allows instructors to teach while they travel as well as to collaborate with other instructors around the world. Along with these advantages, contingent faculty and graduate students bring creativity and value to our online classrooms, as a quick glance at contributors' biographies demonstrates.

Yet we wonder if individuals in these groups are adequately rewarded for and supported in the groundbreaking work they are doing. When we posed our questions about staff cutbacks, we suspected that most online faculty members were not well-prepared for the work. We were heartened to discover, however, the variety of mentoring models our contributors have developed to support individuals who have little or no online teaching experience. While some educators see online learning as an extension of face-to-face learning, the two are not interchangeable; consequently, supporting those who lack teaching experience in online environments has increased the need for training and mentoring support. Texas State Technical College's Mentor2Mentor program, University of Cincinnati's communities of practice, and University of Nevada at Las Vegas's classroom support pages are among the examples of such mentoring and training this collection describes. We see an increasing need for institutions to devote resources to instructor support if they want to maintain a high quality of instruction in online classes. Eaton's list of characteristics of successful online instructors, according to the graduate students she surveyed, provides a way for instructors to evaluate whether online instruction is for them. We contrast this list to the many examples of surveys available online that provide students with means of predicting their own success in online environments, and we think it is about time that someone was as frank about the qualities of good online instructors and asks, "What does it take to teach successfully online?"

While postsecondary institutions have increased their online courses in response to budgetary reductions, lean times have also made online education more attractive to a wider student population, notably nontraditional students who return to school because they are unemployed or underemployed, professionals who want increased job security through graduate degree attainment, and former students who want to complete their degrees but no longer live near their original institutions. The numbers of international students who seek learning from U.S. institutions has also increased, as Popham and Thrush, and Tesdell note. Eaton's chapter describes the increased age of graduate students and the changed characteristics of online graduate students since her last survey. However, because students come to us from both urban and rural settings, their ability to access technology may be more challenging for them, as Martinez and Gibson discuss. Tesdell also describes international differences in connectivity that can affect students attending U.S. classes from international locations.

Another outcome of these changes is that programs and departments that offer multiple sections of courses taught by geographically dispersed or temporary instructors need a way to maintain consistency of instruction and outcomes as well as assessment. Predesigned courses (PDCs), course templates, and scaffolding are possible approaches described in this collection to ensure consistency across sections. At the same time, balancing the need for consistency with the need to afford instructor creativity is among the foremost issues facing this generation of online instructors and program directors.

Technological Questions: The technological context in which we teach online has simplified online instruction through the use of standardized and institutionalized classroom management systems, but it has also complicated our work if we choose to employ social networking, virtual worlds, or mobile technologies. Why and how are we using these newer developments in our classes, and to what end?

We have been impressed with the variety of technologies our contributors have described. While we have some contributors using common content management systems, also called learning or learner management systems, such as Blackboard Vista and Design2Learn, we have many contributors who have modified and changed their delivery methods, creating instructional sites that move beyond the printed page and correspondence-type delivery to harness the power of Web 2.0's new media formats and virtual worlds for educational purposes. Cason and Jenkins demonstrate how instructors can employ the Internet's capabilities and modify their course materials to make them more accessible and interesting to students who use them. Likewise, Jones describes how unconventional use of common CMS features can better support student learning, and Fagerheim provides multiple approaches for successfully embedding—or at least incorporating—library services into course activities. Stillman-Webb cautions instructors to consider privacy and ethical concerns as we design instruction and engage our students in online learning activities and assignments. Tucker's replication study demonstrates that students are gaining, if not new then additional, communication literacies in Web-based games and bringing those into the classroom. Contrary to popular belief, she argues that online gaming teaches students to collaborate and construct knowledge. Scopes and Carter demonstrate how virtual worlds can open up authentic learning spaces and provide unique opportunities to engage students culturally and technologically with others.

At the same time, Gibson and Martinez advise online instructors to integrate technologies carefully and considerately in their online classes. They argue that the digital divide remains a concern for online instructors, so instructors must provide learning environments that will allow access and learning opportunities to all students, regardless of their network's robustness and speed. Tillery and Nagelhout's discussion of their decision to remain well behind the technology curve with their courseware provides an excellent example of Gibson and Martinez's advice in practice.

These answers to our technological questions leave us with insights into where tomorrow's classroom may be situated in virtual spaces—both in games and virtual worlds—but also remind us that tomorrow is not yet here. As instructors, we must recognize our students' abilities and needs and evaluate the fit of our technologies to those students' needs. The "cool" factor may allow us occasionally to experiment with technologies on the bleeding edge of technology, but our classrooms should be accessible to students, wherever and however we connect to them. On the other hand, we also need to find ways to accommodate the needs and expectations of increasing numbers of digital natives in our classes, lest what we teach become increasingly detached from their lives and the work they will need to do after graduation. Online instructors may need to develop creative ways to span wider ranges in technological literacy and in access to technology among their online students. Some of our students are already technologically way ahead of us, while others may lag too far behind to be able to catch up in the course of one class.

Theoretical Questions: Have we moved beyond the theory-building stage we described in our first book to a more theory-based instruction? If so, what theories are we using, and which ones work best in application?

As we worked with our collections' authors, we wondered if the essays would ultimately allow us to answer this question, and we wondered what theoretical themes would weave through the collection. We could see, as chapters developed, that our contributors sometimes echoed each other as they discussed the theoretical assumptions that underpin their work in the online classroom. In general, we found contributors using theories as either scaffolds on which they built their online courses or explanatory lenses through which they could view and understand their online courses and students.

Not surprisingly, we identified rhetoric, particularly as a means of understanding audiences, to be a touchstone theory that our contributors apply in their essays. They rely on it to understand online student populations: for example, Eaton's identification and description of the needs of technical communication graduate students in the United States, Thrush and Popham's discussion of the implications of a globally diverse student population in online classes, and Gibson and Martinez's cautionary analysis of the still-present digital divide and its effects on students' ability to participate in online classes. Other contributors use rhetorical theory to understand the needs of online faculty (Dutkiewicz, Holder, & Sneath; Tillery & Nagelhout; Jaramillo-Santoy & Cano-Monreal) and to evaluate the effectiveness of online course delivery technologies (Tillery & Nagelhout). Expanding our view of audience beyond the confines of online faculty and students, Stillman-Webb cautions us about the porous boundaries of online classes and warns that we must consider client intellectual property and privacy when we engage our students in projects with and for outside organizations.

Several of our contributors also engage rhetorical theory to describe how both students and teachers build ethos in the online classroom. For example, Jones recommends introductions to construct instructor ethos, while Eaton recommends strategies for recruiting and sustaining enrollment in online programs. The interplay of rhetorical and genre theories is also apparent in Tucker's argument that online gaming experience is changing the shape and patterns of online discussions, and Cason and Jenkins' description of the evolution of their online teaching materials.

Like rhetorical theory, social construction of knowledge is a theory often associated with technical communication pedagogy. Our contributors engaged social construction almost as frequently as rhetorical theory. How to engage students as they construct knowledge in our classes—whether we are designing courses or activities—was a common theme. Jones discusses the importance of instructor participation in online discussion. Too often, online instructors disengage from discussions, resulting in students who feel rudderless or alienated from the group. Fagerheim explores the challenges of student research in online settings, and she suggests that embedding library services within our online courses can help students construct knowledge through improved instruction in how to access, evaluate, and integrate research in their projects. Tucker's chapter argues that students with gaming experience have learned to construct knowledge through participation in group gaming activities; these experiences, she argues, enrich and support their construction of knowledge in course discussions. Scopes and Carter extend this argument, contending that virtual worlds like Second Life are ideally suited for social construction of knowledge. Not only do these worlds allow students to meet across distances, but they also promote student collaboration and social interaction to fulfill course requirements.

The role of communities of practice in online instruction was another common theoretical thread identified in the collection. Communities of practice are an extension of social construction theory. From a faculty viewpoint, Meloncon and Arduser describe their relationship as a community of practice that helped them to develop and sustain their first online courses. Although other chapters throughout the collection may not mention communities of practice per se, they effectively describe the use of communities of practice to negotiate course development and consistency, to create course materials, and to usher new instructors into their first online course experiences. Two chapters discuss student communities of practice: Scopes and Carter argue that students interacting in virtual worlds can lead to the development of communities of practice, and Tesdell illustrates how online courses can result in communities that expand across geographic and spatial boundaries. As we consider this theory in light of our own experiences, we find that it well describes our own discussions about our online classes over the years as well as the knowledge we've gained from engaging with contributors to our collections.

In addition to rhetorical, social construction, and communities of practice theories, two final kinds of theories are prevalent in this collection: instructional design theories and critical theories of technology. Our contributors draw on both kinds of theories to understand and adapt to online education's reliance on and employment of technology to deliver instruction. Of the two, instructional design theory is the more instrumental. Our contributors called on instructional design to explain why and how consistent course design supports student learning. Whether they describe consistency in terms of predesigned courses or course templates, instructional design theories guide the way instructors integrate course outcomes into their activities or think about scaffolding activities to actuate student learning. Instructional design theories have also informed contributors when they are adding headings or advance organizers to their course Web sites, integrating navigational links within their courses, or integrating new media to deliver instruction. Finally, best practices, such as the Quality Matters guidelines, derive from instructional design research across disciplines engaged in online education.

A collection like this will tend to attract contributors whose ultimate response to online education is positive, but we hope that we will not collectively be seen as uncritical cheerleaders for online education. Our contributors are aware that the affordances of delivery technologies are not universal and may come at a cost. They have experimented with many technologies to find the combination that best supports their students' learning, but they recognize that, as in face-to-face instruction, experimentation can result in both successes and failures, and sometimes failures have consequences on student learning. To examine and weigh the costs of teaching online, many of our contributors have engaged the final kind of theory we identify in this collection—critical theories of technology. They explore such questions as these:

- When we design our instruction for online learning, what is gained and what is lost?
- When instruction is delivered online, whose interests are best served?
- When instruction is delivered online, who can access it and who cannot?

We believe that online teachers should continue to ask critical questions about the uses of technology in education and not look to technology as a panacea for educational delivery problems. Technology, while solving some problems, will always present its own set.

However, while we believe that online educators should continue to look at technology with a critical eye, we don't see much to be gained from perpetuating the debate about online education's validity—the question of whether it is an acceptable alternative to on-site education. Nevertheless, we'll review some of the issues here once again to make the point that neither online nor on-site education is clearly better; they just have different strengths.

The arguments that online education is poorer than on-site typically dwell on the loss of what are often called the "intangible," synergistic benefits of on-site interaction, such as the rapid-fire give and take of ideas in a lively face-to-face discussion and the stimulating energy, inspiration, and creativity that can result; the nuances of meaning that can be communicated by tone of voice, facial expression, and body language when a class is physically present in the same room; the warmth and camaraderie, the shared laughter, or even the shared food. We have all experienced these things, though not, we hasten to add, in every face-to-face class we have taught (we can recall on-site classes that have been a little short on conviviality). Although some of these benefits can happen in online classes too, we agree that interpersonal qualities like those listed above are probably the most obvious advantages of face-to-face instruction (when it's going really well). These benefits seem to be what people mean when they talk about the "richness" of face-to-face instruction that they don't find in online instruction.

However, against those advantages, we would submit those of online instruction that contribute to *its* richness, which is of a different kind. For instance, assuming Internet access, students and instructors can participate in an online class at almost any time of day or night and from almost any location. This access advantage alone is huge when compared with the traditional class that meets for only about 3 hours per week in the same physical location, since the expanded access allows for more diverse groups of students to come together in a class; but it's not the only source of richness in online classes.

In the traditional seminar class, students may discuss topics in small groups for some of the time, but for most of the time it's likely that only one of them—or the instructor—will be talking at any given moment while the rest listen and await their brief turns. The hypothetical transcript of a semester's worth of such class meetings would be relatively short, and it would be filled with the hesitations and imprecisions typical of impromptu oral discussions. What sounded good at the time may not look quite so erudite when seen transcribed.

By contrast, the transcript of an online class that uses asynchronous discussion forums (where all members of the class can post simultaneously over an extended period, and where multiple conversations can take place concurrently) would not only be many times longer, but the posts would also tend to be better expressed, even more thoughtful, the authors having had time to consider and revise their written comments before posting them. This, at least, has been our experience. Also, in such an online class, there actually *is* a transcript of everything that has been posted, and students can review or even print out everything that has been "said" in the class. Synchronous audio and video discussions also have the advantage of audio transcripts, and MOO- or chat-based synchronous meetings have text-based transcripts of discussions. In a face-to-face class, there is seldom a transcript to review. Most of what is said in the meetings lives on only in a few notes and the memories of those who were present.

We could go on, but our argument boils down to this: the pros and cons of each instructional medium result in differences but not in an obvious advantage for either medium. Both of us continue to teach online and on-site classes. When we teach in one medium, we may miss the advantages of the other, but we don't go so far as to lament their loss or cite the loss as sufficient reason to reject the medium. Rather, we enjoy teaching in either medium (or using a combination of the two in the same class), and we celebrate the advantages of each.

Some classes may be better suited either to online or to face-to-face instruction, but we argue that online education should not be seen, as a whole, as any "less rich" than face-to-face. It's simply rich in different ways. We suspect that many of the critics who take the conservative line that online classes are invariably poor substitutes for traditional face-to-face classes have not experienced online education at its best. This collection has tried to continue the work of our previous one (*Online Education: Global Questions, Local Answers*), aiming to show some of the possibilities and potential for success—as well as the challenges—of online education in technical communication.

CONCLUSION

We began collecting the essays in this book with questions about how online instruction has matured in the past 10 years. We are happy to report that it is alive and well. Online instructors are developing a sound theoretical basis that informs our teaching and our use of teaching technology. Furthermore, based on our reading of these essays, we are convinced that online teaching is grounded in theory, not unexamined practice. The more we practice teaching in online environments, the more able we are to explain why we are doing what we do.

We also have found ways to weather the fiscal leanness of the recessionary years in spite of cuts in our human resource budgets and increases in our teaching loads and expectations. We predict that online instruction will continue to grow in popularity among students and instructors in the coming years, although we expect that, just as our ways of knowing and teaching face-to-face supported our preliminary investigations in online learning, online instruction will soon repay the favor. As our enrollments—both online and on-site—are increasingly filled with digital natives, we expect to see knowledge of online instructional best practices beginning to inform on-site instruction. Our willingness to incorporate elements of online life—from social media to games and virtual worlds—may well lead the way.

Effective online teaching, we believe, is not just face-to-face teaching delivered through neutral technology that requires no new pedagogical skills. To teach well online requires training, mentoring, and practice. It thrives when instructors who experiment with new approaches reflect upon and share what they learn with those who follow. We believe the contributors to this collection are among this avant-garde, and their contributions demonstrate the reflexivity that marks quality instruction. As we noted in the introduction, we hope, too, that they have inspired and engaged you in thinking about what online learning is and what it can be.

Contributors

Lora Arduser is an Assistant Professor of Professional and Technical Writing at the University of Cincinnati, where she teaches graduate and undergraduate courses in the Professional Writing program. Her research interests focus on examining how people collaborate to build knowledge in online communities and how patients enact rhetorical agency in medical contexts.

University of Cincinnati   lora.arduser@uc.edu
Department of English
P.O. Box 210069
248 McMicken Hall
Cincinnati, OH 45221-0069

Gina Cano-Monreal is a Senior Instructor in the Biology Department at Texas State Technical College in Harlingen, Texas. In addition to teaching in the face-to-face classroom, she has developed and delivered anatomy and physiology distance learning courses. She has served as Department Chair for Academic Distance Education and assisted in the development and implementation of Mentor2Mentor, a training program to support faculty new to distance learning course development and instruction. Gina received her Ph.D. in microbiology and immunology from St. Louis University School of Medicine and is a member of the Texas Distance Learning Association.

Texas State Technical College Harlingen   glcano-monreal@tstc.edu
1902 North Loop 499
Harlingen, TX 78550

Bryan Carter is an Associate Professor of literature at the University of Central Missouri. He specializes in African-American literature of the 20th century, with a primary focus on the Harlem Renaissance, and has a secondary emphasis on visual culture. He has published numerous articles on his doctoral project, Virtual Harlem, and has presented it at locations around the world.

400 Grampian Drive   bc7@mac.com
Columbia, MO 65203

Jacqueline Cason is an Associate Professor of English at the University of Alaska Anchorage and an affiliate faculty member of Environmental Studies. She coordinates the English Department's composition program and teaches a variety of genre and discipline-specific courses-essay, narrative nonfiction, scientific and technical writing, advanced composition, and public science writing. Her research areas include online pedagogy and dialogic spaces, public science writing, and deliberative rhetoric.

3211 Providence Dr.   jecason@uaa.alaska.edu
University of Alaska Anchorage
Department of English
Anchorage, AK 99508

Barbara J. D'Angelo is Assistant Clinical Professor of Technical Communication at Arizona State University. She received her PhD in Technical Communication and Rhetoric from Texas Tech University and her MSLIS from the University of Illinois at Urbana-Champaign. She teaches courses in technical communication, business communication, health communication, and intellectual property. Her research interests include writing assessment; the impact of assessment on curriculum development, outcomes, and pedagogy; electronic portfolios; and information literacy.

1442 N. Sierra Heights   bdangelo@asu.edu
Mesa, AZ 85207

Keri Dutkiewicz has been developing online learning tools and teaching online since the mid-1990s. During this time, she has worked as an instructional designer, e-learning consultant, and large-scale online learning systems designer for clients in academia and the Fortune 100. She currently serves as the Director of Faculty Learning at Davenport University, a multi-campus professional school that prepares students for careers in Business, Technology, and Healthcare. In this role, Dr. Dutkiewicz aligns university-wide development initiatives with academic needs to provide professional development opportunities for faculty in all stages of their careers. She also teaches online courses in Professional Writing, Literature, and Global Cultures.

Davenport University   kdutkiewicz@davenport.edu
220 East Kalamazoo
Lansing, MI 48933-2197

Angela Eaton is an Associate Professor of Technical Communication and Rhetoric in the Department of English at Texas Tech University, where she teaches in their online and onsite Master's and PhD programs. She teaches and researches technical editing, grant and proposal writing, pedagogical methods, and quantitative research methods. She is the co-author of *Technical editing*, 5th ed., with Carolyn Rude. She is also President of Angela Eaton & Associates, LLC, a grantwriting and editing firm.

Department of English   angela.eaton@ttu.edu
Texas Tech University
Lubbock, TX 79409-3091

Britt Fagerheim is the Coordinator of Library Services for Regional Campuses and Distance Education at Utah State University's Merrill-Cazier Library. She is the subject specialist for departments in the Jon M. Huntsman School of Business. Before coming to USU, she spent 6 years with the Bill & Melinda Gates Foundation, developing curriculum for a computer training program in public libraries. She received an undergraduate degree from Mount Holyoke College in International Relations and a Master's degree in Library and Information Science from the University of Washington.

Utah State University   britt.fagerheim@usu.edu
3000 Old Main Hill
Logan, UT 84322

Keith Gibson has taught at Auburn University and Utah State University and is a technical writer, editor, and user experience researcher in the greater Salt Lake City area. He researches the intersections of science and public policy and the rhetoric of science and technology, especially as it influences the teaching of technical communication.

keith.evan.gibson@gmail.com

LuAnne Holder taught Professional Writing for Davenport University for almost 3 years and served as Course Coordinator for 2 years. After completing her PhD in Instructional Design for Online Learning at Capella University, she took a position as Associate Dean, Distance Education Programs for Notre Dame College in Ohio, where she oversees new online course development projects.

6165 Crabapple Drive   luanneholder@wowway.com
Troy, MI 48098

Janie Jaramillo-Santoy has over 18 years experience as an educator. She has taught high school, community college, and university level courses. Her distance education experience ranges from ITV, hybrid, and fully online asynchronous to fully online synchronous courses. She served as Chair for the English Department at Texas State Technical College for 6 years. She was active in the college's Distance Education Committee for 3 years, serving as chair for one. She is currently a faculty member in the language and Communications department at Western Governors University and completing her PhD from Texas Tech University.

34503 Island Estate   janie.santoy@gmail.com
San Benito, TX 78586

Patricia Jenkins is an Associate Professor of English at the University of Alaska Anchorage, where she teaches a variety of composition courses, including online technical writing and online professional writing. Her research areas include online pedagogy, Alaska Native ways of teaching and learning, and the effects of unionizing.

4722 Mills Drive   pmienkins@uaa.alaska.edu
Anchorage, AK 99508

Dan Jones, a Professor of English at the University of Central Florida, has taught a wide variety of technical communication courses for the past 32 years. He has taught numerous online courses for the past 15 years, including developing and teaching the first online sections of the introductory technical communication course at UCF. His publications include three books: *Technical writing style* (Allyn and Bacon, 1998); *The technical communicator's handbook* (Allyn and Bacon, 2000); and *Technical communication: Strategies for college and the workplace* (Longman, 2002), co-authored with Karen Lane. He is also a Fellow of the Society for Technical Communication.

804 Palmetto Terrace   dan. jones@ucf.edu
Oviedo, FL 32765

Barry Maid is a Professor, and for ten years was program head, of Technical Communication at Arizona State University. Previously, he taught at the University of Arkansas at Little Rock where, among other things, he helped in the creation of the Department of Rhetoric and Writing. For more than 15 years, he has been actively participating in online communities and using them as teaching/learning spaces. Along with numerous articles and chapters focusing on technology, independent writing programs, and program administration, he is a co-author, with Duane Roen and Greg Glau, of *The McGraw-Hill guide: Writing for college, writing for life.*

2637 N. Layton Circle
Mesa, AZ 85207

barry.maid@asu.edu

Diane Martinez is an assistant professor of professional and technical communication at Western Carolina University. She also taught composition and technical communication full-time online for over 8 years. Her research interests include studying the effects of globalization in technical communication.

English Department
305 Coulter Building
Western Carolina University
Cullowhee, NC 28723

dlmartinez@email.wcu.edu

Lisa Meloncon is an Associate Professor of Professional and Technical Writing at the University of Cincinnati, where she teaches graduate and undergraduate courses in the Professional Writing program. She is the editor of *Rhetorical accessibility: At the intersection of technical communication and disability studies.* Beyond accessibility issues, her research interests include medical rhetoric and technology, programmatic issues in technical and professional communication and environmental/health communication.

22 St. Nicholas Place
Fort Thomas, KY 41075

meloncon@tek-ritr.comkelli

Ed Nagelhout is an Associate Professor at the University of Nevada, Las Vegas, where he teaches graduate and undergraduate courses in rhetoric, professional writing, and linguistics. He has edited two collections, published 17 articles, and presented more than 80 papers on a variety of topics, including writing program administration, teaching in digital environments, writing in the disciplines, and contrastive rhetoric. His current research projects examine academic program design and the impact of social media on technical communication.

9617 Big Man St.
Las Vegas, NV 89123

ed.nagelhout@unlv.edu

Susan L. Popham is an Associate Professor at the University of Memphis, where she teaches professional writing and composition. She earned a PhD in Rhetoric and Composition from the University of Louisville in 2002 before coming to the University of Memphis. She conducts research in writing program administration, online pedagogies, and medical rhetoric. She currently serves as the Director of English Undergraduate Studies. Her research often focuses on the ways in which communicative tools function within activity systems and workplaces to conscript students, authors, agents, or other administrators into pre-defined roles.

3517 Philsdale Ave.   spopham@memphis.edu
Memphis, TN 38111

Lesley Scopes is the author of the Model of Cybergogy of Learning Archetypes and Learning Domains, which emanates from her 2009 master's dissertation at The University of Southampton, UK, where she is a visiting fellow. She is a faculty developer for Online Education at Drury University, Springfield, MO. She is a consortium member in a European Union project where the Model of Cybergogy underpins the virtual teaching aspects. Her theory of cybergogy is profiled in the Kapp and O'Driscoll (2010) book, *Learning in 3D*, and she has a chapter in the Hinrichs and Wankel (2011) book, *Transforming Virtual World Learning*.

University of Southampton   l.scopes@soton.ac.uk
School of Education
Building 32, University Road
Southampton, UK
SO17 1BJ

Wayne D. Sneath is an Assistant Professor in the College of Arts & Sciences at Davenport University. He teaches composition and professional writing in the university's online program and serves as the Program Director for Experiential Learning. In this role, he supports the development of academic service learning, internships, and course-based business and industry projects. Dr. Sneath holds a degree in American Culture Studies from Bowling Green State University with an emphasis in American Literature, Sociology, and Popular Culture. He has also worked in administrative roles at non-profit agencies in Detroit and Cincinnati collaborating with youth and the elderly on community development projects.

Program Director Experiential Learning   wayne.sneath@davenport.edu
College of Arts & Sciences
Davenport University
6191 Kraft Avenue SE
Grand Rapids, MI 49512

Natalie Stillman-Webb holds a PhD in English from Purdue University. She is an Associate Professor/Lecturer in the University Writing Program at the University of Utah, where she teaches technical and business communication, usability testing, and visual rhetoric. Her research interests include digital rhetoric, intellectual property, and writing in the disciplines.

University Writing Program   natalie.stillman-webb@utah.edu
University of Utah
255 S. Central Campus
Dr. Rm. 3700
Salt Lake City, UT 84112

Lee S. Tesdell is an Associate Professor in the English Department at Minnesota State University, Mankato and a graduate of Iowa State University's Rhetoric and Professional Communication program. After completing his degree, he first worked in industry as a technical writer and now teaches courses (both face-to-face and online) in the technical communication program at MSU Mankato. His teaching and research interests are in documentation, online pedagogy, cross-cultural technical communication, and new media writing. One of Lee's current projects is to build an international online learning consortium linking instructors and students at universities around the world.

Department of English   lee.tesdell@mnsu.edu
230 Armstrong Hall
Minnesota State University, Mankato
Mankato, MN 56001

Emily A. Thrush is a Professor in the Professional Writing and Applied Linguistics programs at the University of Memphis and coordinates the Composition and Professional Writing programs. She served as a Senior Fulbright Scholar in Mexico in 2000-2001 and has conducted teacher training in Brazil, China, Germany, Italy, Mexico, Lebanon, the Czech Republic, and Slovakia. Her research interests include international and multicultural issues in technical communication. She has been teaching online classes since 1998.

2382 Eastover Dr.   ethrush@memphis.edu
Memphis, TN 38119

Denise Tillery is an Associate Professor at the University of Nevada–Las Vegas, where she has directed both the professional writing certificate and the business writing program. She has regularly developed and taught online courses since 2005. Her research focuses on environmental rhetoric and gender and the history of scientific rhetoric, and she has published articles in *Technical Communication Quarterly, Rhetoric Review,* the *Journal of Technical Writing and Communication,* and *IEEE Transactions on Professional Communication.*

English Department   denise.tillery@unlv.edu
University of Nevada, Las Vegas
4505 Maryland Parkway, Box 455011
Las Vegas, NV 89154-5011

Virginia Tucker is Director of Interdisciplinary Studies and Program Coordinator for the Interdisciplinary Studies degree in Professional Writing at Old Dominion University. She has taught courses in technical and scientific writing, digital writing, composition, and electronic portfolios since 2004. As a distance educator, she is interested in how web users communicate and learn online and the ways in which those practices can be adapted in the distance classroom. Presently, she is working toward a PhD in Technical Communication and Rhetoric at Texas Tech University.

35 Old Fox Hill Rd.   vmtucker@odu.edu
Hampton, VA 23669

Index